Simulation-Based Learning in Communication Sciences and Disorders

Moving From Theory to Practice

Simulation-Based Learning in Communication Sciences and Disorders

Moving From Theory to Practice

EDITORS

CAROL C. DUDDING, PHD, CCC-SLP, F-ASHA, CHSE
James Madison University
Harrisonburg, Virginia

SARAH M. GINSBERG, EDD, CCC-SLP, F-ASHA
Eastern Michigan University
Ypsilanti, Michigan

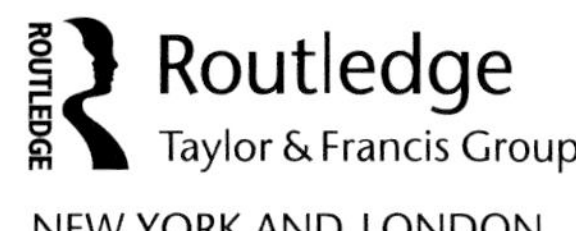

NEW YORK AND LONDON

First published 2023 by SLACK Incorporated

Published 2024 by Routledge
605 Third Avenue, New York, NY 10158

and by Routledge
4 Park Square, Milton Park, Abingdon, Oxon, OX14 4RN

Routledge is an imprint of the Taylor & Francis Group, an informa business

Library of Congress Cataloging-in-Publication Data

Names: Dudding, Carol C., editor. | Ginsberg, Sarah M., 1966- editor.
Title: Simulation-based learning in communication sciences and disorders : moving from theory to practice / [edited by] Carol C. Dudding, Sarah M. Ginsberg.
Description: Thorofare, NJ : SLACK Incorporated, [2023] | Includes bibliographical references and index.
Identifiers: LCCN 2023010716 (print) | ISBN 9781638220008 (paperback)
Subjects: MESH: Speech-Language Pathology--education | Simulation Training--methods | Audiology--education | BISAC: MEDICAL / Audiology & Speech Pathology
Classification: LCC RC428 (print) | NLM WL 18 | DDC 616.85/50071--dc23/eng/20230505
LC record available at https://lccn.loc.gov/2023010716

Cover Artist: Tinhouse Design

ISBN: 9781638220008 (pbk)
ISBN: 9781003526421 (ebk)

DOI: 10.4324/9781003526421

Dedication

This book is dedicated to all those educators who believe that
"education is not the learning of facts but training the mind to think" (Albert Einstein).

Contents

Acknowledgments

The editors wish to express our gratitude to all of the contributing authors who are on the leading edge of simulations in communication sciences and disorders. This book would not be possible without the assistance of Mary Kate Foley, Patrick Massey, and Rachel Tinsley, students at James Madison University.

About the Editors

Carol C. Dudding, PhD, CCC-SLP, F-ASHA, CHSE, is a professor at James Madison University, Harrisonburg, Virginia. She has presented and published nationally and internationally on e-supervision, telepractice, distance education, and simulation. She served in several leadership positions of the Council of Academic Programs in Communication Sciences and Disorders (CAPCSD). Carol is a Certified Healthcare Simulation Educator (CHSE). She serves on the American Speech-Language-Hearing Association Board of Directors as Vice President for Standards and Ethics for Speech-Language Pathology.

Sarah M. Ginsberg, EdD, CCC-SLP, F-ASHA, is a full professor of Communication Sciences and Disorders at Eastern Michigan University. She was the founding editor of *Teaching and Learning in Communication Sciences & Disorders* (*TLCSD*). She is also the editor of *Xerostomia: An Interdisciplinary Approach to Managing Dry Mouth* and co-editor with Jennifer C. Friberg and Colleen F. Visconti of *Evidence-Based Education in the Classroom.* She is co-author of *Scholarship of Teaching and Learning in Speech-Language Pathology and Audiology: Evidence-Based Education.* Her work has appeared in the *Journal of Scholarship of Teaching and Learning, The Teaching Professor, Contemporary Issues in Communication Science and Disorders, To Improve the Academy*, and *The ASHA Leader*. Her research focus has been primarily on issues of teaching and learning in communication sciences and disorders.

Contributing Authors

Meredith L. Baker-Rush, PhD, MS, CCC-SLP/L, CHSE, FNAP (Chapters 3 and 8)
Associate Program Director
Interprofessional Healthcare Studies
College of Health Professions
Interprofessional Faculty Lead
DeWitt C. Baldwin Institute for
Interprofessional Education
Rosalind Franklin University of Medicine and Science
North Chicago, Illinois

David K. Brown, PhD, CCC-A (Chapters 4 and 6)
Professor and Director
Audiology Simulation Lab
School of Audiology
Pacific University
Hillsboro, Oregon

Erin S. Clinard, PhD, CCC-SLP, CHSE (Chapter 5)
Assistant Professor
Department of Communication Sciences and Disorders
James Madison University
Harrisonburg, Virginia

Julie M. Estis, PhD, CCC-SLP (Chapter 6)
University of South Alabama
Mobile, Alabama

Sue McAllister, PhD, FSPA (Chapter 2)
The University of Sydney and Flinders University
Adelaide, South Australia, Australia

Suzanne Moineau, PhD, CCC-SLP (Chapter 7)
Professor
California State University San Marcos
San Marcos, California

Kevin Phaup, MFA (Chapter 9)
Associate Professor of Industrial Design
James Madison University
Harrisonburg, Virginia

Alison R. Scheer-Cohen, PhD, CCC-SLP (Chapter 7)
Associate Professor
California State University San Marcos
San Marcos, California

Richard I. Zraick, PhD, CCC-SLP, F-ASHA, CHSE (Chapter 3)
Professor
School of Communication Sciences and Disorders
University of Central Florida
Orlando, Florida

Introduction

This book is designed to be a guide useful to any clinical educator or classroom educator who is interested in learning more about the use of simulation-based learning in communication sciences and disorders. Simulation-based learning is a useful learning strategy that can improve the impact of your teaching, no matter what context you teach in. The use of simulation in the learning context should always be seen as a learning approach that can help provide a solution to a challenge or improve a learning outcome. While it is novel and engaging, it should not be used without clear thinking regarding the benefits and need for the technology in the specific learning context for which it is being considered. We hope that all readers, from those who are simulation curious to simulation experienced, can find new content that will help you move to the next level in your teaching and learning with simulation.

The book is organized into three parts. The first part, "Foundations in Clinical Simulations," provides an overview of simulation-based learning and principles of teaching and learning in higher education. Here you will find concepts related to simulation modalities as well as foundational theories that will be useful to you in planning your teaching with simulation. Additionally, this part will help you identify when and how simulations can be used within your courses and your programs.

"Clinical Simulation Learning Experiences" is the second part of the book and will explore in greater detail the various forms of simulation available for teaching. Here you will also learn more about the best practices for implementing simulations for learning in your environment. This part will also help you identify ways to incorporate simulation-based learning into your curriculum, including effectively assessing and evaluating learners' performances.

The last part, "Professional Issues and Advocacy," moves the reader to the next level of knowledge. In this part, you will learn more about how to expand your simulation teaching. This part may be useful to those who are looking to not only grow their own skills but to develop the skills of colleagues on their campus as well. For those interested in developing research around the simulation-based learning experience, particularly for the scholarship of teaching and learning, you will find this part useful.

We wish you every success as you explore the use of simulation-based learning for your courses and programs.

PART I

Foundations in Clinical Simulations

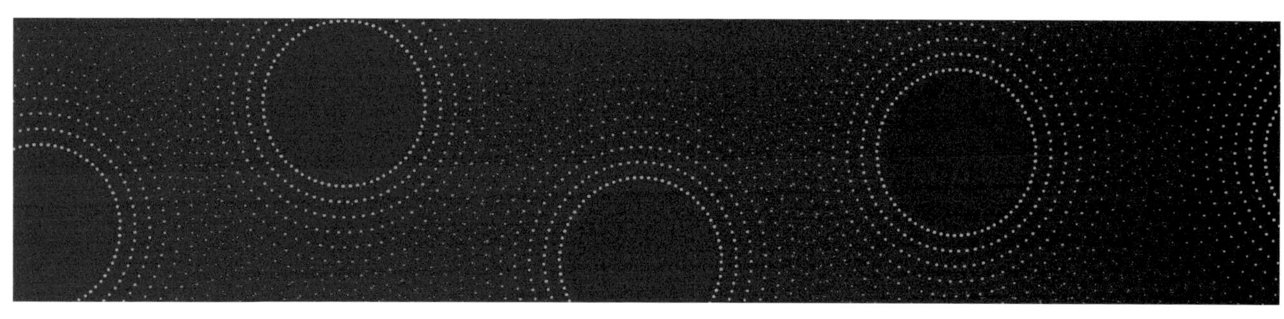

Introduction to Simulation-Based Learning

Carol C. Dudding, PhD, CCC-SLP, F-ASHA, CHSE

Education is not the learning of facts but training the mind to think.
—Albert Einstein (Frank, 1947)

This book is intended for academic and clinical educators interested in exploring ways to supplement current methods of clinical education. It is intended for those unfamiliar with simulation practices, as well as those who have some experience but wish to know more. It provides a framework for thinking about simulation education that is built on learning theories and strategies familiar to the educator. It provides a summary of the evidence in support of clinical simulation and identifies gaps in our current practices.

Simulation-Based Learning and Clinical Education Practices in Communication Sciences and Disorders

Graduate programs in audiology and speech-language pathology in the United States are required to provide students with a wide range of knowledge, clinical skills, and professional skills in order to qualify for entry into the professions. Speech-language pathology students are required to earn 375 clock hours providing direct clinical care to qualify for certification from the Council for Clinical Certification in Audiology and Speech-Language Pathology (CFCC; 2018). While graduate students in audiology are not required to obtain a specified number of clinical clock hours, they are required to demonstrate specific clinical and professional skills across the scope of practice (Accreditation Commission for Audiology Education, 2016; CFCC, 2018). For this reason, graduate programs in both audiology and speech-language pathology have employed a 1:1 apprentice model of training that relies heavily on external sites and clinical educators (i.e., supervisors and preceptors) for student training. While multitudes of students have been successfully trained using the apprenticeship model of clinical education, there are a number of recognized problems with this model.

Dudding, C. C., & Ginsberg, S. M. (Eds.).
Simulation-Based Learning in Communication Sciences and Disorders: Moving From Theory to Practice. (pp. 3-16).

Current Model of Clinical Education

The current model of clinical education for graduate students in communication sciences and disorders (CSD) places a significant burden on graduate programs and clinical educators, both on and off campus. On-campus clinical educators are tasked with securing quality experiences for their students while faced with an increasing number of students, an expanding scope of practice, and fewer clinical placement sites. While a number of CSD programs have an on-campus clinic, most programs cannot provide the students with all the necessary clinical experiences without relying on off-campus placements (i.e., practicum, externships, internships). Another limiting factor of this model of clinical education is that not all students are guaranteed access to the same types of patients and disorders. Think about the acute hospital setting that provides experiences in diagnostics but few opportunities for developing therapeutic skills. Consider a private audiology practice that primarily dispenses hearing aids with no exposure to vestibular rehabilitation. To combat this, many programs require students to enroll in several placements in different settings (e.g., public schools, hospitals, private practice, skilled nursing facilities). Yet, this still does not guarantee equal access to a wide range of experiences within our clinical scopes of practice (e.g., transgender voice therapy, accent modification, cochlear implant mapping). Not to mention the time and resources required of programs in order to secure these placements.

Graduate programs in audiology and speech-language pathology rely heavily on off-campus clinical educators to provide the needed time, attention, and education to our students, while still maintaining all the responsibilities of the work setting. These allies are always balancing the learning needs of the students while prioritizing the welfare of the patient. Going beyond the range of experiences, we must consider the quality of the learning experiences. "See one, do one, teach one" is a mantra often heard in medical training programs. It supposes that in order to learn, the student must first observe an experienced professional conducting a procedure before performing the procedure themselves. The student will then demonstrate their knowledge and skill by "teaching back" (i.e., demonstrating) to the experienced professional. These types of learning experiences are perpetuated daily within the clinical practicum experiences of speech-language pathology and audiology students. This type of training, while effective, is resource intensive. It requires a 1:1 pairing of the teacher and learner. It also assumes that the clinical educator is knowledgeable about supervision and is instructing based on evidence-based practice (EBP), and that the student will have the opportunity to engage in observation and performance.

In the past, it had been assumed that good clinicians made good supervisors. Our own personal experiences may have taught us otherwise. A lack of clear expectations, limited or inconsistent feedback, and variability in assessment are all possible negative consequences of an untrained clinical educator. In recent years there has been an emerging recognition of supervision as a distinct area of clinical practice in CSD. It is only since 2020 that the CFCC has required training in supervision for clinical educators engaged in the supervision of graduate students and clinical fellows in speech-language pathology and audiology (CFCC, 2018).

These challenges, along with the anecdotally reported decrease in the number of available placements and increasing numbers of students in our graduate programs, make this model unsustainable as our primary method of clinical education. Clinical educators are thoughtfully seeking alternate approaches to clinical training to address the increasing difficulty in securing the necessary clinical placements for graduate students that provide diverse experiences across the expanding scope of clinical practice (McAllister, 2005; Ward et al., 2015).

Critical Thinking

The roles and responsibilities of clinical educators, whether on or off campus, go beyond teaching specific clinical skills and include additional responsibilities, such as clarifying concepts, conducting performance evaluations, mentoring, modeling professional behavior, and assisting in the development of critical thinking (Dudding & Pfeiffer, 2018). Teaching students to think critically and to seek answers based on evidence is the cornerstone of programs in higher education charged with the training of future health care professionals. Critical thinking is described as "an intellectual process of active conceptualization, application and synthesis of information gained through observation, experience and reflection" (Müller-Staub, 2006, p. 275). Finn, Brundage, and DiLollo (2016) offer the following to support the importance of critical thinking for communication sciences professionals:

- Critical thinking helps to minimize professional and personal biases.
- Future practitioners will need to be able to critically evaluate the quality of an expanding clinical knowledge base.
- Critical and clinical thinking are essential for EBP.
- Critical thinking is a core competency for collaborative and interprofessional endeavors.

Clinical decision making (CDM) is a process that, while informed by critical thinking, involves "an ongoing series of decisions where data are gathered, interpreted, and evaluated in order to make an evidence-based decision" (Tiffen et al., 2014, p. 399). It is the ability to engage in CDM that allows health care practitioners to perform accurate differential diagnosis and provide appropriate treatment to people with communication disorders. The ability to think critically and clinically extends beyond the ability to diagnose and treat; it includes the ability to thoughtfully consider and balance issues related to ethics, consent, and patient-centered care. A clinician's decision-making skills impact patient outcomes (Norman, 2005; Wainwright & McGinnis, 2009) and are the foundation for the development and implementation of high-quality clinical care (American Speech-Language-Hearing Association, 2005).

Few clinical educators in CSD would disagree on the importance of developing a student's critical and clinical thinking abilities; however, there is an assumption among many educators in higher education that bright, degree-seeking students will develop CDM through coursework and clinical experiences (Arum & Roksa, 2011; Crebbin et al., 2013). Research both within CSD and in related disciplines suggests that this is not the case and that more explicit instruction is needed for novice clinicians to develop these skills (Abrami et al., 2015; DeAngelo et al., 2009; Dudding & Pfeiffer, 2018; Finn, 2011; Ginsberg et al., 2016).

There is limited research literature on how to effectively teach critical thinking and CDM; however, a review of literature gives us important first steps as we move forward in this area. Abrami and colleagues (2015) conducted a meta-analysis of research related to teaching critical thinking. They determined that learners at all educational levels and across disciplinary areas can develop skills in critical thinking using a number of teaching strategies. These teaching strategies include the following:

- Critical discussion/dialogue (teacher and/or group led)
- Authentic or situated learning environments
- Mentorship, including 1:1 coaching, tutoring, and apprenticeship models

As we move through this book, you will recognize opportunities to include these educational strategies as part of a quality simulation-based learning experience (SBLE).

Factors Impacting Simulation-Based Learning in Communication Sciences and Disorders

In recent years, graduate programs in CSD have begun exploring clinical simulation as a way of supplementing current clinical education experiences. This interest is partly in response to the demands and challenges facing our clinical education programs, including availability of clinical placements, expanding scope of practice, and clinic closings due to a pandemic. The Council of Academic Programs in Communication Sciences and Disorders (CAPCSD) laid the foundation for simulation in CSD through the work of two task forces. The first task force explored the feasibility of simulations in CSD (CAPCSD, 2013), and the second task force produced an ebook outlining best practices in simulation (Dudding et al., 2019). A survey conducted in 2015 (Dudding & Nottingham, 2018) revealed that 51% of 136 responding programs in CSD reported using simulation in clinical education. Programs using simulations reported most often using standardized patients (SPs) and/or computer-based simulation. Barriers to using simulation included a lack of knowledge, limited financial resources, undertrained faculty, and little guidance from accrediting bodies. A number of respondents agreed with the statement that simulated experiences could account for up to 25% of required direct clinical hours in speech-language pathology and audiology (Dudding & Nottingham, 2018).

In 2016, American Speech-Language-Hearing Association's CFCC voted to modify the implementation language for Speech-Language Pathology Standard V-B to allow up to 20% of the required 375 direct clinical hours to be obtained through simulation (CFCC, 2018). Audiology standards allow for up to 10% of the students' clinical experiences to be obtained through simulation.

Along with an increase in interest in clinical simulation comes an increase in presentations, publications, and webinars. Research articles on the topic have begun to appear in peer-reviewed journals. The journal *Teaching and Learning in Communication Sciences and Disorders* (*TLCSD*) published a special topic issue showcasing the research being conducted in CSD specific to simulation.

The pandemic of 2020 forced many training sites and university programs to close down and/or switch to virtual formats to continue the clinical education of students enrolled in graduate programs. The lasting impact of the forced transition to telepractice and virtual simulations has yet to be seen in CSD.

Background in Simulation-Based Learning

History of Simulation

The use of simulation for medical training is not new. More than 150 years ago, visionaries in the fields of nursing and medicine saw the opportunity to revolutionize student training through use of clinical simulation. The literature mentions the use of a "mechanical dummy" as early as 1847 to give nursing students practice in bandaging limbs (Hayden et al., 2014, p. S4). In the 1960s, faced with combat mortality rates of 24%, the U.S. military began applying their simulation methods used for strategic combat training to medical and nursing training (Eubanks et al., 2020). In 1997, the Tactical Combat Casualty Care program was developed by the military with simulation at its core. The goal was to train frontline medics using medical simulation technologies. The combat-related death rate dropped from 90% to 10%, proving the success of simulation training (Eubanks et al., 2020).

The use of simulation for medical and nursing training, sometimes referred to as *health care simulation*, continued to grow throughout the 1990s and into the new millennium. During this period, patient health care had become more complex, which resulted in a corresponding increase in medical errors. Calls for improved patient safety, advancement in simulation technologies, and limited availability of preceptors and clinical supervisors prompted an increased use of high-fidelity health care simulation in civilian nursing and medicine (Hayden et al., 2014). In his history of medical simulation, Bradley (2006) describes the societal, political, and professional factors that led to the rapid increase in the use of simulation. These factors include (a) failures of the traditional training methods, (b) reduced availability of training sites, (c) increases in licensing regulations and calls for safety, and (d) mandates for interprofessional training. These challenges should sound familiar to those engaged in clinical education in CSD. A corresponding increase in advanced technologies, such as computers, virtual reality (VR), and artificial intelligence, has allowed for growth in the types and availability of technologies available for simulation for health care training (Bradley, 2006). As simulation-based learning became more prevalent in the medical and nursing schools, allied health professionals, such as physical therapists, respiratory therapists, dentists, audiologists, and speech-language pathologists, began to take notice and consider the benefits of simulation for education for all students pursuing degrees in health care professions.

Research Evidence

It was these successes in the military that prompted medical and nursing programs throughout the United States to incorporate simulation into the clinical education of health care professionals. In turn, the effectiveness of simulation in related health care disciplines, such as nursing and medicine, has been well studied (Cook et al., 2011; Hayden et al., 2014; Sherwood & Francis, 2018). In an often-cited study, Cook and colleagues (2011) examined the effectiveness of simulation for student training across nursing, medicine, and allied health professions. They conducted a meta-analysis of more than 600 articles from the fields of medicine, nursing, dentistry and other health professions. The researchers concluded that "technology-enhanced simulation training in health professions education is consistently associated with large effects for outcomes of knowledge, skills, and behaviors and moderate effects for patient-related outcomes" (Cook et al., 2011, p. 978). In a similar study looking at physical therapy students, researchers found that replacing up to 25% of traditional clinical experiences with simulated experiences did not affect student performance on an examination of clinical skills when compared to a control group of students who participated in traditional clinical training (Watson et al., 2012). These results suggest that the use of simulation in the training of allied health students is a viable alternative to traditional hands-on practice with real patients.

In a landmark study published in 2014 in the *Journal of Nursing Regulation,* Hayden et al. investigated the use of simulation in prelicensure nursing education using a randomized controlled study that included 666 students across 10 programs. The control group received all clinical education through traditional means, while treatment groups replaced 25% or 50% of traditional clinical education with simulation. Participants were assessed using a variety of measures. Findings revealed no significant differences between the control group and treatment groups in the measures of clinical competency, critical thinking, and preparedness to practice as a registered nurse.

The field of nursing has been prolific in its research of health care simulation and serves as a solid foundation for allied health fields, such as CSD, in moving forward with simulation with confidence. The International Nursing Association for Clinical Simulation and Learning (INACSL) has published a series of best practices in health care simulation, as shown in Table 1-1. The articles are readily available for viewing at https://www.inacsl.org and include a rationale and criteria for each of the best practices.

Research Evidence in Communications Sciences and Disorders

There is a long-standing body of literature supporting the use of SPs in CSD education (Alanazi et al., 2017; Hill et al., 2013; Naeve-Velguth et al., 2013; Syder, 1996; Zraick, 2002, 2020; Zraick et al., 2003). Studies on the use of task trainers (Benadom & Potter, 2011), high-fidelity manikins (Alanazi et al., 2016; Clinard & Dudding, 2019; Estis et al., 2015; Potter & Allen, 2013; Ward et al., 2015), and computer-based game scenarios (Lieberth & Martin, 2005) specific to CSD can be found in the literature. These studies indicate that simulated learning environments increase learners' levels of comfort and confidence in performing various techniques. Some studies report that learners gained foundational knowledge in working with a variety of different disorder groups.

The number and types of research being conducted to the use of simulation in CSD is growing. Hill and colleagues (2020) conducted a randomized controlled trial with 325 speech-language pathology students enrolled in six university programs in Australia. For the treatment group, approximately 20% of the total clinical hours were replaced by 5 days of simulation. The results support findings of other disciplines in that simulation can replace face-to-face learning while yielding similar learning outcomes.

TABLE 1-1

A Summary of International Nursing Association for Clinical Simulation and Learning Best Practices in Simulation

STANDARD	STATEMENT	CRITERIA
Professional Development	Professional development is necessary for the simulationist to stay current with simulation-based education.	• Develop an educational needs plan based on self-reflection, assessment of current knowledge, and future goals. • Attend and participate in professional development activities at local, regional, national, and international levels. • Revise the educational plan on an ongoing basis.
Professional Integrity	Professional integrity is demonstrated and upheld by all involved in SBLEs.	• Uphold the Healthcare Simulationist Code of Ethics, as well as the standards of practice and ethics of one's profession. • Practice inclusion by respecting equity, diversity, and inclusivity. • Require confidentiality of the performances and scenario content.
Simulation Design	SBLEs align with identified objectives and optimize the achievement of expected outcomes.	• Design the SBLE in consultation with content experts and those knowledgeable of best practices in simulation education, pedagogy, and practice. • Base the design on a needs assessment and include objectives that build upon the learner's foundational knowledge. • Provide the context for the SBLE in order to create the required perception of realism. • Use a learner-centered facilitative approach. • Include a plan for prebriefing, feedback, and evaluation of the learner and the experience. • Pilot test of the SBLE before implementation.
Outcomes and Objectives	All SBLEs begin with clearly written, measurable objectives designed to achieve expected behaviors and outcomes.	• Create objectives based on needs of the learners, that are measurable and appropriately scaffolded to learner knowledge, skills, and attributes (KSAs). • Define outcomes based on formative or summative evaluation. • Select simulation modality and level of fidelity to meet the learning objectives/outcomes. • Include guidelines for the facilitation of the SBLE.
Prebriefing: Preparation and Briefing	Prebriefing prepares learners for the SBLE.	• Prepare learners for the educational content of the SBLE. • Convey ground rules for the SBLE.
Facilitation	Facilitation guides participants to work cohesively, comprehend learning objectives, and develop a plan to achieve desired outcomes.	• Requires specific skills and knowledge in simulation pedagogy. • Provide facilitation approach appropriate to the level of learning, experience, and competency of the participants. • Include preparatory activities and a prebriefing. • Deliver cues to assist participants in achieving expected outcomes. • Support participants in achieving expected outcomes.

(continued)

TABLE 1-1 (continued)

A Summary of International Nursing Association for Clinical Simulation and Learning Best Practices in Simulation

STANDARD	STATEMENT	CRITERIA
Debriefing Process	SBLE activities must include a planned debriefing process. This debriefing process may include any of the activities of feedback, debriefing, and/or guided reflection.	• Incorporate the debrief into the SBLE to guide the achievement of the desired learning objectives and outcomes. • Construct, design, and/or facilitate the debrief using a person/people competent in providing appropriate feedback, debriefing, and/or guided reflection. • Promote self, team, and/or systems analysis. • Structure based on theoretical frameworks and/or evidenced-based concepts.
Evaluation of Learning and Performance	SBLEs include evaluation of the learner.	• Determine evaluation and learning performance measures and methods before the SBLE. • Consider use of formative, summative, or high-stakes evaluation.
Operations	All simulation-based education programs require systems and infrastructure to support and maintain operations.	• Coordinate and align resources to achieve goals. • Provide personnel with appropriate expertise. • Manage space, equipment, and personnel resources. • Secure and manage the financial resources to support stability, sustainability, and growth. • Use process for effective systems integration. • Create policies and procedures to support, sustain, and/or grow the program.
Simulation-enhanced IPE (Sim-IPE)	Sim-IPE enables learners from different health care professions to achieve shared objectives and outcomes.	• Base on a theoretical or conceptual framework. • Utilize best practices in the design and development. • Recognize and address potential barriers to Sim-IPE. • Include an evaluation plan for Sim-IPE.

Adapted from INACSL Standards Committee. (2021). INACSL healthcare simulation standards of best practice (4th ed.). https://www.inacsl.org/healthcare-simulation-standards

A keyword search using the words "simulation," "audiology," and "speech-language pathology" yields an exciting list of peer-reviewed articles. These keyword searches offer information regarding frameworks for simulated learning in CSD (Clark & Lombard, 2020; Hewat et al., 2020a, 2020b; Stead et al., 2020), the effectiveness of simulated learning environments as learning tools (Carter, 2019; Vinney et al., 2016), effective integration of simulated learning into the curriculum (MacBean et al., 2013), learning outcomes in specific disorder types (e.g., hearing detection, dysphagia, feeding and transnasal endoscopy; Alanazi & Nicholson, 2019; Broadfoot & Estis, 2020; Ward et al., 2015), and evaluation and assessment practices (Clinard, 2020). There is also information on professional competencies (Wolford & Wolford, 2020).

Clinical Simulation as a Technique

Mention the word *simulation* and thoughts of expensive simulation centers filled with high-tech manikins and hospital equipment and a technology team worthy of a space launch fills our heads. We soon feel defeated, thinking that our own programs could never afford a simulation program, let alone know what to do with one. What is key to realize is that simulations are "a technique—not a technology—to replace or amplify real experiences with guided experiences that evoke or replicate substantial aspects of the real world in a fully interactive manner" (Gaba, 2004, p. i2). With that assurance, our minds begin to wonder about ways we can provide opportunities for our students to engage in real-world experiences. Perhaps you have a list of challenges facing your clinical education program. Clinical simulation can help address some of those challenges; whether it is a need to provide students with training in a specific skill or task, as an evaluation tool to assess clinical competencies, or as an experiential learning opportunity for students.

Clinical simulation is a form of simulation designed to represent a real-life clinical event for the purpose of "practice, learning, evaluation, testing, or to gain understanding of systems or human actions" (Lopreiato, 2016, p. 15). It is designed to provide learners the opportunity to perform clinical skills, demonstrate a wide range of competencies, and learn to collaborate with other professionals. The term *clinical simulation,* also known as *health care simulation,* is most often associated with the medical setting—nursing, medicine, and allied health professionals, such as physical therapists, audiologists, occupational therapists, and speech-language pathologists. However, the use of simulation as a technique is not limited to medical situations and can be applied to any clinical practice setting, including school-based settings.

Simulation-Based Learning Experiences

The SBLE refers to the collection of carefully planned educational methods and procedures that make up a quality SBLE (Rudolph et al., 2014). In other words, SBLE is more than a simulation; it is a process. An SBLE requires additional steps of the prebrief and debrief in order to create a successful learning event. This goes along with the earlier definition of simulation as a technique and not a technology (Gaba, 2004). Most often, SBLE is described as consisting of three stages: the prebrief, the simulation experience, and the debrief. Prior to engaging in the simulation experience, the learners are oriented to the technology, introduced to the clinical case, and assigned roles for the simulation. This is referred to as the *prebrief.* In order to encourage a safe learning environment, it is recommended that the prebriefing include a discussion of expectations of performance, including learning objectives and evaluation measures (Dieckmann et al., 2007; Gaba, 2004; Jeffries, 2005). As part of the prebrief, learners may be asked to share their initial thoughts relative to their clinical hypothesis and plan for assessment and/or intervention, much like what takes place between the student and the clinical educator in a traditional clinical experience.

After completion of the prebriefing, the learners will engage in the *simulation experience.* In designing the simulation, much consideration is given to the scenario. The scenario can be thought of as the script for the simulation experience and can vary in length and complexity, depending on the learning objectives. The learning objectives for a given simulation should address all domains of knowledge (cognitive), skills (psychomotor), and attributes (characteristics of the learner). These domains are often identified collectively as KSAs. Typical simulation experiences are 20 to 30 minutes in duration, excluding the prebrief and debrief. The simulation experience should include opportunities for CDM, as well as the acquisition of knowledge and skills. The experienced clinical educator will determine the expected level of learner participation (e.g., student led or instructor led), types of evaluation and assessment, and the level of fidelity or realism required of the experience, as well as the physical setup of the room/environment, equipment, and supporting documentation. For a full discussion of developing learning objectives and development of a scenario for simulation, the reader is directed to Chapter 5 as well as the work of Alinier (2011) and Jeffries et al. (2015). Chapter 6 provides the rationale and practical guidance in developing a comprehensive assessment plan as part of the early stages of simulation design.

The final step in the SBLE process is the *debrief.* The debrief is often cited as the most critical learning component of the simulation learning experience. The debrief, which typically occurs immediately following the simulation experience, is led by an experienced facilitator, such as an academic or clinical educator, who has observed or participated in the SBLE. During this time, the participants receive feedback and are encouraged to engage in reflective thinking, while various clinical aspects of the simulation are discussed. The debrief is key in learner assimilation and transfer of learning to future situations, which is ultimately the goal of SBLE (Jeffries et al., 2015). There are many models of debriefing in the literature (e.g., Debriefing with Good Judgment, PEARLS, Diamond).

Organizations such as the Society for Simulation in Healthcare (SSH) and the INACSL highlight the importance of training for those engaged in the simulation debrief. Refer to Chapter 5 for a full discussion of the prebrief, simulation experience, and the debrief. Chapter 7 is written for those interested in professional development and training in this area of clinical education.

Simulation Technologies

Now that we have spent considerable time addressing simulation as a technique, it is time to consider the technologies employed. It is only after identifying the learning objectives and designing the scenario that the educator will determine the types of simulation modalities and technologies to best meet the learning objectives and needs of the learners. There are a number of technologies employed in simulation-based education. Each of these technologies varies according to the level of fidelity and/or realism. Commonly used forms of clinical simulation include SPs, task trainers, high-tech manikins, computer-based programs, and virtual/augmented reality (AR). Definitions and examples of each type of technology to follow. Simulations that include more than one modality, such as an SP wearing a false tracheostomy tube,

BOX 1-1

Models of Debriefing in Simulation

Debriefing with Good Judgment	Rudolph, J. W., Simon. R., Dufresne, R. L., & Raemer, D. B. (2006). There's no such thing as "nonjudgmental" debriefing: A theory and method for debriefing with good judgment. *Simulation in Healthcare, 1*(1), 49-55.
Promoting Excellence and Reflective Learning in Simulation (PEARLS)	Bajaj K., Meguerdichian M., Thoma B., Huang S., Eppich W., & Cheng A. (2018). The PEARLS healthcare debriefing tool. *Academic Medicine, 93*(2), 336.
Plus Delta	Sawyer, T. L., & Deering, S. (2013). Adaptation of the US Army's After-Action Review for simulation debriefing in healthcare. *Simulation in Healthcare, 8*(6), 388-397.
Diamond	Jaye, P., Thomas, L., & Reedy, G. (2015). "The Diamond": A structure for simulation debrief. *Clinical Teacher, 12*(3), 171-175.

are referred to as a *hybrid model of simulation*. The reader should be aware that a higher level of realism does not guarantee improved learning outcomes and so should not be the main determinant when designing a simulation experience.

Standardized Patient

An SP may be an able-bodied individual trained to simulate a patient's illness or may be a patient trained to present their disease. The part of the label *standardized* means that the SP performs and responds in a consistent manner within each simulation experience, thus ensuring the experience is the same across learners.

An SP encounter can be a simulated patient encounter, such as portraying someone with a communication disorder, but a simulated patient encounter is not necessarily standardized (Adamo, 2003). SPs are well suited for SBLEs that require interpersonal and professional communication skills. SPs are often used in a performance-based clinical assessment called the *Objective Structured Clinical Examination* (OSCE). The OSCE has become a well-accepted method of summative clinical skills assessment requiring students to perform specific tasks within a prescribed period in a highly structured encounter (Harden, 1988). The pharmacy profession worldwide, like that of medicine, has moved toward requiring all applicants for licensure to successfully pass a standardized, high-stakes OSCE. The OSCE requires applicants to demonstrate competencies in a number of clinical and professional areas, and there is emerging evidence supporting its use in speech-language pathology and audiology (Hill et al., 2013; Nickbakht et al., 2013).

Task Trainer

Task trainers are a form of simulation technology frequently used in training students in speech-language pathology and audiology. Task trainers are especially effective in allowing the learner to practice psychomotor skills repeatedly until the point that the skill is acquired. Task trainers can be either life-like models of different body parts, such as an ear or head/neck region, or nonanatomical devices/mechanical models, such as an audiometer, used to teach function, pathologies, or testing concepts. Task trainers break down a specific psychomotor skill into its discrete action steps. An example of this technology is an otoscopy trainer OtoSim 2. This is a computer-based trainer, consisting of an artificial ear and otoscope, through which the student can learn about the anatomy of the tympanic membrane and practice identifying a variety of tympanic and middle ear pathologies. Task-trainers have entered a new stage of wearable technologies. An example of a wearable task trainer is Avtrach (Avkin). Avtrach is a prosthetic chest with a trach tube that is worn by an SP. The Avtrach provides a realistic trach-suctioning experience, allows learners to listen to lung sounds, and alerts the learner if they are endangering the patient. Coupled with the behavioral responses of a well-trained SP, the use of wearable technologies is a powerful tool in establishing an interactive and lifelike environment. The appropriate pairing of a wearable task trainer and an SP would be considered a hybrid simulation.

High-Tech Manikin

The next type of simulation technology includes manikins. Manikins vary in the level of realism and technology. It is worth noting that not all manikins employ technology. Educators often employ dolls to practice feeding and positioning for infants. Digitized manikins are high-fidelity simulators or computerized manikins that allow learners to practice conducting tests or procedures. These life-size simulators are designed to be realistic and are available in a variety of preterm, infant, child, and adult models. High-fidelity simulators simulate physiologic functions, such as cardiac function, pulse rate, respiratory patterns, pupil dilation, muscle tone, electroencephalogram, and cochlear hair cell movement (Damassa & Sitko, 2010; Dudding et al., 2019). High-fidelity simulators allow learners to practice complex high-risk, low-incidence procedures in a safe yet realistic and responsive context. Through the computer-controlled manikin, many pathologies or disorders can be replicated. Learners can practice tests or protocols to aid in diagnosis. For example, otoacoustic emissions or auditory brainstem response testing can be conducted on a lifelike infant manikin (Brown, 2017). High-fidelity preterm manikins have been used to train clinical and nonclinical students to assess oral feeding skills in preterm infants (Broadfoot & Estis, 2020; Clinard & Dudding, 2019; Ferguson & Estis, 2018). High-fidelity manikins are well suited for training in collaborative and interprofessional practice (otherwise known as *simulation-enhanced interprofessional education*). High-fidelity manikins equipped with a tracheostomy tube and a speaking valve have been used to prepare speech-language pathology, respiratory therapy, and nursing students for interprofessional collaborative practice (Estis et al., 2015).

Computer-Based Programs and Virtual/Augmented Reality

There are an increasing number of computer-based and VR simulations being developed across the simulation health care industry. The advent of the COVID-19 pandemic and the demand for virtual clinical learning has surely hastened development in this area. Computer-based simulations model real-life processes, usually with minimal levels of realism. As the name implies, they are usually associated with a monitor and a keyboard. Those in the field of speech-language pathology and audiology will recognize Simucase as the predominant company offering computer-based simulation designed and produced specifically for the training of students in our professions. There are a range of cases, both diagnostic and intervention, across a number of disorders (e.g., articulation, phonation, traumatic brain injury, voice, swallowing). Computer-based simulations are learner centered in that they allow the learner to "create their own adventure" based on their responses. Once the learner has logged in to a simulation, they can start and stop the simulation at will. The cases are designed to step learners through a clinical procedure and allow the learner to make choices based on their clinical knowledge and skill. The learner receives both formative and summative feedback about their performance in real time. Learners quickly become skilled in monitoring the points awarded for various decisions, view their progress toward completion, or receive a final grade based on their performance. It is for these and other reasons that this category of simulation is sometimes referred to as *gamification*. This term is often avoided in clinical education given its association with recreational video gaming; however, when based on a strong pedagogical basis as described in this book, such computer-based simulations are effective learning tools.

VR is the latest technology that holds promise in the realm of simulation. VR simulation is defined as real people controlling a simulated experience (Lopreiato, 2016). VR, in the broad sense, refers to a three-dimensional experience, created by computer technologies, in order to create an immersive, interactive environment that simulates real life (Dudding et al., 2019). Examples of virtual simulations include flight simulators, surgical simulators (e.g., laparoscopic surgery), and vestibular testing. In some cases, the interaction takes place in the form of a three-dimensional computer-generated persona, known as an avatar. In other cases, interaction takes place with use of game controllers, motion detectors, haptic gloves, or even hand motion. Many of the technologies employed in VR come from the world of gaming, social media, and business, and are adapted for the creation of virtual health care simulations. AR is seen by some as an exciting next step in clinical simulation. Some of you have experienced this application in your online retail experiences. For example, AR will allow you to use your cellphone to virtually try on a pair of designer glasses by superimposing them on a photo of your face. There is great anticipation about the future of AR as it makes its way into the educational arena. Refer to Chapter 4 for a full description of the modalities and technologies being employed as part of the SBLE.

Best Practices in Simulation-Based Learning

The best practices described earlier and that follow in the subsequent chapters of this book are grounded in educational philosophies and learning theories; some are specific to simulated learning, but many have long standing in the area of teaching and learning. They are rooted in the domains of behaviorism, constructivism, and cognitive science. Chapter 2 will provide an in-depth exploration of key learning theories as they relate to CDM, competency development, and learning. This section serves to introduce you to some of the relevant learning theories in order to provide a framework as you move forward in your consideration of the role of clinical simulation as part of clinical education in CSD.

Let's begin with a discussion of what constitutes a quality simulation learning experience. Kneebone (2005) lists several characteristics of quality SBLEs:

- They allow for deliberate practice.
- They are learner centered.
- They provide expert facilitation.
- They are designed to be similar to real life (realism).

Let's explore each of these criteria.

Deliberate Practice

Deliberate practice (DP) is when learners actively practice a skill or task to improve their current level of proficiency (Clapper & Kardong-Edgren, 2012). DP must be immediate, be specific, offer informative feedback, allow for problem solving and evaluation, and provide opportunities for repeated performance. DP allows for repeated practice without the risk of harm to the patient. Simulation is well suited for skill development, such as passing a videoscope through the nasal passage, preparing ear molds, and programming a cochlear implant device.

Learner Centered

The second of Kneebone's criteria states that the experience should be learner centered. Learner-centered approaches come out of the constructivist model and are based on the idea that learners construct meaning through integration of new knowledge and their own experiences (Weimer, 2013). Learner centered means that students assume responsibility for their learning by engaging themselves in the experience and reflecting on their experience. Experiential learning theory is an example of a learner-centered approach. Kolb's experiential learning theory proposes that learning takes place as a result of "grasping and transforming experience" (Kolb, 1984, p. 51). Importantly, the learners are responsible for the direction of the SBLE as they move through a learning cycle consisting of four stages: concrete experience, abstract conceptualization, reflective observation, and active experimentation. A learner-centered approach dictates a change in the way we view ourselves as teachers and educators.

Expert Facilitation

The role of the academic and/or clinical educator is to function as a facilitator to guide students in their learning and help them to make meaningful connections between prior and new knowledge and to reflect on the learning process (Bada, 2015). Facilitators should possess a clear understanding of the characteristics of learners and teachers, be familiar with learning styles, foster experiential learning, and support critical thinking and metacognition.

Fidelity

In order to meet all of Kneebone's criteria for a quality SBLE, the SBLE must be designed in a way to mimic real life. In the world of clinical simulation, this is often referred to as *fidelity*. Fidelity refers to how closely the SBLE replicates the real-world experience and allows the learner to immerse themselves and suspend disbelief (Wilson & Wittmann-Price, 2015). The design elements that influence fidelity as well as the importance of fidelity for student learning are up for debate (Dieckmann et al., 2007). There are three types of simulation fidelity:

1. Physical or environmental
2. Conceptual
3. Psychological (Dieckmann et al., 2007; INACSL Standards Committee, 2016)

Physical or environmental fidelity, as the name implies, refers to how closely the physical context of the simulation reflects the real-life environment. Physical fidelity includes the simulator, equipment, and related props. Many nursing and medical education programs have a simulation center or lab. These often include a number of rooms made to look like actual spaces within the health care system (e.g., patient hospital room, operating room, consultation room). The rooms are outfitted with all the furniture and medical equipment that you would find in the real-world environment. The space is designed to allow learners to physically interact with the tools and/or devices that mimic an aspect of clinical care (Lopreiato, 2016). Within these spaces, learners will often encounter high-tech manikins that closely replicate human functioning such as breathing, eye movement, circulation, sweating, and bleeding. The students may encounter a high-tech manikin, such as SimMan (Laerdal), dressed in a hospital gown and lying in a hospital bed surrounded by monitors. In the case of a pediatric SBLE, Baby HAL (Gaumard) may be found in an incubator with an arterial line and apnea monitor in place. SPs may don make-up, known as *moulage*, replicating an open and bleeding wound.

Another type of simulation fidelity is conceptual fidelity, which ensures that all elements of the scenario or case relate to each other in a realistic way and comply with actual standards of practice (INACSL Standards Committee, 2016). For example, in designing an SBLE around a person with aphasia following a stroke, the materials and reports provided to the learner should be consistent with best practices in patient care and reflect what the learner is likely to experience in the real-world situation. In fact, many SBLEs are designed with an actual patient as the basis for the scenario. It is recommended that the case scenario and supporting documentation be reviewed by subject matter experts and piloted before use in order to support conceptual fidelity.

Psychological fidelity seeks to replicate the psychological and/or emotional demands under which the simulation takes place. For example, an SP serving in the role of a parent begins to cry as you explain to them that their newborn has failed the newborn hearing screening. Other ways to enhance psychological fidelity is to include other health care team members, add an element of time pressure, and introduce competing priorities (e.g., patient experiences respiratory arrest while trialing a speaking valve). Research also suggests that psychological fidelity enhances carry over and generalization of skills (Kozlowski & DeShon, 2004). The overall aim of these efforts is to produce an immersive experience in which participants are willing to suspend disbelief and accept falsehoods and inconsistencies in order to fully engage in the experience.

It is a commonly held belief that the higher the level of fidelity, the better the simulation learning experience. There is an expectation that a $140,000 high-tech simulator housed within a multimillion-dollar simulation center will provide learners with exceptional learner outcomes. For those of us who do not have access to simulation centers and high-tech manikins, it is important to note that research has not shown a direct link between the level of fidelity and learning outcomes when measured as soon as 1 week post simulation (Dieckmann et al., 2007; Sherwood & Francis, 2018). More recent research suggests that fidelity is not proportional to the effectiveness of the simulation and suggests that mid-level fidelity has the most utility in health care student training (Kim et al., 2016; Sherwood & Francis, 2018; Shin et al., 2015).

Ethical, Legal, and Regulatory Considerations

Hopefully you have formulated some ideas about the role that clinical simulation education has to play in our clinical education programs—specifically in the development of high-quality professionals who are able to effectively, efficiently, and compassionately serve those with communication disorders. A well-designed SBLE goes beyond drill and practice of skill development and offers a unique opportunity to develop the learner's sense of professional identity and integrity (MacBean et al., 2013). This section will introduce the ethical, legal, and regulatory requirements that will help to ensure the safety of both the patients and the learners engaged in simulation education.

The learner–educator relationship is critical to the success of clinical simulation learning. Throughout this book, you will hear mention of the importance of creating a safe environment for the learner in order to establish trust between the learner and the educator. Some would argue that it applies to all types of learning environments. It is by design that learner safety and trust are established in the context of simulation for clinical education. Among those factors to be considered are providing the learners with (a) clear expectations, including codes of conduct; (b) an evaluation process that is fair and transparent and linked to learner objectives; and (c) stated policies on confidentiality. This would also include a policy on the use of deception in simulation (Calhoun, 2020; Haupt & Meakin, 2015).

In January 2018, an international group of simulation educators gathered to create a code of ethics to guide those engaged in clinical simulation. The resulting Healthcare Simulationist Code of Ethics (Park et al., 2018) is available to readers through the SSH website (https://www.ssih.org/SSH-Resources/Code-of-Ethics). The key principles in this guiding document include the aspiration values of integrity, transparency, mutual respect, professionalism, accountability, and results orientation. They encompass all of the factors contributing to both patient and student safety. These principles, described in Table 1-2, are in alignment with other standards of conduct, including the INACSL Standards for Professional Integrity (INACSL Standards Committee et al. 2021), and should be familiar to those engaged in simulated learning.

You will read about the importance of integrating simulation learning into the existing curriculum. In doing so there may be additional regulatory considerations that are specific to the institution and/or learning environment. For example, what are the policies regarding documentation and Health Insurance Portability and Accountability Act compliance that might impact the SBLE? What is required in terms of institutional approval when using simulation learning as part of research? What is the institution's policy of the use of deception? In the unlikely event that a learner is harmed, either physically or emotionally, what are the requirements for incident reporting? These questions are not meant to dissuade or frighten anyone away from the use of simulation-based learning but are meant to inform, and thereby support, the development of high-quality, safe learning experiences.

Summary

Clinical simulation allows students to begin the process of integrating knowledge and skills acquired in the classroom to the real-life application of clinical skills in a safe, risk-free environment. A strategic and thoughtful integration of clinical simulation into university training programs offers students access to a range of learning opportunities that may not be available in every clinical setting. The students can repeat a simulation until they have reached a level of competency. They can develop clinical skills in a safe and controlled environment without risk to the patient or themselves. A well-trained simulation educator provides detailed and immediate feedback to the learner, taking advantage of the teachable moments. Additionally, the simulation experience can be customized to the learner. Clinical simulation is also an effective assessment tool.

Moving beyond procedural skill development and practice, clinical simulations are also effective in developing professional behaviors, such as teamwork, interprofessional collaboration, and ethical decision making. This book will build on the best practices for simulation design, implementation, and evaluation. It will offer examples that are applicable to programs in CSD and that employ a range of technologies. You will be reminded in many ways throughout this book, both subtle and direct, that simulation is "a technique—not a technology" (Gaba, 2004, p. i2).

TABLE 1-2

Standards of Professional Integrity and Ethical Behavior

STATEMENT	CRITERIA
INACSL Standard Professional Integrity Professional integrity refers to the ethical behaviors and conduct expected of all involved in simulation-based experiences. These standards apply to facilitators, learners, and participants.	Uphold the SSH Code of Ethics, and the code of ethics of their professional association. Follow standards of best practice, guidelines, and principals of the profession. Create and maintain a safe learning environment. Respect diversity, inclusion, and equity. Follow guidelines for confidentiality.
Healthcare Simulationist Code of Ethics This Simulationist Code of Ethics aims to promote, strengthen, and support an ethical culture among all individuals and organizations engaged in health care simulation. It has been adopted by many institutions and organizations.	Value I. Integrity Healthcare Simulationists shall maintain the highest standards of integrity including honesty, truthfulness, fairness, and judgment in all matters affecting their duties. Value II. Transparency Healthcare Simulationists shall perform all healthcare simulation activities in a manner that promotes transparency and clarity in the design, communication, and decision-making processes. Value III. Mutual Respect Healthcare Simulationists shall respect the rights, dignity, and worth of all. They shall practice empathy and compassion to support beneficence and non-maleficence toward all involved in simulation activities. Value IV. Professionalism Healthcare Simulationists shall conduct themselves in a manner that upholds the professional standards inherent in healthcare simulation. Value V. Accountability Healthcare Simulationists shall be accountable for their decisions and actions in fulfilling their duties and responsibilities. Value VI. Results Orientation Healthcare Simulationists shall serve to support activities that enhance the quality of the profession and healthcare systems. Outcomes are inclusive of all parts of the process of healthcare simulation and are not exclusive to a final product.

Adapted from Park, C. S., Murphy, T. F., & the Code of Ethics Working Group. (2018). Healthcare Simulationist Code of Ethics. Society for Simulation in Healthcare, http://www.ssih.org/Code-of-Ethics and INACSL Standards Committee, Bowler, F., Klein, M. & Wilford, A. (2021). Healthcare Simulation Standards of Best Practice Professional Integrity. *Clinical Simulation in Nursing, 58*, 45-48. https://doi.org/10.1016/j.ecns.2021.08.014

References

Abrami, P. C., Bernard, R. M., Borokhovski, E., Waddington, D. I., Wade, C. A., & Persson, T. (2015). Strategies for teaching students to think critically: A meta-analysis. *Review of Educational Research, 85*(2), 275-314. https://doi.org/10.3102/0034654314551063.

Accreditation Commission for Audiology Education. (2016). *Accreditation standards for the doctor of audiology program*. https://acaeaccred.org/wp-content/uploads/sites/1543/2016/07/ACAE-Standards-5.11NEW-WEB-2.pdf

Adamo, G. (2003). Simulated and standardized patients in OSCEs: Achievement and challenges 1993-2003. *Medical Teacher, 25*(3), 262-270. https://doi.org/10.1080/0142159031000100300

Alanazi, A. A., & Nicholson, N. (2019). Audiology and speech-language pathology simulation training on the 1-3-6 early hearing detection and intervention timeline. *American Journal of Audiology, 28*(2), 348-361. https://www.doi.org/10.1044/2019_AJA-18-0185

Alanazi, A. A., Nicholson, N., Atcherson, S. R., Franklin, C., Anders, M., Nagaraj, N. K., Franklin, J., & Highley, P. (2016). Use of baby ISAO simulator and standardized parents in hearing screening and parent counseling education. *American Journal of Audiology, 25*, 211-223. https://pubs.asha.org/doi/abs/10.1044/2016_AJA-16-0029

Alanazi, A. A., Nicholson, N., Atcherson, S. R., Franklin, C., Nagaraj, N. K., Anders, M., & Smith-Olinde, L. (2017). Audiology students' perception of hybrid simulation experiences: Qualitative evaluation of debriefing sessions. *Journal of Early Hearing Detection and Intervention, 2*(1), 12-28. https://digitalcommons.usu.edu/jehdi/vol2/iss1/3/

Alinier, G. (2011). Developing high fidelity health care simulation scenarios: A guide for educators and professionals. *Simulation and Gaming, 42*(1), 9-26. https://doi.org/10.1177/1046878109355683

American Speech-Language-Hearing Association. (2005). *Evidence-based practice in communication disorders.* https://www.asha.org/policy/ps2005-00221/

Arum, R., & Roksa, J. (2011). *Academically adrift: Limited learning on college campuses.* University of Chicago Press.

Bada, S. O. (2015). Constructivism learning theory: A paradigm for teaching and learning. *Journal of Research & Method in Education, 5*(6), 66-70.

Benadom, E. M., & Potter, N. L. (2011). The use of simulation in training graduate students to perform transnasal endoscopy. *Dysphagia, 26*, 352-360. http://doi.org/10.1007/s00455-010-9316-y

Bradley, P. (2006). The history of simulation in medical education and possible future directions. *Medical Education, 40*, 254-262. https://doi.org/10.1111/j.1365-2929.2006.02394.x

Broadfoot, C., & Estis, J. (2020). Simulation-based training improves student assessment of oral feeding skills in preterm infants. *Teaching and Learning in Communication Sciences & Disorders, 4*(3). https://ir.library.illinoisstate.edu/tlcsd/vol4/iss3/8

Brown, D. K. (2017). Simulation before clinical practice: The educational advantages. *Audiology Today, 29*(5), 16-25. https://www.audiology.org/news-and-publications/audiology-today/articles/simulation-before-clinical-practice-the-educational-advantages/

Calhoun, A. W. (2020). Guidelines for the responsible use of deception in simulation. *Simulation in Healthcare, 15*(4), 7.

Carter, M. D. (2019). The effects of computer-based simulations on speech-language pathology student performance. *Journal of Communication Disorders, 77*, 44-55. https://doi.org/10.1016/j.jcomdis.2018.12.006

Clapper, T. C., & Kardong-Edgren, S. (2012). Using deliberate practice and simulation to improve nursing skills. *Clinical Simulation in Nursing, 6*(1), e7-e14.

Clark, E., & Lombard, L. (2020). Developing an acute care simulation lab and practicum. *Teaching and Learning in Communication Sciences & Disorders, 4*(3). https://ir.library.illinoisstate.edu/tlcsd/vol4/iss3/5

Clinard, E. (2020). Assessing outcomes of simulation in communication sciences and disorders. *Teaching and Learning in Communication Sciences & Disorders, 4*(3). https://ir.library.illinoisstate.edu/tlcsd/vol4/iss3/7

Clinard, E. S., & Dudding, C. C. (2019). Integrating simulations into communication sciences and disorders clinical curriculum: Impact of student perceptions. *American Journal of Speech-Language Pathology, 28*(1), 136-147. https://doi.org/10.1044/2018_AJSLP-18-0003

Cook, D. A., Hatala, R., Brydges, R., Zendejas, B., Szostek, J. H., Wang, A. T., Erwin, P. J., & Hamstra, S. J. (2011). Technology-enhanced simulation for health professions education: A systematic review and meta-analysis. *Journal of the American Medical Association, 306*(9), 978-988. https://doi.org/10.1001/jama.2011.1234

Council for Academic Programs in Communication Sciences and Disorders. (2013). *Preparation of speech-language pathology clinical educators* [White paper].

Council for Clinical Certification in Audiology and Speech-Language Pathology. (2018). *2020 standards for the certificate of clinical competence in audiology.* American Speech-Language-Hearing Association. www.asha.org/certification/2020-Audiology-Certification-Standards/

Crebbin, W., Beasley, S. W., & Watters, D. A. K. (2013). Clinical decision making: How surgeons do it. *ANZ Journal of Surgery, 83*(6), 422-428. https://doi.org/10.1111/ans.12180

Damassa, D. A., & Sitko, T. (2010). *Simulation technologies in higher education: Uses, trends, and implications.* EDUCAUSE Center for Applied Research. http://www.educause.edu/ecar

DeAngelo, L., Hurtado, S., Pryor, J. H., Kelly, K. R., Santos, J. L., & Korn, W. S. (2009). *The American college teacher: National norms for the 2007-2008 HERI faculty survey.* Higher Education Research Institute, UCLA. https://heri.ucla.edu/publications-fac/

Dieckmann, P., Gaba, D., & Rall, M. (2007). Deepening the theoretical foundations of patient simulation as social practice. *Simulation in Healthcare, 2*(3), 183-193. https://journals.lww.com/simulationinhealthcare/fulltext/2007/00230/Deepening_the_Theoretical_Foundations_of_Patient.5.aspx

Dudding, C. C., Brown, D., Estis, J. M., Szymanski, C., & Zraick, R. (2019). *Best practices in healthcare simulations in communication sciences and disorders.* Council of Academic Programs in Communication Sciences and Disorders. https://wordpressstorageaccount.blob.core.windows.net/wp-media/wp-content/uploads/sites/1023/2019/06/eBook-Best-Practices-in-CSD-March-2019.pdf

Dudding, C. C., & Nottingham, E. E. (2018). A national survey of simulation use in university programs in communication sciences and disorders. *American Journal of Speech-Language Pathology, 27*(1), 71-81.

Dudding, C. C., & Pfeiffer, D. (2018). Clinical decision-making in speech-language pathology graduate students: Quantitative findings. *Teaching and Learning in Communication Sciences & Disorders, 2*(1). https://doi.org/doi.org/10.30707/TLCSD2.1Dudding

Estis, J. M., Rudd, A. B., Pruitt, B., & Wright, T. (2015). Interprofessional simulation-based education enhances student knowledge of health professional roles and care of patients with tracheostomies and Passy-Muir Valves. *Journal of Nursing Education and Practice, 5*(6), 123.

Eubanks, A., Volner, K., & Lopreiato, J. O. (2020). *Past, present and future of simulation in military medicine.* StatPearls. http://www.ncbi.nlm.nih.gov/books/NBK553172/

Ferguson, N. F., & Estis, J. M. (2018). Training students to evaluate preterm infant feeding safety using a video recorded patient simulation approach. *American Journal of Speech-Language Pathology, 27*(2), 566-573. http://dx.doi.org/10.1044/2017_AJSLP-16-0107

Finn, P. (2011). Critical thinking: Knowledge and skills for evidence-based practice. *Language, Speech, and Hearing Services in Schools, 42*(1), 69-72. https://doi.org/10.1044/0161-1461(2010/09-0037)

Finn, P., Brundage, S., & DiLollo, A. (2016). Preparing our future helping professionals to become critical thinkers: A tutorial. *Perspectives of the ASHA Special Interest Groups, 1*(10), 43-68. https://doi.org/10.1044/persp1.SIG10.43

Frank, P. (1947). *Einstein: His life and times.* (G. Rosen, Trans.). Knopf.

Gaba, D. (2004). The future vision of simulation in health care. *BMJ Quality & Safety, 13*(1), i2-i10. https://pubmed.ncbi.nlm.nih.gov/15465951/

Ginsberg, S. M., Friberg, J. K., & Visconti, C. F. (2016). Diagnostic reasoning by experienced speech-language pathologists and student clinicians. *Contemporary Issues in Communication Science and Disorders, 43*, 87-97. https://doi.org/10.1044/cicsd_43_S_87

Harden, R. M. (1988). What is an OSCE. *Medical Teacher, 10*, 19-22.

Haupt, B. A., & Meakin, C. H. (2015). Ethical, legal and regulatory implications in healthcare simulation. In L. Wilson & R. A. Wittmann-Price (Eds.), *Review manual for the Certified Healthcare Simulation Educator exam* (pp. 103-110). Springer Publishing Company.

Hayden, J. K., Smiley, R. A., Alexander, M., Kardong-Edgren, S., & Jeffries, P. R. (2014). The NCSBN national simulation study: A longitudinal, randomized, controlled study replacing clinical hours with simulation in prelicensure nursing education. *Journal of Nursing Regulation, 5*(2), S3-S40.

Hewat, S., Penman, A., Davidson, B., Baldac, S., Howells, S., Walters, J., Purcell, A., Cardell, E., McCabe, P., Caird, E., Ward, E., & Hill, A. E. (2020a). A framework to support the development of quality simulation-based learning programmes in speech-language pathology. *International Journal of Language & Communication Disorders, 55*(2), 287-300. https://doi.org/10.1111/1460-6984.12515

Hewat, S., Walters, J., Caird, E., Aldridge, D., Penman, A., Cardell, E., Davenport, R., Davidson, B., Howells, S., McCabe, P., Purcell, A., Ward, E., & Hill, A. (2020b). Clinical educators' perceptions of students following a simulation-based learning program. *Teaching and Learning in Communication Sciences & Disorders, 4*(3). https://ir.library.illinoisstate.edu/tlcsd/vol4/iss3/9

Hill, A. E., Davidson, B. J., & Theodoros, D. G. (2013). Speech-language pathology students' perceptions of a standardised patient clinic. *Journal of Allied Health, 42*(2), 84-91.

Hill, A. E., Ward, E., Heard, R., McAllister, S., McCabe, P., Penman, A., Caird, E., Aldridge, D., Baldac, S., Cardell, E., Davenport, R., Davidson, B., Hewat, S., Howells, S., Purcell, A., & Walters, J. (2020). Simulation can replace part of speech-language pathology placement time: A randomised controlled trial. *International Journal of Speech-Language Pathology, 23*(1), 92-102. https://doi.org/10.1080/17549507.2020.1722238

INACSL Standards Committee. (2016). INACSL standards of best practice: Simulation simulation design. *Clinical Simulation in Nursing, 12*, S5-S12. http://dx.doi.org/10.1016/j.ecns.2016.09.005.

INACSL Standards Committee, Bowler, F., Klein, M. & Wilford, A. (2021). Healthcare Simulation Standards of Best Practice Professional Integrity. *Clinical Simulation in Nursing, 58*, 45-48. https://doi.org/10.1016/j.ecns.2021.08.014

Jeffries, P. (2005). A framework for designing, implementing, and evaluating simulations used as teaching strategies in nursing. *Nursing Education Perspectives, 26*(2), 96-103. https://pubmed.ncbi.nlm.nih.gov/15921126/

Jeffries, P., Dreifuerst, K., Kardong-Edgren, S., & Hayden, J. (2015). Faculty development when initiating simulation programs: Lessons learned from the national simulation study. *Journal of Nursing Regulation, 5*(4), 17-23. http://www.sciencedirect.com/science/article/pii/S2155825615300375

Kim, J., Park, J.-H., & Shin, S. (2016). Effectiveness of simulation-based nursing education depending on fidelity: A meta-analysis. *BMC Medical Education, 16*(1), 152. https://doi.org/10.1186/s12909-016-0672-7

Kneebone, R. (2005). Evaluating clinical simulations for learning procedural skills: A theory-based approach. *Academic Medicine*, 80(6), 549-553.

Kolb, D. A., (1984). *Experiential learning: Experience as the source of learning and development*. Prentice-Hall. https://search.library.wisc.edu/catalog/999550475402121

Kozlowski, S. W. J., & DeShon, R. P. (2004). A psychological fidelity approach to simulation-based training: Theory, research, and principles. In E. Salas, L. R., Elliott, S. G. Schflett, & M. D. Coovert (Eds.), *Scaled worlds: Development, validation, and applications* (pp. 75-99). Ashgate Publishing.

Lieberth, A. K., & Martin, D. R. (2005). The instructional effectiveness of a web-based audiometry simulator. *Journal of the American Academy of Audiology, 16*(2), 79-84. https://doi.org/10.3766/jaaa.16.2.3

Lopreiato, J. O. (2016). *Healthcare simulation dictionary*. Agency for Healthcare Research and Quality.

MacBean, N., Theodoros, D., Davidson, B., & Hill, A. E. (2013). Simulated learning environments in speech-language pathology: An Australian response. *International Journal of Speech Language Pathology, 15*(3), 345-357. https://doi.org/10.3109/17549507.2013.779024

McAllister, L. (2005). Issues and innovations in clinical education. *Advances in Speech Language Pathology, 7*(3), 138-148. https://doi.org/10.1080/14417040500181239

Müller-Staub, M. (2006). Clinical decision making and critical thinking in the nursing diagnostic process. *Pflege, 19*(5), 275-279. https://pubmed.ncbi.nlm.nih.gov/17051512/

Naeve-Velguth, S., Christensen, S. A. & Woods, S. (2013). Simulated patients in audiology education: Student reports. *Journal of the American Academy of Audiology, 24*(8), 740-746. https://www.thieme-connect.de/products/ejournals/abstract/10.3766/jaaa.24.8.10

Nickbakht, M., Amiri, M., & Latifi, S. M. (2013). Study of the reliability and validity of Objective Structured Clinical Examination (OSCE) in the assessment of clinical skills of audiology students. *Global Journal of Health Science*, 5(3), 64-68. https://doi.org/10.5539/gjhs.v5n3p64

Norman, G. (2005). Research in clinical reasoning: Past history and current trends. *Medical Education, 39*(4), 418-427. https://doi.org/10.1111/j.1365-2929.2005.02127.x

Park, C. S., Murphy, T. F., & the Code of Ethics Working Group. (2018). *Healthcare simulationist code of ethics*. Society for Simulation in Healthcare. http://www.ssih.org/Code-of-Ethics.

Potter, N. L., & Allen, M. (2013). Clinical swallow exam for dysphagia: A speech pathology and nursing simulation experience. *Clinical Simulation in Nursing, 9*(10), e461-e464. http://doi.org/10.1016/j.ecns.2012.08.001

Rudolph, J. W., Raemer, D. B., & Simon, R. (2014). Establishing a safe container for learning in simulation: The role of the presimulation briefing. *Simulation in Healthcare: Journal of the Society for Simulation in Healthcare, 9*(6), 339-349. https://doi.org/10.1097/SIH.0000000000000047

Sherwood, R. J., & Francis, G. (2018). The effect of mannequin fidelity on the achievement of learning outcomes for nursing, midwifery and allied healthcare practitioners: Systematic review and meta-analysis. *Nurse Education Today, 69*, 81-94. https://doi.org/10.1016/j.nedt.2018.06.025

Shin, S., Park, J. H., & Kim, J. H. (2015). Effectiveness of patient simulation in nursing education: Meta-analysis. *Nurse Education Today, 35*(1), 176-182. https://doi.org/10.1016/j.nedt.2014.09.009

Stead, A., Lemoncello, R., Fitzgerald, C., Fryer, M., Frost, M., & Palmer, R. (2020). Clinical simulations in academic courses: Four case studies across the medical SLP graduate curriculum. *Teaching and Learning in Communication Sciences & Disorders, 4*(3). https://ir.library.illinoisstate.edu/tlcsd/vol4/iss3/6

Syder, D. (1996). The use of simulated clients to develop the clinical skills of speech and language therapy students. *European Journal of Disorders of Communication, 31*, 181-192.

Tiffen, J., Corbridge, S., & Slimmer, L. (2014). Enhancing clinical decision making: Development of a contiguous definition and conceptual framework. *Journal of Professional Nursing, 30*(5), 399-405. http://www.sciencedirect.com/science/article/pii/S8755722314000349

Vinney, L. A., Howles, L., Leverson, G., & Connor, N. P. (2016). Augmenting college students' study of speech-language pathology using computer-based mini quiz games. *American Journal of Speech-Language Pathology, 25*(3), 416-425. https://doi.org/10.1044/2015_AJSLP-14-0125

Wainwright, S. F., & McGinnis, P. Q. (2009). Factors that influence the clinical decision-making of rehabilitation professionals in long-term care settings. *Journal of Allied Health, 38*(3), 143-151.

Ward, E. C., Hill, A. E., Nund, R. L., Rumbach, A. F., Walker-Smith, K., Wright, S. E., Kelly, K., & Dodrill, P. (2015). Developing clinical skills in paediatric dysphagia management using human patient simulation (HPS). *International Journal of Speech-Language Pathology, 17*(3), 230-240. https://doi.org/10.3109/17549507.2015.1025846

Watson, K., Wright, A., Morris, N., McMeeken, J., Rivett, D., Blackstock, F., Jones, A., Haines, T., O'Connor, V., Watson, G., Peterson, R., & Jull, G. (2012). Can simulation replace part of clinical time? Two parallel randomised controlled trials. *Medical Education, 46*(7), 657-667. http://doi.org/10.1111/j.1365-2923.2012.04295.x

Weimer, M. (2013). *Learner-centered teaching: Five key changes to practice* (2nd ed.). Jossey-Bass.

Wilson, L., & Wittmann-Price, R. A. (Eds.). (2015). *Review manual for the Certified Healthcare Simulation Educator (CHSE) exam*. Springer Publishing Company.

Wolford, L., & Wolford, G. (2020). Comparing in vivo versus simulation training for transnasal endoscopy skills. *Teaching and Learning in Communication Sciences & Disorders, 4*(3). https://ir.library.illinoisstate.edu/tlcsd/vol4/iss3/3

Zraick, R. (2002). The use of standardized patients in speech-language pathology. *Perspectives on Issues in Higher Education, 5*, 14-16. http://doi.org/10.1044/ihe5.1.14

Zraick, R. I. (2020). Standardized patients in communication sciences and disorders: Past, present and future directions. *Teaching and Learning in Communication Sciences and Disorders, 4*(3), 4.

Zraick, R., Allen, R., & Johnson, S. (2003). The use of standardized patients to teach and test interpersonal and communication skills with students in speech-language pathology. *Advances in Health Sciences Education*, 8, 237-248. http://www.ncbi.nlm.nih.gov/pubmed/14574048

Foundational Theory for Simulation-Based Learning Experiences

Sue McAllister, PhD, FSPA and Carol C. Dudding, PhD, CCC-SLP, F-ASHA, CHSE

In this chapter we are inviting you to move beyond the attractive, immediate, and compelling surface features of simulated learning-based experiences (SBLEs) toward developing a deeper scholarly and considered approach to designing SBLEs that effectively support the development of the learners' professional practice. As Anderson et al. (2008) identified very early in the history of the use of simulation in curricula, we must use educational theory to ensure we use simulation effectively, including centralizing the needs and development of the learner in our educational practice and design:

> Our challenge is to use not only the available technology, but also the knowledge, theory, and collective clinical experience around us to create needs-based goal-oriented curricula that will equip our learners with the ability to use forward reasoning and reflective practice to advance their expertise and ultimately improve the outcomes of their patients. (p. 600)

We will identify the steps for a scholarly approach to designing SBLEs as a controlled and planned representation of real-world professional activities, paired with educational methods and procedures (Rudolph et al., 2007) as depicted in Figure 2-1. Our aim is to provide you with an evidence-based theoretical and practical framework to enable you to design, select, and implement quality SBLEs and avoid being distracted by the attractive but irrelevant characteristics of the technologies. We will discuss the principles and educational theories underpinning a quality design and implementation process and provide examples throughout for both audiologists and speech-language pathologists.

Learning Theories for Simulation-Based Learning Experiences

Those new to designing simulations should resist the urge to skip over the sections of this chapter devoted to learning theory and instructional design. Instructional design informed by both theory and evidence is critical for effective incorporation of simulated learning experiences maximizing both efficiency and quality. Cook et al. (2013) conducted a systematic review and meta-analysis of instructional designs used in simulation-based education and found that the impact of the modality used in an SBLE varied widely. They noted that focusing on the *what*, or type of technology used,

Dudding, C. C., & Ginsberg, S. M. (Eds.).
Simulation-Based Learning in Communication Sciences and Disorders: Moving From Theory to Practice. (pp. 17-34).

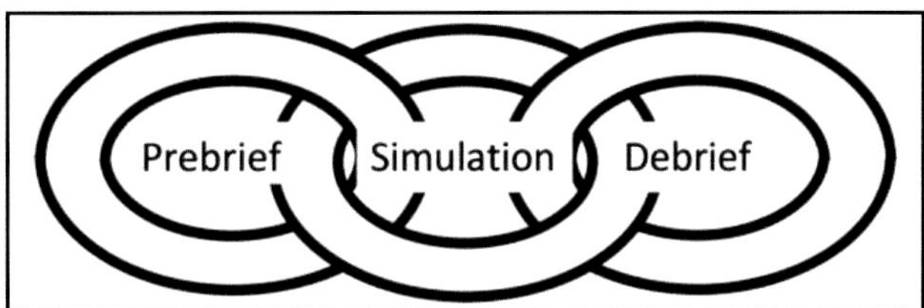

Figure 2-1. Components of an SBLE.

is less productive for quality SBLE practices than focusing on the *why* and *how* through theory-informed instructional design. Furthermore, this theory-based approach enables us to more effectively integrate emerging simulation tools and technologies into our SBLEs and curricula and stay focused on ensuring these tools are used in service of curriculum and not the other way around.

The role of learning theory in health professional education has received more attention in the past decade as attending to theory enables us to develop and test educational activities and distill principles for application beyond a specific subject or local circumstances (Schuwirth & Durning, 2018; Schuwirth & van der Vleuten, 2011). A scholarly approach based on theory-informed educational principles empowers us as educators to design and effectively use SBLEs. We can effectively address the competency-based learning outcomes we are targeting for our students, using the resources available to us in the context of our own programs. Learning theories enable us to identify what aspects of the design are critical for success.

Clinical educators and practitioners should be encouraged, because this reasoned approach to SBLEs is like how we approach evidence-based practice. Theory-informed instructional design frameworks assist us in designing SBLEs in the same way that evidence-informed practice guidelines assist us in designing quality therapeutic interventions. Attending to the theory helps us understand why our SBLE did or did not enable students to develop the targeted competency-based outcomes and what we should consider changing in the next iteration.

Knowledge, Skills, and Attributes

An important step in the understanding of learning theories and the development of professional competency is a broadened understanding of what is meant by the terms *knowledge*, *skills*, and *attributes* (KSAs). Knowledge encompass everything we know and includes propositional knowledge such as theory, facts, and principles; know-how; and insights gained through experience (Carter, 1985; Higgs & Jones, 2000; Higgs & Titchen, 2001; McAllister et al., 2011). Skills are what we can do, but this extends beyond psychomotor skills to include metacognitive skills, such as reflection and analysis, as well as emotional/social skills, such as effective interactions with others. Attributes are characteristics of the learner that influence their performance. This can include cognitive styles, such as creativity, resilience, and initiative, as well as attitudes and values that are congruent with ethical practice. See Table 2-1 for examples related to communication sciences and disorders.

The following sections will outline relevant learning theories and how they are linked to design and implementation of quality SBLEs. As shown in Table 2-2, learning theories as they apply to SBLEs fall into one of three broad categories: behaviorist, constructivist, and cognitive theory.

Behavioral Learning and Deliberate Practice

Behaviorist theories posit that all behaviors are learned through interactions with environmental stimuli and that learning is based on observable behaviors and conditioning (Skinner, 1974). Behaviorist learning theories in simulations would be best applied when the learning objectives target skills or professional tasks requiring consistent skill sets and behaviors, such as passing of a nasoscope, administering an oral mechanism exam, or mapping a digital hearing aid.

You may be familiar with the old joke about the musician who travels to New York City for the first time. The musician asks a stranger on the streets, "How do I get to Carnegie Hall?" The stranger responds, "Practice." There is truth and wisdom in this humor. In a now-famous study conducted with a group of violinists it was found that those deemed as expert violinists had put in more than 10,000 hours of practice—2,500 to 5,000 hours more than their less accomplished counterparts (Ericsson, 2004). While no one is proposing that learners spend 10,000 hours in SBLE to develop their skills, this and other studies support the importance of deliberate practice (DP; Ericsson, 2004; McGaghie et al., 2016; McGaghie et al., 2010).

DP enables key skills or tasks to become automated process schema that no longer require conscious attention, freeing up cognitive resources for more complex professional action (McGaghie et al., 2010, 2016). DP provides learners with opportunities to maintain and/or improve their current level of proficiency (Clapper & Kardong-Edgren, 2012; Ericsson, 2004). DP requires:

- Repetitive performance of cognitive or motor skills
- Rigorous assessment of those skills
- Specific, instructional feedback on performance (Ericsson, 2004)

Skills suitable for DP are well defined and will become one part of a competent performance (van Merriënboer & Kirschner, 2018). For example, the removal of cerumen from an ear canal is only one aspect of competent cerumen management.

TABLE 2-1

Knowledge, Skills, and Attributes

	INCLUDES	EXAMPLES
Knowledge Things I know	**Propositional**—Theory, facts, and principles learned through educational activities. **Practice**—Knowing how something is done. **Personal**—Theory, facts, and principles learned through prior personal experience.	• Knowing how sound is converted to nerve impulses and processed in the brain. • Knowing how routine hearing screenings are conducted. • Knowing about autism spectrum disorder through the experience of a sibling.
Skills Things I can do	**Psychomotor**—Implementing professional skills and technologies. **Metacognition**—Using thinking about before, during, and/or after action to influence or change outcome. **Emotional/social**—Implementing strategies for effective professional interactions with patients/clients and colleagues.	• Conducting a standardized language assessment. • Reflecting on the environmental factors that might be influencing a child's behavior during testing. • Reassuring a child who is anxious about the standardized language assessment process.
Attributes Things about me that influence my performance	**Cognitive style**—Preferences regarding how to solve problems. **Interpersonal style**—Personal characteristics that influence responses. **Integrity**—Attitudes/beliefs/values that support ethical practice and actions that are congruent.	• Becoming defensive when a parent challenges your diagnostic impression. • Appearing confident when conducting hearing screening. • Modifying instructions explained with patience and without patronizing tone. Reacts positively and with curiosity regarding causes of a child's uncooperative behavior during assessment.

Constructivist Theories

Another category of learning theory highly relevant to simulation and health care education is constructivist theory. In a general sense, constructivist learning theory is based upon the tenet that learners actively construct their own new knowledge based on their experiences and active engagement in the learning process. This theory positions what the learner does is central to learning, rather than what the teacher does. A constructivist view holds that the teacher becomes a facilitator of the learners' knowledge development rather than an imparter of knowledge (Biggs, 1999). This theory first gained notice in the 1970s with the work of Piaget (1957), Vygotsky (1978), and Bruner (1971). Constructivist theories popularized the concepts of developmental stages of learning and the importance of scaffolding support to maximize learning. The constructivist theory of learning continues in today's classrooms in the form of active learning strategies and student-centered teaching strategies, such as problem-based learning, team-based learning, and flipped classrooms. These active and learner-centered constructivist strategies are evidence of the movement to improve student outcomes and promote competency development as well as serve as a natural foundation for the design and implementation of SBLEs.

Experiential Learning Theory

Experiential learning theory (ELT) is widely used in simulation education and is learner centered and focusses on how the learner constructs their knowledge through experience. Kolb's (1984) ELT proposes that learning takes place as a result of "grasping and transforming experience." The central focus of the learning process is the learning outcome and involves both the learner and the educator. Kolb's ELT consists of four stages, concrete experience, abstract conceptualization, reflective observation, and active experimentation, as shown in Figure 2-2. Learners engage in each of these four stages throughout the SBLE experience.

The ELT framework is readily applicable to the prebrief, simulation experience, and debrief experiences as part of the SBLE. According to Kolb (1984), the concrete experience stage allows the learner to actively engage in a new or different learning experience. This would occur as a matter of course as learners engage in the simulation experience.

TABLE 2-2

Overview of Learning Theories Relevant to Simulation Design

LEARNING THEORY	KEY CONCEPTS	APPLICATION TO BEST PRACTICES SIMULATION DESIGN
Behaviorism	• DP • Learner is responding to stimuli, acquiring new or changing current behaviors	• Provide opportunities for repeated practice with feedback
Constructivism	• ELT • Reflection on and in action • Situated learning • Learner is interpreting new information based on their personal reality/world experiences	• Design an immersive learning environment that replicates substantial aspects of the real world in an interactive fashion
Cognitive science	• Cognitive load • Learner is processing and organizing new information	• Match the task to the learner's level of expertise • Support and prepare the learner before and during the SBLE • Allow learners to generate solutions in a safe, risk-free environment

Adapted from Ahlbrand, A. (2017). Learning theories and law: Behaviorism, cognitivism, constructivism. RIPS Law Librarian Blog. https://ripslawlibrarian.wordpress.com/2017/03/14/learning-theories-and-law-behaviorism-cognitivism-constructivism

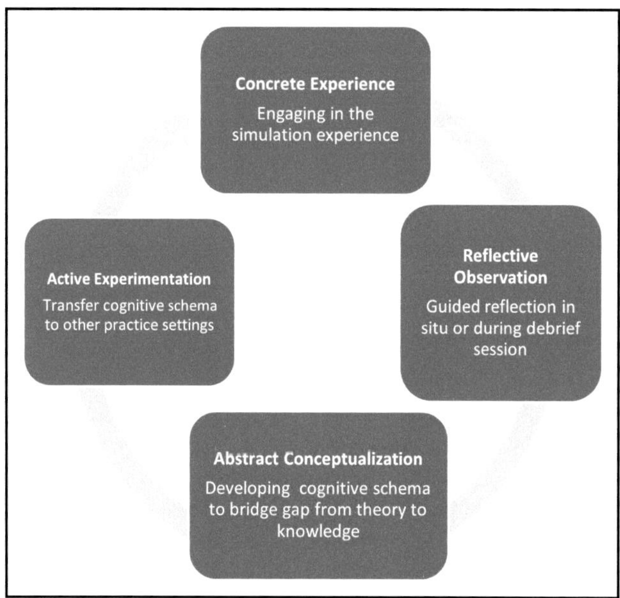

Figure 2-2. Kolb's ELT applied for simulation-based experiences. (Adapted from Kolb, D. A. [1984]. *Experiential learning: Experience as the source of learning and development*. Prentice-Hall and Poore, J. A., Cullen, D. L., & Schaar, G. L. [2014]. Simulation-based interprofessional education guided by Kolb's Experiential Learning Theory. *Clinical Simulation in Nursing, 10*[5], e241-e247. https://doi.org/10.1016/j.ecns.2014.01.004)

The second and third stages of ELT, reflective observation and abstract conceptualization, involve reflective practices that are a cornerstone of SBLE. In these stages, the educator guides the learner by providing feedback and questioning to promote reflection. This process is ongoing and occurs during the simulation (in situ) and later as part of the debrief process. The debrief is where schema that facilitate active experimentation or transfer are constructed and elaborated.

In the final stage of ELT, active experimentation, learners are guided in their ability to transfer what is learned and apply it to other practice settings. The design of the SBLE may allow the learner to move through a single or multiple learning cycles.

Reflective Thinking

ELT has at its core the concept of reflective thinking. As early as the 1930s, John Dewey introduced the notion of reflection as it applies to learning. In the 1980s, Schön extended this thinking to include "reflection-in-action" and "reflection-on-action" in order to engage in a process of continuous learning (Schön, 1983). *Reflection-in-action* refers to the immediate thinking during the experience and can be thought of as thinking on your feet. *Reflection-on-action* refers to the later analysis of the events in considering what went well and what did not (Schön, 1983). King and Kitchener (2004) extended the process of reflection to include prereflection that recognizes the importance of engaging in reflection prior to the experience. This occurs as part of the prebrief and serves as an opportunity for the learner to connect what they already know and can do to what they are about to learn through participation in the SBLE. Reflection-in-action requires immediate feedback and may occur as a planned part of the simulation experience in which the health care simulation educator may stop the scenario to allow learners the opportunity to discuss and share feelings, thoughts, and planned actions. Reflection-on-action is integral in most debriefing scenarios occurring after the simulation activity. These forms of reflection are key to the development of more sophisticated process and pattern-based schema and support the ongoing development of professional competency and transfer across different aspects of professional practice.

Situated Learning Theory

Another learning theory to be addressed under the umbrella of constructivist theories is that of situated learning. Situated learning theory proposes that knowledge needs to be presented in authentic contexts that are embedded within the activity, context, and culture in which it will be used (Lave, 1988). Situated learning theory includes engagement, social interaction, and collaboration as essential components of the learning process. These components are integral to a well-developed simulation as simulation attempts to replicate whole or parts of real-world professional practice. The power of situated learning can be recruited in two ways: (a) by providing the context as to when and where the KSAs are learned and ultimately integrated into performance and (b) by allowing interaction and collaboration between learners and educators to enable learning for professional practice to occur.

Design of the SBLE should consider the physical, psychological, and sociological environment to effectively recruit the benefits of situated learning. However, it should not be assumed that all SBLEs need to be hyperrealistic to be effective—the degree and type of fidelity (physical, psychological, and sociological) should be determined in relation to learning outcomes and learner stage (Naismith et al., 2020). See Chapter 4 for more detail. A particular benefit of SBLEs is that they more closely align with how learning happens in the workplace through collaboration as part of a health care team, as opposed to how learning may occur in the classroom that results in competition among students (Bohmer & Edmonson, 2001; Le Maistre & Pare, 2004). For example, consider the ways learners traditionally learn how to administer a standardized test. They may learn the terminology such as standard score, norm-referenced, validity, and reliability in a classroom lecture; read about administration protocols in a textbook; or perhaps check out a standardized test from the clinic and read the manual prior to administration. The enlightened professor may even pair the students and have them to practice the test on one another as a skills lab. These activities are important steps in the learning process but do not meet the criteria of situated learning. Now consider the important learning that occurs in an SBLE where the administration of a standardized assessment is situated in the context of a complex professional task of assessing a person trained to respond as someone with aphasia within a room that is designed to look like a treatment room. In this case, the students' learning is situated in a context that more closely mirrors the complexities of professional practice and shifts their focus from mastering only the technical aspects of administration to learning how to do this while also interacting with a real person and managing the assessment process in a real environment.

Cognitive Load Theory

Having explored how both behaviorist and constructivist learning theories inform quality SBLE design, we are left to examine cognitive theories that apply to the use of simulations in education. Cognitive science is an interdisciplinary scientific study of the mind that seeks to construct models of thinking and learning, which can guide SBLE design and practice. Cognitive load theory is particularly important when considering how to design learning tasks and experiences such as SBLEs (van Merriënboer & Kirschner, 2018; van Merriënboer & Sweller, 2005). Cognitive load theory proposes that new information is first dealt with by our working memory before being consolidated into long-term memory. Working memory is limited in its ability to handle complex tasks by the amount of information that it can hold as well as the length of time that it can retain that information without rehearsal (< 2 seconds). Failure to consolidate information from working memory to long-term memory means an opportunity for learning is lost. Cognitive load theory seeks to identify strategies to make the encoding and consolidation of new knowledge into schema more efficient (van Merriënboer & Sweller, 2005). Cognitive load theory distinguishes between three types of load: (a) intrinsic, (b) extraneous, and (c) germane (van Merriënboer et al., 2006). The *intrinsic load* refers to the inherent difficulty of the task or problem in combination with the expertise of the learner, such as the intrinsic difficulty of making a well-fitting accurate ear mold impression when the learner has never done this before. *Extraneous cognitive load* refers to how the task is structured and positioned within an instructional procedure. Extraneous cognitive load is not necessary for learning and, if not carefully considered, might have a negative impact on learning. Extraneous load should be kept as low as possible, so not to overwhelm the cognitive resources of the learner, and carefully considered in learning design as the learner develops their expertise. The third type of load, *germane load*, allows for long-term storage of information. This happens when the SBLE includes strategies such as guided self-reflection and debriefing that engage the learner in making the effort to integrate newly gained knowledge and skill into new or existing schema. The continued development of such schema enable learners to move from novice to expert. How we consider the various forms of cognitive load is case dependent. For example, introducing an uncooperative patient into a scenario may not be appropriate for a novice learner and would be considered extraneous cognitive load; however, the introduction of an uncooperative patient for an intermediate level increases the difficulty of the task, making it an intrinsic cognitive load. These nuances should be fully considered in the design and execution of SBLEs (van Merriënboer & Sweller, 2005).

Educators creating SBLEs should be aware how learning tasks that contribute to cognitive load will vary according to the experience level of the learners. For example, introducing an uncooperative patient into a scenario may be considered extraneous cognitive load for a novice student. Yet for an intermediate-level student who has a higher level of expertise, an uncooperative patient may be considered as intrinsic. The process of actively engaging with this scenario will generate a germane load that will contribute to further development of their schema regarding fitting ear molds to this more challenging patient scenario. These nuances should be carefully considered in the design and execution of SBLEs (van Merriënboer & Kirschner, 2018).

Competency-Based Education

There would be no argument that the aim of our educational programs is to graduate competent speech-language pathologists and audiologists, but there is little agreement as to what competent means and even less agreement on how to determine that a sufficient level of competency has been achieved. Tables 2-3 and 2-4, respectively, offer a competency-based framework and an example of professional tasks related to cerumen management. Successful execution of professional tasks, such as the steps for conducting an oral motor examination, are not equivalent to professional competency. Professional competency includes the competent selection of professional tasks, knowing when and why they should be used in practice, and adapting them to contexts of professional practice such as steps of oral motor examination with a child vs. an adult (Heywood et al., 1992; ten Cate, 2005). Developing professional competence requires a competency-based education model. Such an educational model requires a careful and focused approach beginning with the development of learning objectives that encompass the necessary KSAs and align with the learners' place in the curriculum. A competency-based education model also requires competency-based outcomes and assessments that support the development of professional competency. Professional competency is the desired outcome of audiology and speech-language pathology curricula.

Conceptualization of Professional Competency

General competency is commonly viewed as being able to demonstrate a specific technical skill, such as analyzing a language sample or administering a pure tone threshold hearing assessment. However, competent practice also requires integrating these skills with capabilities, such as clinical reasoning, communication, lifelong learning, and professionalism (Gonczi, 1994; McAllister et al., 2011). Focusing on technical competence often leads to atomistic and exhaustive lists of skills intended to cover every aspect of professional practice but fails to capture wholistic integration with key professional capabilities that leads to quality professional practice (Beckett, 2004; Cowan et al., 2005; Gonczi, 1994; Hager, 1994). Furthermore, these lists of skills look backward, in that they quickly become outdated as new technologies or evidence lead to new practices, rather than looking forward and ensuring that our students graduate as capable of advancing their professional practice.

A competent professional can demonstrate performances of complex professional tasks by integrating professional skills with capabilities, both of which draw on key KSAs. They are able to demonstrate this competency across a wide variety of patients/clients in contexts of varying complexity (Heywood et al., 1992; Higgs & Bithell, 2001). Therefore, professional competency involves the competent exercise of complex professional judgment to inform action across all tasks and contexts of professional practice (Hager, 2000; McAllister et al., 2011). This definition of professional competency allows the individual to develop their expertise through transferring and applying their competency across their professional practice as they gain experience.

Professional competency develops through interactions between the learner with the practice context, including patients, colleagues, student peers, educators, workplaces, and communities. It includes the way in which the learner combines KSAs to solve professional problems. SBLE design that draws on this richer conceptualization of competency allows the educator to design and incorporate SBLEs into the curriculum in a way that moves the learner beyond completing a lengthy checklist of skills or professional tasks performed in an isolated manner.

By moving toward a more integrated and comprehensive understanding of competence, we can begin to think about these isolated skills and professional tasks in the fuller

TABLE 2-3

Competency-Based Frameworks

TERM	DEFINITION
Competency	Ability to exercise professional judgment and action across all tasks and contexts of professional practice (McAllister et al, 2011).
Competencies	Broad categories of occupational and professional activity that underpin professional competency and support transfer across contexts of practice (McAllister et al, 2011). Competency is inferred based on observations of performances, which can include performance of professional tasks and explanations of one's internal through processes (e.g., why I selected particular formal and/or informal assessment elements).
Occupational competencies	What we do as speech-language pathologists and audiologists. For example, we gather data to assess the communication, swallowing, and/or hearing problem; we analyze and interpret this data; we use this interpretation to plan an intervention.
Professional competencies	How we work as speech-language pathologists and audiologists. For example, we demonstrate reasoning, lifelong learning, communication, and professionalism. These competencies operate in combination with the occupational competencies. Also known as generic competencies.
Professional tasks context	Specific professional activities that draw on KSAs from which competency can be inferred.
Professional competency needs to be demonstrated across a range of contexts and levels of complexity. Context includes people (e.g., patient/client, family, community, colleagues) and service environments (e.g., funding, type of service, policy) and the communication, swallowing, or hearing issue being addressed.	

TABLE 2-4

Example of a Professional Task and Relationship to Competencies and Knowledge/Skills/Attributes

PROFESSIONAL TASK: CERUMEN REMOVAL		
Example Activities Within Professional Task	*Example Competencies That Could Be Inferred From Performance of the Professional Task*	*Example Knowledge, Skills, and Attributes Integrated During This Performance*
Patient understands procedure and feels safe	Communication	Knowledge—Personal Skills—Emotional/social Attribute—Integrity
Cerumen is removed	Intervention	Knowledge—Propositional and practice Skills—Psychomotor and metacognitive
Preventative education of patient	Communication	Knowledge—Propositional Skills—Metacognitive and emotional/social Attribute—Integrity

context of professional practice. We can then design SBLEs that support the learner to develop the ability to make quality professional judgments and undertake quality professional actions and provide opportunities for them to demonstrate this competency (Hager, 2000; McAllister et al., 2010).

Knowledge, Skills, and Attributes

As mentioned, an understanding of KSAs is paramount to the development and understanding of professional competency. It is well accepted that knowledge and skills underpin professional practice. Consideration of the role of attributes has become more common; however, professional practice is complex and dynamic, and a wide range of characteristics are considered to be important for the development

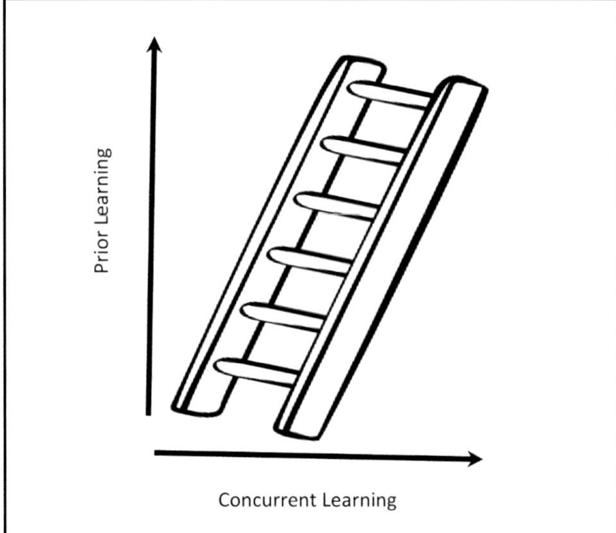

Figure 2-3. Vertical and horizontal alignment within the curriculum.

and maintenance of expertise. For example, recognizing that knowledge alone is not sufficient for quality practice underpins the shift over the past 50 years to competency-based outcomes vs. focusing only on acquisition of knowledge (Carraccio et al., 2002; Davidoff, 2008). At the same time, new understandings regarding other types of skills and personal qualities underpin expertise, in combination with different types of knowledge, have developed. The following taxonomy draws on this background with a particular debt to Carter's (1985) taxonomy of objectives for professional education and the work of Higgs and Jones (2000) and Higgs and Titchen (2001), which in turn informed research in speech pathology on the key elements that should be assessed on placement (McAllister et al., 2011). The latter research refers to knowledge, skills, and personal qualities, but the third category is now named "attributes" to acknowledge the range of characteristics that can be included.

This KSA taxonomy is based on the principles that growth and change can occur across all three categories and that quality professional practice arises from the ongoing and simultaneous development, integration, and coordination of KSAs. This taxonomy only focuses on the individual and should be considered in combination to the ways in which competent performance may or may not be facilitated by the context in which the individual works. Well-designed SBLEs attend to and facilitate the learner's development, integration, and coordination of KSAs to support development of professional competency.

Mapping Competency Development Across Curricula

Students' ability to draw on relevant KSAs and integrate these into competent performance of professional tasks develops across their program. Therefore, when deciding on competency-based learning objectives for SBLEs, it is critical to determine the stage of the learners in context of the curriculum for their program. This understanding of the learner drives the development of the SBLE and expectations of performance on the competencies being assessed (see next section). Curricula have both vertical and horizontal continua, which is illustrated in Figure 2-3 (Al-Eyd et al., 2018; Brown et al., 2012). Vertical continua relate to the learner's sequential progression through the curriculum and considers how prior learning can be recruited for new learning and how achievement of the current learning outcomes will support the next stage of competency development. For example, an academic program requires a course in normal language development as a prerequisite to a course related to speech-language disorders in children. Horizontal continua relate to what the student is learning right now across concurrent subjects and how these opportunities can be recruited and integrated across the current learning activities. Recruiting a student's learning experiences occurring as part of a concurrent clinical placement to inform their learning in an SBLE is an instance of horizontal integration. It is important that we make this horizontal and vertical aspect of curriculum explicit to the learners who, as novices, are not always able to identify what learning is most relevant and is applicable to the new learning experience (transfer). We see evidence of this when novice learners separate their knowledge by course subject. For example, graduate students may consider phonological disorders and developmental language disorders as two discrete entities because they were taught the content in two distinct courses. A well-designed SBLE that is effectively integrated into our curricula will maximize its impact on our students' professional development over time, particularly if it considers both learning objectives and assessment and how these facilitate achievement of competency-based learning outcomes.

Integration Into the Curriculum

A well-designed SBLE will not build competency unless it is effectively integrated into the curriculum (McGaghie et al., 2010). Ideally, SBLEs are positioned within a curriculum that is both goal and learner oriented (Anderson et al., 2008). As stated earlier, our position is that a goal-oriented curriculum addresses competency-based outcomes that are focused on the big picture of graduating competent health professionals and considers the interactions between these outcomes, assessment, and learning strategies (Biggs, 1999; Wiggins & McTighe, 2005). A learner-oriented curriculum accepts that learning is constructed by the learner rather than transmitted to them by the teacher (Biggs, 1999; Hager, 2004). A curriculum that is designed to be learner oriented embraces the active learning opportunities enabled through experiential learning strategies employed in SBLEs, such as cycles of feedback and practice.

As we craft competency-based learner outcomes for our SBLEs, it is important that we think about where the SBLE is positioned in the curriculum (Secheresse & Nonglaton, 2019). Curricula in audiology and speech-language pathology courses inherently aim to move students along a continuum of expertise from novice to entry-level professionals. It considers what KSAs need to be developed and when and how they are integrated. For example, in audiology training programs, KSAs related to audiologic assessment precedes instruction of KSAs related to recommendations regarding types of hearing aids. The curriculum further considers how these KSAs are related to performance of professional tasks and requires transitioning of these tasks into solving real-world problems for patients, clients, and communities as the student develops their professional and occupational competencies Therefore, the positioning of the SBLE in the curriculum will determine the level of performance on competency-based outcomes (KSAs, professional tasks, and competencies) that will be reflected in the learning objectives guiding the development, implementation and assessment of an SBLE. Refer to Chapter 5 for more detail.

Competency-Based Outcomes and Assessments

A competency-based outcomes approach to curriculum focuses on outputs vs. inputs and is underpinned by a learner-oriented curriculum that draws on current learning theories and practices described earlier in this chapter. In other words, a competency-based outcomes approach focuses on demonstrated competency or ability to practice (output) vs. accumulating hours of supervised experience (input). Moving to a competency-based outcomes approach may require a significant shift from more common approaches to curriculum that prioritize inputs such as learning activities, teacher behaviors, and dissemination of content (Biggs, 1999; Wiggins & McTighe, 2005). The teacher should no longer be preoccupied only with the learning environments they are designing within their own subject area. Rather, they should maximize opportunities to facilitate students' development of competency through integration of prior and current learning across the program's curriculum.

An outcomes-based curriculum, whether at the program or course level, begins with the end in mind to guide the articulation of learning outcomes. Once learning outcomes are determined, then follows the development and facilitation of the learning and assessment process (Biggs, 1999; Wiggins & McTighe, 2005). An outcomes-based curriculum, whether at the program or course level, must clearly articulate the specific outcomes and performance levels that the student must demonstrate. This approach assures us that the learner can use what they are learning to explain phenomena, create new understandings, and/or solve problems and develop their professional practice (Wiggins & McTighe, 2005). The end or desired outcome of audiology and speech-language programs is professional competency.

A competency-based outcomes curriculum ensures that learning outcomes are closely connected to problems students will encounter in professional practice. It is learner oriented and constructivist in that the focus is on what the learner does as they build their professional competency rather than what the teacher does. The teacher, therefore, is the facilitator of learning, rather than imparter of learning (Biggs, 1999). The goal of a competency-based outcomes curriculum is to enable students to:

- Develop quality pattern-based schema, so they can identify a problem.
- Effectively employ the related process schema, to gather information to accurately characterize the problem, determine, and implement an appropriate course of action.
- Integrate and apply the KSAs throughout this process to ensure quality and compassionate care.

Thus, a competency-based outcomes approach is focused on what the student does as a learner as they develop their competency—that is, their ability to undertake quality professional judgments and actions (McAllister et al., 2011). The SBLE is, therefore, a tool in service of these outcomes rather than a discrete learning activity or input.

An integrated wholistic conceptualization of professional competency also leads us to consider how to best evaluate competency in learners. A critical distinction regarding assessment in a competency-based outcomes curriculum is assessment *for* learning rather than assessment *of* learning. The former focuses on designing assessments that support ongoing development of expertise, whereas the latter only assesses and marks what has been demonstrated at a particular point of time, often only assessing aspects that are readily quantified or articulated rather than the deep and complex learning that underpins professional practice (Schuwirth & van der Vleuten, 2020). Assessment for learning is motivating and challenging for the learner as it simulates learning as part of the assessment process and develops self-assessment skills critical for developing expertise with experience (Boud & Soler, 2016; Price et al., 2011). SBLEs are rich with opportunities for high-quality formative and summative assessment.

Formative assessment in SBLEs is facilitated through feedback from peers, facilitators, and/or the simulation technology, such as computer simulations, virtual worlds, manikins, and standardized patients. If learners are clear about what they need to demonstrate to pass their subject (competency-based outcomes), then they are in a better position to actively engage in their development through comparing their performance in the SBLE against these criteria. This allows them to effectively use feedback to change their performance. Active engagement in self-evaluation and effective use of feedback are both critical components for development of lifelong learning skills (Boud & Soler, 2016; Hattie, 2015; Tai et al., 2018). Summative assessments identify what matters for learners, and if they are clearly linked to both the formative assessments, feedback cycles, and learning objectives, then the outcome should be no surprise to the learner. Teaching to the test, or well-designed summative assessment tasks, in the case of a competency-based curriculum is not only allowed—it is highly desirable. Chapter 6 provides a full discussion of assessment practices in simulation education.

TABLE 2-5

COMPASS© Competencies

Occupational competencies	• Assessment • Analysis and interpretation • Planning evidence-based speech pathology practice • Implementation of speech pathology practice • Planning, providing, and managing speech pathology services • Professional and supervisory practice • Lifelong learning and reflective practice
Professional competencies	• Reasoning • Communication • Learning • Professionalism

Data sources: McAllister, S., Lincoln, M., Ferguson, A., & McAllister, L. (2013a). *COMPASS©: Competency assessment in speech pathology* (2nd ed.). Speech Pathology Australia and Speech Pathology Australia. (2011). *Competency-based occupational standards for speech pathologists: Entry level.* Author.

COMPASS© (Competency Assessment in Speech Pathology; McAllister et al., 2013a) provides an example of an assessment that exemplifies the key points we have made in this chapter related to SBLEs and competency-based outcomes and frameworks. This includes incorporating key learning theories, an integrated and wholistic conceptualization of competency, and considering the learner's position in the curriculum. Its fitness for purpose was validated through a research program (see Speech Pathology Australia, https://www.speechpathologyaustralia.org.au/; Ferguson et al., 2010; McAllister et al., 2010, 2011, 2013b). COMPASS© is an online assessment tool that is used internationally to judge a student's performance, or development of competency, in the workplace. It is used to guide judgment of the student's ability to apply the occupational competencies developed by the Australian speech pathology profession (The Speech Pathology Association of Australia Ltd Staff, 2017) in combination with an additional four professional competencies (reasoning, communication, learning, and professionalism; Table 2-5). Therefore, COMPASS© is not a set of detailed checklists of professional tasks or skills. Rather, it takes a wholistic approach to competency that can be applied to a broad range of professional tasks and contexts of practice. The educator and student judge the student's ability to integrate and coordinate professional tasks within and across competencies (all of which are underpinned by relevant KSAs as they are applied in different workplace contexts). Behavioral exemplars are provided of the types of performances (novice, intermediate, or entry-level) on professional tasks related to each competency that are opportunities to judge the student's development of expertise. The minimum level of performance is determined in relation to the student's position in the entire program's curriculum. If this is the student's first placement, they may only need to demonstrate a novice level of performance. If it is their last semester, they will need to demonstrate entry-level performance on completion of their placement. This judgment is translated into ratings on a visual analog scale and is based on observed behaviors that are linked to competency-based outcomes. COMPASS© enables the student's development of expertise in integrating, applying, and transferring their competencies to be judged and tracked across different contexts of professional practice (e.g., service delivery models, client groups) and over the course of their program until the they are deemed ready to enter practice (i.e., entry-level performance) and capable of ongoing development post-graduation.

Transfer and Expertise

Another strength of SBLEs is the opportunity to develop cognitive schema that support transfer and the development of expertise. The need for learners to bridge the gap between theory and practice is frequently expressed by clinical educators. The transfer of knowledge to professional practice is not so much bridging a gap, or even solely about transferring knowledge. Rather, it is about negotiating an ongoing journey of developing expertise for practice. A SBLE based on best practices, not necessarily expensive equipment, can effectively provide the learner with the opportunity to build quality cognitive schemas that enable transfer into practice and clinical reasoning that supports the application of these schema to decision making and action (Ginsberg et al., 2016; Forsberg et al., 2013; Patel et al., 2000; van Merriënboer & Kirschner, 2018). That is, a well-designed SBLE does more than provide a learner with the KSAs required to perform a specific task. Through careful design and feedback, it can enable the learner to develop schemas (see Box 2-1) that lay the foundation to become a thoughtful problem solver able to adapt experiences to solve novel problems and progress along the continuum of expertise.

There are two types of schemas: process and patterns (van Merriënboer & Kirschner, 2018). They are most commonly discussed in health profession education with regard to the development of clinical reasoning, but they underpin all aspects of cognitive activity and related action (Fraser et al., 2015; van Merriënboer & Sweller, 2005). Process-based schemas are related to algorithms, principles, and heuristics—"rules of thumb" as to how to go about a professional task or solve a professional problem (e.g., inductive and deductive reasoning; Doeltgen et al., 2018). The professional and occupational competencies described in COMPASS© (McAllister et al., 2013a) could be considered process competencies. For example, our students need to know how to go about an assessment, interpreting/analyzing assessment information and planning/implementing interventions. Pattern-based schemas are networks of knowledges that we match to the client's presentation (Croskerry, 2009). For example, these patterns enable us to recognize what is likely to be the nature of the communication problem (diagnosis) and effective strategies to address it (management). This pattern matching happens rapidly and often unconsciously.

Process schemas and pattern schemas act in concert and are critical for ensuring we graduate professionals who know where to start on problems that are new to them (process schema) and are equipped to continue to develop their expertise (pattern schema; Benner et al., 1996; Crespo et al., 2004; Devantier et al., 2009; Patel et al., 2015; Torre et al., 2020). Quality schema enable graduates to tailor their services to the unique combination of issues and circumstances with which a client presents, rather than applying a rigid rule-based recipe—key features of quality evidence-based practice (Dollaghan, 2007).

The development and use of quality schemas is also closely related to the development of expertise over time as the health professional develops richer representations of problems and processes to solve them (Chi et al., 1988). Chi and colleagues assert that quality learning design will enable the learner to identify what features of existing schemas they hold might be relevant (transfer) to a new problem-solving context. This process of automating skills and developing accurate pattern-based schemas is central to why experts make fewer errors than novices—they have better pattern schemas and more working memory available in the moment (Croskerry, 2009; Doeltgen et al., 2018). This also enables prior learning to be connected to and transferred for use in new situations. See Box 2-2 for an example of schemas in practice.

SBLEs are very useful for supporting development of expertise through automating schemas by enabling students to develop general rules for action through procedural guidance in the form of feedback, explanations by the facilitator, and briefing and debriefing strategies (Riviere et al., 2019; van Merriënboer & Kirschner, 2018). They can also be useful for providing opportunities for learners to practice specific professional tasks, so they become more automatic, such as repeated practice passing of a nasoendoscope. This automation decreases cognitive load by freeing up working memory so that the student can gather data while using these professional skills as part of solving more complex problems (Maggio et al., 2015).

The inherent nature of SBLEs provides opportunities for learners to construct their schemas by making the schemas relevant to the SBLE explicit and supporting the learner to inductively construct their own schemas. This is accomplished by providing supportive prompts, models, and examples that make the schemas underpinning decision making explicit (van Merriënboer & Kirschner, 2018). A well-designed SBLE provides a framework for the learner to elaborate on and create quality, detailed schemas as they construct their own mental representations of practice through engagement with authentic tasks for professional practice. This process will be further supported by quality facilitation as part of the prebriefing, feedback during the simulation, and debriefing. SBLEs also provide a variety of problems or cases within an SBLE that assist the student to develop more detailed schemas they can apply to cases that may look different on the surface but share key deep features (Barnett & Ceci, 2002; van Merriënboer & Kirschner, 2018). For those interested, van Merriënboer and Kirschner (2018) provide a very thorough explanation of current theory regarding schemas and their critical role in development and transfer of professional skills and how good curriculum design supports students to construct, automate, and coordinate these schemas.

BOX 2-1

What Are Schemas?

Schemas are the ways in which information has been organized and stored in long-term memory and enable efficient retrieval and use in our working memory and help us manage cognitive load (Fraser et al., 2015). Learners actively construct their schema as they learn through their interactions with the world, including educational activities like simulations. These schemas are stored and automatically applied when solving problems.

There are two types of schema: processes and patterns.

1. Processes—These are schemas about how things are done. For example, learners will develop a simulation schema through prebriefings and set routines which will free up their working memory for learning during the SBLE (Fraser et al., 2015).
2. Patterns—These are networks of knowledges that enable us to recognize phenomena and identify appropriate options for action. For example, identifying patterns in case history material provided in the case notes for the SBLE that suggest a child may have conductive hearing loss.

Instructional Design for SBLEs

There are a handful of systematic instructional design models and best-practice documents in the literature that offer useful insights and guidance and that are applicable to

BOX 2-2

Exemplar of Pattern and Process Schema in Practice

McAllister et al. (2020) found that schemas were central to the clinical reasoning processes engaged in by expert speech-language pathologists when conducting an initial clinical bedside swallow evaluation (CBSE) on patients referred for suspected dysphagia in an acute hospital:

1. Processes—The speech-language pathologists used the same heuristic or overarching process steps in conducting a CBSE: (a) preassessment information gathering, (b) patient subjective interview, (c) incidental observation, (d) physical examination, and (e) initial management planning. They also had heuristics to categorize data gathered throughout these processes to decide on the next step in the CBSE: is the presentation acute or chronic; is the etiology neurological or non-neurological; is aspiration likely or unlikely; how responsive is the patient to instruction; what was the patient's usual diet; and what is the site of the possible swallowing impairment?
2. Patterns—The speech-language pathologists recognized common patterns of presentations and used this to efficiently generate initial hypotheses that were then tested. For example, recognizing from the preassessment information gathering phase that the area affected by the patient's stroke meant that silent aspiration of fluids was a high possibility. They also identified when new information during the assessment did not match the expected pattern and generated new hypotheses to test by systematically collecting and interpreting the implications of new data.

the design and implementation of quality SBLEs. A partial listing includes the Integrated Simulation and Technology Enhanced Learning Framework (Gough et al., 2016), National League of Nursing/Jeffries Framework (Groom et al., 2014; Jeffries, 2005), and the Stepwise Model (Khamis et al., 2020). See Table 2-6 for a summary of major design components of each of these design models. Additionally, practice guidelines such as AMEE's "Simulation in Healthcare Education: A Best Evidence Practical Guide" (Motola et al., 2013) and the International Nursing Association for Clinical Simulation and Learning's (INACSL's) "Standards of Best Practice Simulation Design" (INACSL Standards Committee et al., 2021) offer guidance to the motivated educator.

Another useful framework that we will discuss in more detail is the four-component instructional design (4C/ID) framework developed by van Merrioënboer and Kirschner (2018). The framework outlines 4 components to good instructional design with 10 related steps (Figure 2-4). These 4 components of the 4C/ID framework—learning tasks, supportive information, procedural information, and part-task practice—are integral to many SBLEs.

The 4 components and 10 related steps of the framework can also be readily linked to instructional design models you may already be familiar with and/or are using. The 4C/ID framework is informed by both theory and evidence, and links closely to the key concepts for SBLE design that we have discussed throughout this chapter, including schema building and transfer, development of expertise, skill development, and effective management of cognitive load. The 4C/ID framework enables considerations of designs that develop competency-based outcomes, such as the students' ability to coordinate and integrate professional tasks within competencies as they master complex learning and professional practice. The 4C/ID framework can be applied to any curriculum design regardless of where it is situated (university or workplace) and, therefore, facilitates vertical and horizontal integration across curricula.

The following is a summary of key principles that encompass the major constructs discussed in this chapter:

Principle 1: All learning should occur in a "whole task" environment (i.e., situated learning) that is meaningfully related to professional practice and includes an assessment (formative and summative) that requires the student to demonstrate the required performance, so competency and level of expertise can be inferred.

Principle 2: The learning activity should include learning tasks with recurrent and nonrecurrent aspects. Recurrent aspects are rule-based activities and procedures (process schema) that need to become automated through DP and support professional practice through freeing up working memory (cognitive load theory). Nonrecurrent aspects involve applying schemas to unique problems of professional practice; for example, reasoning and decision making needed for performing a well-targeted clinical bedside swallow assessment for diagnosis and intervention planning for patients who have different presentations.

Principle 3: Learning tasks should include resources and supports to enable the learner to develop mastery of the interrelated recurrent and nonrecurrent tasks (i.e., learner-centered supports). Simulation technologies provide excellent opportunities for providing/activating procedural and supportive information at the time it is needed, thereby facilitating integration and

TABLE 2-6

Design Theories in Simulation

DESIGN THEORIES AND BEST PRACTICE GUIDELINES IN SIMULATION	MAJOR CONSTRUCTS/STEPS
Jeffries, P. R. (2005). A framework for designing, implementing, and evaluating simulations used as teaching strategies in nursing. *Nursing Education Perspectives, 26*(2), 96-103.	• Educational Practices • Teacher • Students • Design Characteristics and Outcomes
Khamis, N., Satava, R., & Kern, D. E. (2020). Stepwise simulation course design model: Survey results from 16 centers. *Journal of the Society of Laparoendoscopic Surgeons, 24*(2). https://doi.org/10.4293/JSLS.2019.00060	• Problem Identification and General Needs Assessment • Targeted Needs Assessment • Goals and Objectives • Educational Strategies • Individual Assessment and Feedback • Program Evaluation • Implementation
Motola, I., Devine, L. A., Chung, H. S., Sullivan, J. E., & Issenberg, S. B. (2013). Simulation in healthcare education: A best evidence practical guide. AMEE guide no. 82. *Medical Teacher, 35*(10), e1511-e1530. https://www.tandfonline.com/doi/full/10.3109/0142159X.2013.818632	• Plan • Implement • Evaluate • Revise
INACSL Standards Committee, Watts, P. I., McDermott, D. S., Alinier, G., Charnetski, M., & Nawathe, P. A. (2021, September). Healthcare Simulation Standards of Best Practice Simulation Design. *Clinical Simulation in Nursing , 58*, 14-21. https://doi.org/10.1016/j.ecns.2021.08.009	1. Consult content experts and simulationists knowledgeable in best practices in simulation education, pedagogy, and practice. 2. Perform a needs assessment. 3. Construct measurable objectives. 4. Structure the format of a simulation based on the purpose, theory, and modality for the simulation-based experience. 5. Design a scenario or case to provide the context for the simulation-based experience. 6. Use various types of fidelity to create the required perception of realism. 7. Maintain a facilitative approach that is participant centered and driven by the objectives, participant's knowledge or level of experience, and the expected outcomes. 8. Begin simulation-based experiences with a prebriefing. 9. Follow simulation-based experiences with a debriefing and/or feedback session. 10. Include an evaluation of the participants, facilitators, the simulation-based experience, the facility, and the support team. 11. Provide preparation materials and resources to promote participants' ability to meet identified objectives.

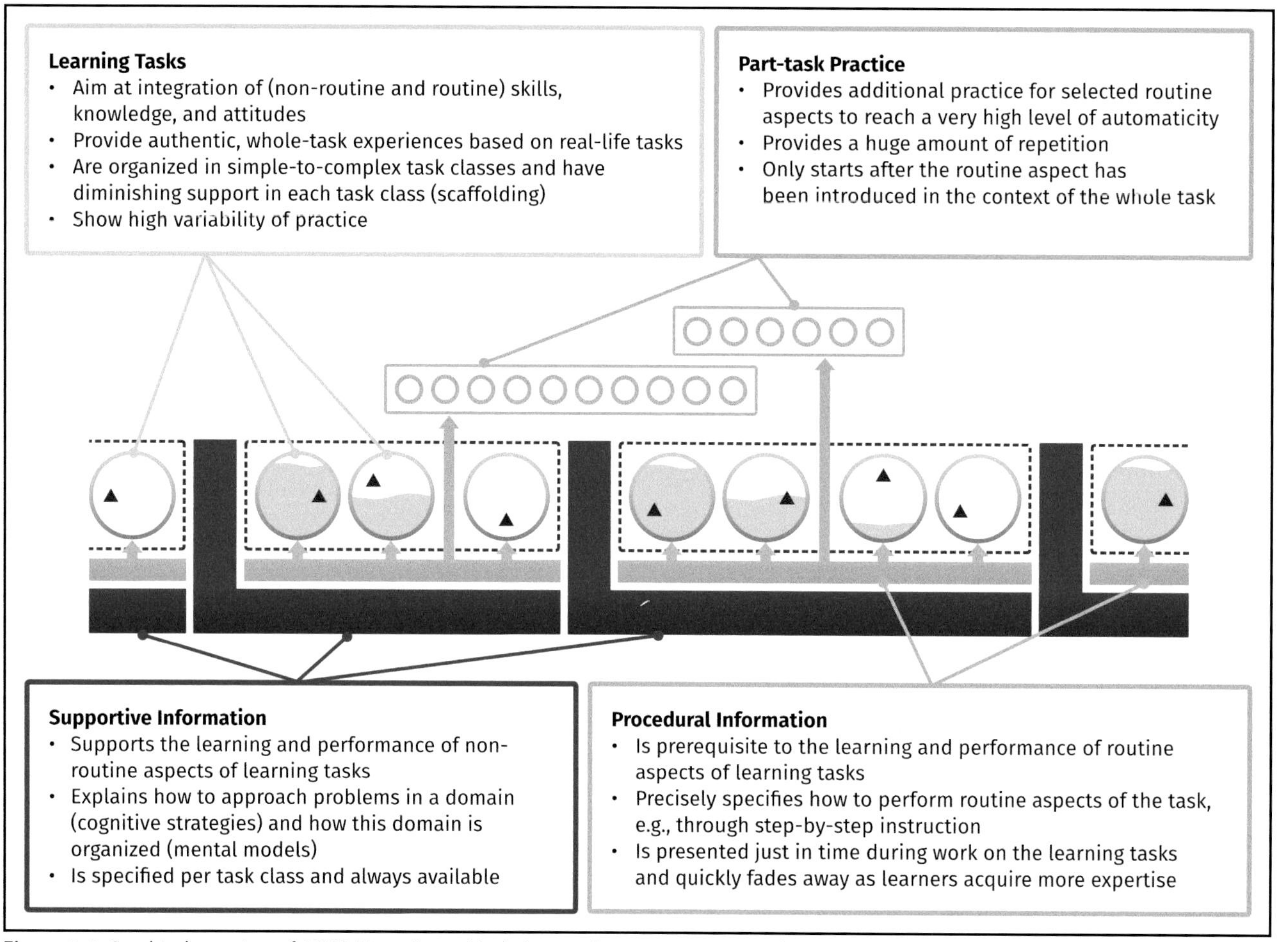

Figure 2-4. Graphical overview of 4C/ID. Note: A graphical view on the 4 components: (a) learning tasks, (b) supportive information, (c) procedural information, and (d) part-task practice. (Reproduced with permission from Van Merriënboer, J. J. G. [2020]. Graphical view on the four components. https://www.4cid.org via NoDerivatives 4.0 International [CC BY-ND 4.0].)

transfer. Simulation technologies support this principle by strategies such as (a) providing procedural information via screen prompts or pop-ups in computer-based or virtual-world simulations, (b) pausing an interaction with a standardized patient in order to provide feedback and redirections, (c) conducting formal debriefings that incorporate quality feedback practices, and (d) reflection among participants as the facilitator enables students to explicitly identify and enrich relevant schema.

Principle 4: Learning is developmental and requires appropriate scaffolding to allow the learner to integrate and apply KSAs and related professional tasks and competencies to increasingly complex problems (McAllister et al., 2011; Wood et al., 1976). A useful framework for analyzing what the student's current level of development is is to consider how well the student's performance indicates that they are managing complexity and integrating and applying the relevant KSAs and competencies, as well as how much support they need to do so (McAllister et al., 2011, 2013a).

The Role of the Educator and Expectations of the Learner

Role of the Educator in SBLE

A learner-centered approach to SBLE is central to a competency-based outcomes curriculum and warrants a paradigm shift in how we view the role of the educator within the learning process. The focus on student learning, or development of competent judgment and action, necessarily pivots the role of the educator responsible for transmitting knowledge through didactic teaching, toward the educator as facilitator of learning (Fink, 2013; Weimer, 2013; Wiggins & McTighe, 2011). To successfully make this shift from teacher to educator, Weimer (2013) suggests that educators need to let students do more of the learning, that is, learner-centered educators ask fewer questions, provide fewer answers, offer fewer examples, and allow the students to organize the materials while striking a balance between offering too much

BOX 2-3

CLEAR

Moulton and colleagues (2016) developed the acronym CLEAR to assist facilitators in meeting best practices.

- **C**ommunication and constructive feedback
- **L**earning partnerships and leader
- **E**nvironment and ensure fidelity
- **A**ccommodation and assessment/evaluation
- **R**eflection

or too little guidance and support or scaffolding (Kirschner et al., 2006; Wood et al., 1976). A well-constructed SBLE facilitates this by enabling learners to direct their own learning as they engage in the simulation, and educators need to allow for this to occur by resisting directing this process. Second, learner-centered educators guide students in how to think, problem-solve, and engage in clinical reasoning through explicit instruction of these learning skills and engagement in metacognition (thinking about their thinking); all of which contribute to students generating their own process schemas as they develop competency (Weimer, 2013). Learner-centered educators will be skilled in providing immediate, specific, and targeted feedback as well as encouraging students to reflect on their own learning via thoughtful facilitation of the debrief process in an SBLE to assist development of process and pattern schemas. Finally, learner-centered educators encourage collaboration within the SBLE promoting behaviors that support the development of professional and occupational competencies necessary in the workforce, such as teamwork and lifelong learning (Le Maistre & Pare, 2004).

The term *facilitator* is often used to specify a particular role of the educator within the realm of simulation education. In this context, the facilitator guides students in their learning and helps them to make meaningful connections between prior knowledge, new knowledge, and the processes involved in learning (Bada, 2015). Facilitators should possess a clear understanding of the characteristics of learners, foster experiential learning, and support critical thinking and metacognition (INACSL Standards Committee, 2016a).

Expectations of the Learners

In order to design an effective SBLE, it is important to consider and inform the expectations of the learners. Many learners have received much of their education through teacher-centered methods, such as lectures and presentations, where learning is transmitted and assessed as if it is a product that can be transferred from the teacher to the learner (Biggs, 1999; Boud & Soler, 2016; Hager, 2004). Learners engaged in activities designed to be learner centered, such as problem-based, team-based, or simulation learning, need to shift their orientation toward learning in order to be successful. This shift in orientation includes a willingness to let students become active participants and to take responsibility for their own learning. It requires a commitment to engagement and reliance on intrinsic motivation rather than extrinsic motivators, such as test grades, and tolerance for the germane cognitive load that is generated as they actively develop their schema (van Merriënboer et al., 2006). Learning for practice also requires the student to move from a competitive to collaborative mindset to successfully develop their competencies (Le Maistre & Pare, 2004). This shift in attitude will also necessitate a change in how they view the role and responsibilities of the educator (Rudolph et al., 2014; Trinidad, 2020).

BOX 2-4

Threats to Learning in an SBLE

- A lack of buy-in to the simulation endeavor
- Failure to suspend disbelief within the simulation
- Defensiveness toward feedback
- Perceived threat to professional identity

It is worth noting that these shifts may be stressful for learners experiencing their first SBLE. Learners are supported in making these shifts in attitudes and expectations through effective use of the prebriefing processes (Rutherford-Hemming et al., 2019). The purpose of the prebriefing is to provide information and instructions to assist learners in achieving learning outcomes and to establish a psychologically safe environment that supports learning (INACSL Standards Committee, 2016b) and to address behaviors and attitudes of the learner that threaten and impede learning within the SBLE (Rudolph et al., 2014).

Rudolph et al. (2014) provide strong evidence for the need to provide learners a safe environment to support learners in their ability to

> (1) tolerate practicing at the edge of their ability, within an unfamiliar and possibly confusing environment; (2) appreciate comprehensive feedback in the context of demanding professional standards; (3) willingly reflect on problems and skills that are new or challenging to them; (4) correct and repeat actions; (5) contemplate and learn from mistakes; and (6) tolerate not knowing the exact answers to complex questions. (p. 339)

Summary

Simulation technologies and tools are seductive and compelling—anyone who has donned a virtual-reality headset or observed students immersed in assessing an actor who is portraying a person with hearing, communication, or swallowing impairment can attest to this. Too often the rich opportunities to develop students' professional practice are lost through neglecting to integrate these technologies into evidence-based and theory-informed SBLEs. The goal for this chapter is to provide a scholarly framework founded in evidence-based education to support the effective integration of SBLEs into the curriculum.

For those interested in designing and implementing quality SBLEs, this and other chapters of this book will guide you in determining how to get there from here. In summary, we offer three touchstones or principles that will serve to guide you as you plan, develop, and implement all the moving parts involved in an SBLE.

- Principle 1: Consider the place of the SBLE in the curriculum sequence and where the learners are in their development of their professional expertise and the implications for the content and processes of your SBLE.
- Principle 2: Determine the learning outcomes to be addressed from a competency-based outcome framework to ensure the students' development of professional expertise is effectively facilitated (Fink, 2013).
- Principle 3: Attend to the evidence and related learning theory when creating or adopting an SBLE.

References

Al-Eyd, G., Achike, F., Agarwal, M., Atamna, H., Atapattu, D. N., Castro, L., Estrada, J., Ettarh, R., Hassan, S., Lakhan, S. E., Nausheen, F., Seki, T., Stegeman, M., Suskind, R., Velji, A., Yakub, M., & Tenore, A. (2018). Curriculum mapping as a tool to facilitate curriculum development: A new school of medicine experience. *BMC Medical Education, 18*(1). https://doi.org/10.1186/s12909-018-1289-9

Anderson, J. M., Aylor, M. E., & Leonard, D. T. (2008). Instructional design dogma: Creating planned learning environments in simulation. *Journal of Critical Care, 23*(4), 595-602. https://doi.org/10.1016/j.jcrc.2008.03.003

Bada, S. O. (2015). Constructivism learning theory: A paradigm for teaching and learning. *Journal of Research & Method in Education, 5*(6), 66-70.

Barnett, S. M., & Ceci, S. J. (2002). When and where do we apply what we learn? A taxonomy for far transfer. *Psychological Bulletin, 128*(4), 612-637. https://doi.org/10.1037//0033-2909.128.4.612

Beckett, D. (2004). Embodied competence and generic skills: The emergence of inferential understanding. *Educational Philosophy and Theory, 36*(5).

Benner, P. A., Tanner, C. A., & Chesla, C. A. (1996). *Expertise in nursing practice: Caring, clinical judgment, and ethics.* Springer Publishing Company.

Biggs, J. (1999). What the student does: Teaching for enhanced learning. *Higher Education Research & Development, 18*(1), 57-75. https://doi.org/10.1080/0729436990180105

Bohmer, R. M. J., & Edmonson, A. C. (2001). Organizational learning in health care. *Health Forum Journal, 44*(2), 32-35.

Boud, D., & Soler, R. (2016). Sustainable assessment revisited. *Assessment & Evaluation in Higher Education. 41*(3), 400-413. https://doi.org/10.1080/02602938.2015.1018133

Brown, T., Bourke-Taylor, H., & Williams, B. (2012). Curriculum alignment and graduate attributes: Critical elements in occupational therapy education. *British Journal of Occupational Therapy, 75*(4), 163-163. https://doi.org/10.4276/030802212x13336366278013

Bruner, J. S. (1971). *Toward a theory of instruction.* The Belknap Press of Harvard University Press.

Carraccio, C., Wolfsthal, S. D., Englander, R., Ferentz, K., & Martin, C. (2002). Shifting paradigms: From flexner to competencies. *Academic Medicine, 77*(5), 361-367. https://pubmed.ncbi.nlm.nih.gov/12010689/

Carter, R. (1985). A taxonomy of objectives for professional education. *Studies in Higher Education, 10*(2), 135-149. https://doi.org/10.1080/03075078512331378559

Chi, M. T. H., Glaser, R., & Farr, M. J. (Eds.). (1988). *The nature of expertise.* Psychology Press. https://doi.org/10.4324/9781315799681

Clapper, T. C., & Kardong-Edgren, S. (2012). Using deliberate practice and simulation to improve nursing skills. *Clinical Simulation in Nursing, 6*(1), e7-e14.

Cook, D. A., Hamstra, S. J., Brydges, R., Zendejas, B., Szostek, J. H., Wang, A. T., Erwin, P. J., & Hatala, R. (2013). Comparative effectiveness of instructional design features in simulation-based education: Systematic review and meta-analysis. *Medical Teacher. 35*(1), e867-e898. https://doi.org/10.3109/0142159X.2012.714886.

Cowan, D., Norman, I., & Coopamah, V. P. (2005). Competence in nursing practice: A controversial concept—A focused review of literature. *Nurse Education Today, 25*(5), 355-362. https://doi.org/10.1016/j.nedt.2005.03.002

Crespo, K. E., Torres, J. E., & Recio, M. E. (2004). Reasoning process characteristics in the diagnostic skills of beginner, competent, and expert dentists. *Journal of Dental Education, 68*(12), 1235-1244. http://www.jdentaled.org/content/68/12/1235.full.pdf

Croskerry, P. (2009). A universal model of clinical reasoning. *Academic Medicine, 84*(8), 1022-1028.

Davidoff, F. (2008). Focus on performance: The 21st century revolution in medical education. *Mens sana monographs, 6*(1), 29-40. https://doi.org/10.4103/0973-1229.37085

Devantier, S. L., Minda, J. P., Goldszmidt, M., & Haddara, W. (2009). Categorizing patients in a forced-choice triad task: The integration of context in patient management. *PLoS ONE, 4*(6), e5881.

Doeltgen, S. H., McAllister, S., Murray, J., Ward, E. C., & Pretz, J. E. (2018). Reasoning and decision making in clinical swallowing examination. *Current Physical Medicine and Rehabilitation Reports, 6*, 171-177. https://doi.org/10.1007/s40141-018-0191-z

Dollaghan, C. A. (2007). *The handbook for evidence-based practice in communication disorders.* Paul H. Brookes.

Ericsson, K. A. (2004). Deliberate practice and the acquisition and maintenance of expert performance in medicine and related domains. *Academic Medicine, 79*(10), 570-581.

Ferguson, A., McAllister, S., Lincoln, M., & McAllister, L. (2010). Becoming familiar with competency-based student assessment: An evaluation of workshop outcomes. *International Journal of Speech-Language Pathology, 16*(6), 545-554.

Fink, L. D. (2013). *Creating significant learning experiences: An integrated approach to designing college courses.* John Wiley & Sons.

Forsberg, E., Ziegert, K., Hult, H., & Fors, U. (2013). Clinical reasoning in nursing, a think-aloud study using virtual patients: A base for innovative assessment. *Nurse Education Today, 34*(4), 538-542. http://dx.doi.org/10.1016/j.nedt.2013.07.010

Fraser, K. L., Ayres, P., & Sweller, J. (2015). Cognitive load theory for the design of medical simulations. *Simulation in Healthcare, 10*(5), 295-307. https://doi.org/10.1097/SIH.0000000000000097

Ginsberg, S. M., Friberg, J. C., & Visconti, C. F. (2016). Diagnostic reasoning by experienced speech-language pathologists and student clinicians. *Contemporary Issues in Communication Science and Disorders, 43,* 87-97. https://doi.org/10.1044/CISCSD_43_S_87.

Gonczi, A. (1994). Competency based assessment in the professions in Australia. *Assessment in Education: Principles, Policy & Practice, 1*(1), 27-44. https://doi.org/10.1080/0969594940010103

Gough, S., Yohannes, A. M., & Murray, J. (2016). The Integrated Simulation and Technology Enhanced Learning (ISETL) framework: Facilitating robust design, implementation, evaluation and research in healthcare. *Physiotherapy, 102*, e27-e28. https://doi.org/10.1016/j.physio.2016.10.039

Groom, J. A., Henderson, D., & Sittner, B. J. (2014). NLN/Jeffries simulation framework state of the science project: Simulation design characteristics. *Clinical Simulation in Nursing, 10*(7), 337-344. https://doi.org/10.1016/j.ecns.2013.02.004

Hager, P. (1994). Is there a cogent philosophical argument against competency standards? *Australian Journal of Education, 38*(1), 3-18. https://doi.org/10.1177/000494419403800101

Hager, P. (2000). Know-how and workplace practical judgement. *Journal of Philosophy of Education, 34*, 281-296.

Hager, P. (2004). Metaphors of workplace learning: More process, less product. *Fine Print, 27*(3), 7-10. https://www.voced.edu.au/content/ngv%3A22796

Hattie, J. (2015). The applicability of visible learning to higher education. *Scholarship of Teaching and Learning in Psychology, 1*(1), 79-91. https://doi.org/10.1037/stl0000021

Heywood, L., Gonczi, A., & Hager, P. (1992). *A guide to the development of competency standards for the professions*. Australian Government Publishing Service.

Higgs, J., & Bithell, C. (2001). Professional expertise. In J. Higgs & A. Titchen (Eds.), *Practice knowledge and expertise in the health professions,* (pp. 59-68). Butterworth-Heinemann.

Higgs, J., & Jones, M. (2000). Clinical reasoning in the health professions. In J. Higgs & M. Jones (Eds.), *Clinical reasoning in the health professions* (2nd ed., pp. 3-14). Butterworth-Heinemann.

Higgs, J., & Titchen, A. (2001). *Practice knowledge and expertise in the health professions.* Butterworth-Heinemann.

INACSL Standards Committee. (2016a). INACSL standards of best practice: Simulation facilitation. *Clinical Simulation in Nursing, 12*, S16-S20. https://www.nursingsimulation.org/article/S1876-1399%2816%2930128-1/fulltext

INACSL Standards Committee. (2016b). INACSL standards of best practice: Simulation simulation glossary. *Clinical Simulation in Nursing, 12*, S39-S47. https://linkinghub.elsevier.com/retrieve/pii/S1876139916301335

INACSL Standards Committee, Watts, P. I., McDermott, D. S., Alinier, G., Charnetski, M., & Nawathe, P. A. (2021, September). Healthcare Simulation Standards of Best Practice Simulation Design. *Clinical Simulation in Nursing, 58*, 14-21. https://doi.org/10.1016/j.ecns.2021.08.009

Jeffries, P. R. (2005). A framework for designing, implementing, and evaluating simulations used as teaching strategies in nursing. *Nursing Education Perspectives, 26*(2), 96-103.

Khamis, N., Satava, R., & Kern, D. E. (2020). Stepwise simulation course design model: Survey results from 16 centers. *JSLS: Journal of the Society of Laparoendoscopic Surgeons, 24*(2). https://doi.org/10.4293/JSLS.2019.00060

King, P. M., & Kitchener, K. S. (2004). Reflective judgment: Theory and research on the development of epistemic assumptions through adulthood. *Educational Psychologist, 39*(1), 18. https://doi.org/10.1207/s15326985ep3901_2

Kirschner, P. A., Sweller, J., & Clark, R. E. (2006). Why minimal guidance during instruction does not work: An analysis of the failure of constructivist, discovery, problem-based, experiential, and inquiry-based teaching. *Educational Psychologist, 41*(2), 75-86.

Kolb, D. A. (1984). *Experiential learning: Experience as the source of learning and development.* Prentice-Hall. https://search.library.wisc.edu/catalog/999550475402121

Lave, J. (1988). *Cognition in practice: Mind, mathematics and culture in everyday life.* Cambridge University Press. https://www.cambridge.org/core/books/cognition-in-practice/2AF0745B4B8636436A1DF8AAF374BB9E

Le Maistre, C., & Pare, A. (2004). Learning in two communities: The challenge for universities and workplaces. *Journal of Workplace Learning, 16*(1), 44-52.

Maggio, L. A., Cate, O. T., Irby, D. M., & O'Brien, B. C. (2015). Designing evidence-based medicine training to optimize the transfer of skills from the classroom to clinical practice: Applying the four component instructional design model. *Academic Medicine, 90*(11), 1457-1461. https://doi.org/10.1097/ACM.0000000000000769

McAllister, S., Lincoln, M., Ferguson, A., & McAllister, L. (2010). Issues in developing valid assessments of speech pathology students' performance in the workplace. *International Journal of Language and Communication Disorders, 45*(1), 1-14. http://informahealthcare.com/doi/pdfplus/10.3109/13682820902745461

McAllister, S., Lincoln, M., Ferguson, A., & McAllister, L. (2011). A systematic program of research regarding the assessment of speech-language pathology competencies. *International Journal of Speech-Language Pathology, 13*(6), 469-479.

McAllister, S., Lincoln, M., Ferguson, A., & McAllister, L. (2013a). *COMPASS®: Competency assessment in speech pathology* (2nd ed.). Speech Pathology Australia.

McAllister, S., Lincoln, M., Ferguson, A., & McAllister, L. (2013b). Validating workplace performance assessments in health sciences students: A case study from speech pathology. *Journal of Applied Measurement, 14*(4), 356-374.

McAllister, S., Tedesco, H., Kruger, S., Ward, E. C., Marsh, C., & Doeltgen, S. (2020). Clinical reasoning and hypothesis generation in expert clinical swallowing examinations. *International Journal of Language & Communication Disorders, 55*(4), 480-492. https://doi.org/10.1111/1460-6984.12531

McGaghie, W. C., Issenberg, S. B., Petrusa, E. R., & Scalese, R. J. (2016). Revisiting "A critical review of simulation-based medical education research: 2003-2009." *Medical Education, 50*(10), 986-991. https://doi.org/10.1111/medu.12795

McGaghie, W. C., Issenberg, S. B., Petrusa, E. R., & Scalese, R. J. (2010). A critical review of simulation-based medical education research: 2003-2009. *Medical Education, 44*(1), 50-63. https://doi.org/10.1111/j.1365-2923.2009.03547.x

Motola, I., Devine, L. A., Chung, H. S., Sullivan, J. E., & Issenberg, S. B. (2013). Simulation in healthcare education: A best evidence practical guide. AMEE guide no. 82. *Medical Teacher, 35*(10), e1511-e1530. https://www.tandfonline.com/doi/full/10.3109/0142159X.2013.818632

Moulton, M., Lucas, L., Monaghan, G., & Swoboda, S. (2016). A CLEAR approach for the novice simulation facilitator. *Teaching and Learning in Nursing, 12*(2), 136-141. https://doi.org/10.1016/j.teln.2016.11.003

Naismith, L. M., Kowalski, C., Soklaridis, S., Kelly, A., & Walsh, C. M. (2020). Participant perspectives on the contributions of physical, psychological, and sociological fidelity to learning in interprofessional mental health simulation. *Simulation in Healthcare, 15*(3), 141-146. https://doi.org/10.1097/SIH.0000000000000425

Patel, R., Sandars, J., & Carr, S. (2015). Clinical diagnostic decision-making in real life contexts: A trans-theoretical approach for teaching: AMEE guide no. 95. *Medical Teacher, 37*(3), 211-227. https://doi.org/10.3109/0142159X.2014.975195

Patel, V. L, Glaser, R., & Arocha, J. F. (2000). Cognition and expertise: Acquisition of medical competence. *Clinical & Investigative Medicine, 23*(4), 256-260.

Piaget, J. (1957). *Construction of reality in the child.* Routledge & Kegan Paul.

Poore, J. A., Cullen, D. L., & Schaar, G. L. (2014). Simulation-based interprofessional education guided by Kolb's experiential learning theory. *Clinical Simulation in Nursing, 10*(5), e241-e247. https://doi.org/10.1016/j.ecns.2014.01.004

Price, M., Carroll, J., O'Donovan, B., & Rust, C. (2011). If I was going there I wouldn't start from here: A critical commentary on current assessment practice. *Assessment & Evaluation in Higher Education, 36*(4), 479-492.

Riviere, E., Jaffrelot, M., Jouquan, J., & Chiniara, G. (2019). Debriefing for the transfer of learning: The importance of context. *Academic Medicine, 94*(6), 796-803. https://doi.org/10.1097/ACM.0000000000002612

Rudolph, J. W., Raemer, D. B., & Simon, R. (2014). Establishing a safe container for learning in simulation: The role of the presimulation briefing. *Simulation in Healthcare, 9*(6), 339-349. https://doi.org/10.1097/SIH.0000000000000047

Rudolph, J. W., Simon, R., & Raemer, D. B. (2007). Which reality matters? Questions on the path to high engagement in healthcare simulation. *Simulation in Healthcare, 2*(3), 161-163. https://doi.org/10.1097/SIH.0b013e31813d1035

Rutherford-Hemming, T., Lioce, L., & Breymier, T. (2019). Guidelines and essential elements for prebriefing. *Simulation in Healthcare, 14*(6), 409-414. https://doi.org/10.1097/SIH.0000000000000403

Schön, D. A. (1983). *The reflective practitioner: How professionals think in action.* Basic Books.

Schuwirth, L. W., & Durning, S. J. (2018). Educational research: current trends, evidence base and unanswered questions. *Medical Journal of Australia, 208*(4), 161-163.

Schuwirth, L. W., & van der Vleuten, C. P. (2020). A history of assessment in medical education. *Advances in Health Sciences Education, 25*(5), 1045-1056. https://doi.org/10.1007/s10459-020-10003-0

Schuwirth L. W., & van der Vleuten, C. P. (2011). Programmatic assessment: From assessment of learning to assessment for learning. *Medical Teacher, 33*(6), 478-485. https://doi.org/10.3109/0142159X.2011.565828

Secheresse, T., & Nonglaton, S. (2019). Theoretical underpinnings of scenario design. In G. Chiniara (Ed.), *Clinical simulation: Education, operations and engineering* (pp. 279-284). Elsevier Science & Technology.

Skinner, B. F. (1974). *About behaviorism.* Random House.

The Speech Pathology Association of Australia Ltd Staff. (2017). *Competency-based occupational standards for speech pathologists—Entry Level.* https://www.speechpathologyaustralia.org.au/SPAweb/SPAweb/Resources_for_Speech_Pathologists/CBOS/CBOS.aspx

Tai, J., Ajjawi, R., Boud, D., Dawson, P., & Panadero, E. (2018). Developing evaluative judgement: Enabling students to make decisions about the quality of work. *Higher Education, 76*(3), 467-481.

ten Cate, O. (2005). Entrustability of professional activities and competency-based training. *Medical Education, 39*, 1176-1177.

Torre, D., Durning, S. J., Rencic, J., Lang, V., Holmboe, E., & Daniel, M. (2020). Widening the lens on teaching and assessing clinical reasoning: from "in the head" to "out in the world". *Diagnosis, 7*(3), 181-190. https://doi.org/10.1515/dx-2019-0098

Trinidad, J. E. (2020). Understanding student-centred learning in higher education: Students' and teachers' perceptions, challenges, and cognitive gaps. *Journal of Further and Higher Education, 44*(8), 1013-1023. https://doi.org/10.1080/0309877X.2019.1636214

Van Merriënboer, J. J. G. (2020). *Graphical view on the four components.* https://www.4cid.org

van Merriënboer, J. J. G, Kester, L., & Paas, F. (2006). Teaching complex rather than simple tasks: Balancing intrinsic and germane load to enhance transfer of learning. *Applied Cognitive Psychology, 20*(3), 343-352.

van Merriënboer, J. J. G., & Kirschner, P. A. (2018). *Ten steps to complex learning: A systematic approach to four-component instructional design* (3rd ed.). Routledge.

van Merriënboer, J. J. G., & Sweller, J. (2005). Cognitive load theory and complex learning: Recent developments and future directions. *Educational Psychology Review, 17*(2), 147-177. https://doi.org/10.1007/s10648-005-3951-0

Vygotsky, L. S. (1978). *Mind in society: The development of higher psychological processes.* Harvard University Press.

Weimer, M. (2013). *Learner-centered teaching: Five key changes to practice.* John Wiley & Sons. http://ebookcentral.proquest.com/lib/jmu/detail.action?docID=1119448

Wiggins, G. P., & McTighe, J. (2005). *Understanding by design* (2nd ed.). Association for Supervision and Curriculum Development.

Wiggins, G. P., & McTighe, J. (2011). *The understanding by design guide to creating high-quality units.* Association for Supervision and Curriculum Development.

Wood, D., Bruner, J., Ross, G. (1976). The role of tutoring in problem solving. *Journal of Child Psychology and Psychiatry, 17*, 89-100. https://doi.org/10.1111/j.1469-7610.1976.tb00381.x

Simulation for Clinical Education in Communication Sciences and Disorders

Meredith L. Baker-Rush, PhD, MS, CCC-SLP/L, CHSE, FNAP and
Richard I. Zraick, PhD, CCC-SLP, F-ASHA, CHSE

Background in Simulation for Clinical Education

Health care simulation can be used to train health care professionals to perform clinical skills and to work in teams with the goal of improved patient safety (MacKinnon, 2011; Mills et al., 2019). Simulation may involve a variety of technologies including, but not limited to, manikin, task trainer, virtual reality (VR), standardized patient (SP), standardized participant, or a mix. Each technology has its own advantages and disadvantages and should be selected based on learning objectives and skill level of the learners. Refer to Chapter 4 for an in-depth discussion of the typology of simulation methodologies, including modality, mode of delivery, and consideration related to fidelity.

Simulation has been used in the clinical education of students across disciplines, including communication sciences and disorders (CSD). Simulation-based learning experiences (SBLEs) include techniques to replace or amplify real experiences with guided experiences that evoke or replicate substantial aspects of the real world in a fully interactive manner (Gaba, 2004). To put it simply, simulation allows a learner to experience, engage in action, think, process, and reflect. Simulation can be thought of as another tool available to academic and clinical educators to assist learners in developing clinical knowledge and skills. SBLEs offer an opportunity to supplement opportunities for clinical education experiences in different work settings and with different populations. It also serves as a way of ongoing assessment and remediation of learners' knowledge, skills, and attributes (KSAs).

Research in Simulation for Clinical Education

Simulation for clinical education has a research history going back over 100 years (Owen, 2016). Quantitative, qualitative, and mixed methods research approaches have been utilized in investigations that have been descriptive, experimental, evaluative, exploratory, and explanative in nature (see Chapter 8). Researchers come from diverse backgrounds and disciplines including clinical health care, social and behavioral sciences, educational science, health care informatics and technology, and public health.

Dudding, C. C., & Ginsberg, S. M. (Eds.).
Simulation-Based Learning in Communication Sciences and Disorders: Moving From Theory to Practice. (pp. 35-51).

The drive by professional organizations and university training programs to incorporate health care simulation into clinical education programs has yielded a call for accountability and evidence in the form of proven outcomes. A review of health care simulation articles published between 2013 and 2015 in the journal *Simulation in Healthcare* revealed that the majority of research articles published during that period focused on how to use SBLEs, improve the simulation experience, and develop and evaluate new simulation systems (Scerbo, 2016). The research has led in part to the development of frameworks, guidelines, and standards of best practice in medicine and nursing.

Research on the use of simulation in CSD goes back to the early 1990s and began with the use of simulated patients presenting with communication disorders to students in the classroom. The field has evolved in its use of simulation as a clinical education tool to include a variety of simulation modalities and technologies, including task trainers, computer-based simulations, and high-tech manikins in order to enhance student learning and assess student skills (Zraick, 2020). Dzulkarnain and colleagues (2015) conducted a systematic review of research related to SBLEs in audiology. It was evidenced that learners engaged in SBLEs showed a significantly higher post-training score compared to other methods of training. Dzulkarnain and colleagues (2015) concluded with caution that SBLE training is an effective tool and can be used for basic clinical audiology training.

The remainder of this chapter will explore best practices and application of clinical simulation for clinical education in CSD. It includes practical examples and considerations for implementation of quality simulation learning experiences in the coursework, clinic, and simulation lab.

Specifically, it will address the use of simulation for the following:

- Obtaining guided observation and clinical clock hours
- Formative and summative assessment, including a discussion of competency-based assessment
- Interprofessional education (IPE) and interprofessional collaborative practice (ICP)

Simulation for Clinical Education in Communication Sciences and Disorders

CSD has been slow to adopt the use of simulation for clinical education. A 2015 survey of simulation use in graduate programs in CSD showed that 51% of responding programs reported using some form of simulation in clinical education (Dudding & Nottingham, 2018). The most used simulation modality was the use of SPs, followed closely by computer-based simulations. Simulations were most frequently used to address clinical skills development and assessment. Some programs reported using simulation to supplement clinical training opportunities in the face of declining number and variety of clinical placements. As one survey respondent indicated, "the use of simulation allows students to practice before interacting with real clientele" (Dudding & Nottingham, 2018). This survey, conducted prior to the 2019 worldwide COVID-19 pandemic, highlighted the burgeoning acceptance of simulation in CSD.

There has been a recent increase in the number of publications related to best practices in clinical simulation in CSD. The Council of Academic Programs in Communication Sciences and Disorders gathered a group of experts to publish an ebook titled *Best Practices in Healthcare Simulations: Communication Sciences and Disorders* (Dudding et al., 2019). While this document focuses on health care education, the principles apply to the use of simulation in educational practice settings. In another publication, Hewat and colleagues (2020) provide a summary of the process and considerations required in the development of an SBLE for programs in speech-language pathology. The authors provide a framework for the development of simulation-based learning programs for university programs and/or workplace training in speech-language pathology. Table 3-1 presents perceived advantages and disadvantages to using SBLEs in CSD.

The use of simulation in clinical education in CSD has been upheld and/or encouraged by accreditation and certification boards in the professions. The Accreditation Commission for Audiology Education encourages the use of multiple methods on instruction and evaluation, including simulation, as part of Standard 21 (Accreditation Commission for Audiology Education, 2016). The American Academy of Audiology (2016) stated their support of students and the use of simulation as part of their response to the global pandemic. They identified the use of simulation, especially virtual simulation, as a way to supplement traditional clinical experiences and develop clinical competence. In 2016, the American Speech-Language-Hearing Association's (ASHA's) Council for Clinical Certification (CFCC) voted to modify the implementation language for Speech-Language Pathology Standard V-B to allow up to 20% of the required 375 direct clinical hours to be obtained through simulation (CFCC, 2014). In 2021, the CFCC revised and upheld the Audiology certification standards giving AuD students the option of obtaining up to 10% supervised clinical experience through clinical simulation. Those engaged in simulation for clinical education are advised to check with state and applicable licensing boards to ensure that there are no limitations on the use of simulation in meeting requirements (ASHA, 2021).

Guided Clinical Observation

While not meeting all the requirements of an SBLE, the use of simulation technology is helpful in obtaining guided clinical observation opportunities for students. Those

TABLE 3-1

Perceived Advantages and Disadvantages of Simulation for Clinical Training

PERCEIVED ADVANTAGES	PERCEIVED DISADVANTAGES
• Exposure to a wider range of clinical scenarios • Provision of a safe, controlled learning environment • Attainment of uniform educational outcomes, despite different rates of trainee progress • Reproducibility of standardized educational experiences, enabling assessment of clinical skills across students on identical scenarios	• Reduced complexity of the simulation • Failure to completely replicate a real-life scenario • Uncertainty regarding accreditation of SBLEs to establish competency • Limited funding and other resources • Suitability of scenarios beyond early stages of learning • Fear that SBLEs may reduce the need for real-world clinical placements

Adapted from MacBean, N., Theodoros, D., Davidson, B., & Hill, A. E. (2013). Simulated learning environments in speech-language pathology: An Australian response. *International Journal of Speech-Language Pathology, 15*(3), 345-357 and Theodoros, D., Davidson, B., Hill, A., & MacBean, N., (2010). Integration of simulated learning environments into speech pathology clinical education curricula: A national approach. Health Workforce Australia. https://www.academia.edu/6618513/Integration_of_simulated_learning_environments_into_speech_pathology_clinical_education_curricula_A_national_approach

BOX 3-1

Is It a Simulation?

Example 1: An educator talks students through a video of modified barium swallow examination as part of a class activity. The educator presents the case history at the beginning and solicits feedback from the students as part of a debriefing session. Watching and discussing a video in a class setting does not meet the criteria of an SBLE even though it may include a prebrief and debrief guided by the instructor. The reason is that watching a recorded video or live session in a group setting does not allow the learner to interact with the material and/or immerse themselves in the learning process. However, that is not to say that videos cannot be incorporated into an SBLE.

seeking ASHA certification upon completion of a graduate program in CSD are required to participate in a minimum of 25 guided observation hours. Guided observation requires that there is communication between a clinical educator who is accredited by ASHA's CFCC and a student observer. Traditionally, students obtained these hours by observing clinicians live in actual practice settings. More recently, these observation experiences have occurred asynchronously (not in real time) using videos, under the supervision of an ASHA-certified clinical educator. Videos can be obtained from the personal archives of the clinical educator or from video sharing sites such as YouTube. Educators are cautioned about violating confidentiality and privacy laws. Additionally, there are commercially available services that provide opportunities for virtual guided clinical observation (e.g., Simucase and Master Clinician Network). The guided observation can take many forms (e.g., live discussion, review of written reflection, individual or group) and closely models the debrief stage of SBLEs. Clinical educators may want to borrow from simulation to inform best practice in debriefing as well as the use of certain simulation technologies for this purpose.

Simulation for Supervised Clinical Experience

As mentioned, both ASHA and American Academy of Audiology allow for a portion of a student's required clinical experiences to be earned through simulation. The activity must meet all the elements of a quality simulation including that it replicates real-world experiences, is guided by an experienced facilitator, and allows the learner to engage with the experience in an interactive manner (Gaba, 2004). A knowledgeable clinical educator trained in best practices in simulation is charged with facilitating the learning experience. It is critical to ensure that the experience meets the definition of a simulation and includes all stages of the SBLE, including the prebrief, simulation, and debrief. Without these criteria, the experience is a learning activity, but not a simulation. This is an important distinction for those seeking certification, in that learning activities that do not meet the criteria for simulation cannot be counted as clinical clock hours. See Chapter 5 for an in-depth discussion on the components of a quality SBLE.

BOX 3-2

Is It a Simulation?

Example 2: An educator offers an open skills lab for learners to independently practice tracheostomy tube suction skills on a full-sized manikin. If the experience does not include a prebrief and/or debrief, the experience may not be considered an SBLE. This activity still has value in that it offers repeated practice. However, it would not be considered an SBLE merely because it was conducted in a simulation lab and with manikins.

BOX 3-3

Is It a Simulation?

Example 3: A graduate student conducts a bedside clinical swallowing evaluation using a manikin while a trained standardized participant portrays a family member. Prior to this activity, the student engages with an educator in a prebrief that includes expectations in terms of roles and an understanding of learning objectives and assessment measures. Following the simulation activity, the student participates in a debrief with the clinical educator and SP. This learning activity meets criteria for a simulation.

It is beyond the scope of this book to advise on the specifics related to what does and does not count toward clinical clock hours per the standards of any organization or licensing board. Best practices in simulation-based education suggest that clinical educators should be trained in all aspects of simulation, abide by codes of ethics, and be familiar with all standards and practices guiding the use of simulations for clinical education.

Simulation for Formative and Summative Assessment

Assessment is a key part of SBLEs just as they are with any quality learning activity. Chapter 6 offers in-depth information on best practices in assessment and evaluation in SBLEs. This section will focus on the ways that simulation-based clinical education can be incorporated into clinical education programs. It will specifically address the use of SBLEs for various forms of formative and summative assessment. Those applications include the use of simulation for learner assessment, remediation, and competency-based assessment. It will include information on Objective Structured Clinical Examinations (OSCEs) as they may apply to CSD.

Clinical education often employs both formative and summative assessment. Anson (2015) explains that assessment can be formative (i.e., assessing learning throughout the teaching processes) or summative (i.e., assessing learning at the completion of a class/course/program). Formative assessment can occur in various ways in SBLEs, such as by providing immediate feedback during or after a simulation in a debrief, coaching, facilitating reflection, or providing supplemental activities for further development. The feedback can be completed in real time, synchronously, or after the activity, asynchronously. It may occur in-person or virtually. Feedback may take many forms including verbal reports, checklists, rubrics, and/or written narrative (e.g., self-reflection). Formative assessment is not just the job of the clinical educator. The Association for Standardized Patient Educators (ASPE) Standards of Best Practices suggest that SPs participate in the formative assessment of learners (Lewis et al., 2017). ASPE provides a framework for SPs to be trained in assessment and feedback. Refer to ASPE Standards of Best Practices Principal 3.3 Training for Feedback for additional details (Lewis et al., 2017).

In contrast to formative assessment, summative assessment is, as the name implies, an assessment of the sum of learning. Summative assessments are high-stakes assessments in that they include a level of evaluation and comparison of performance to a standard or benchmark. Summative assessment allows for the learner to demonstrate the skills in the knowing and showing aspects of learning (Anderson & Krathwohl, 2001, Krathwohl, 2002, Miller, 1990). In a summative assessment, the learner is expected to pull together all the pieces of the training and demonstrate a level of competence regarding predetermined criteria or objectives. This allows for a determination of competence regarding a predetermined set of skills.

Summative assessments can take many forms, such as final exams, state or national boards, or pass/fail frameworks or OSCE. The disciplines of audiology and speech-language pathology are familiar with the concept of a comprehensive assessment. That is, graduate students are required to demonstrate a specified level of performance for specific KSAs to meet requirements for the degree. These high-stake summative assessments sometimes take the form of comprehensive written and oral examinations, portfolios, and/or capstone projects. Given the high-stakes nature, the reliability and validity of the assessment tools must be established prior to the use of the tools. Similar to formative assessments, well-trained SPs can play a key role in summative assessment by providing summative feedback on a learner's demonstration of KSAs directly related to the learning objectives.

Competency-Based Assessment

Simulation-based education has specific application within the realm of competency-based assessment and student remediation. There is an emerging interest in the use of simulation as it applies to learner assessment—specifically as a measure of professional competency. It is important to have a shared understanding of the KSAs that contribute to the discussion of competency.

Each of these constructs are discussed in-depth in Chapter 2. Knowledge (K) is the act of knowing and may include cognitive aspects such as memory, abstraction, critical thinking, and application of learned facts. It is important to recognize the distinction between perceived and real knowledge. Perceived knowledge is what an individual believes they know, while real knowledge is the factual objective measure of concepts and constructs. Simulation allows an opportunity for individuals to bridge any gaps between real vs. perceived knowledge and gain additional insights for growth and learning (Baker-Rush, 2016). Skills (S) are the application of knowledge and the demonstration of how the knowledge applies in each situation (Miller, 1990). Attributes (A) refers to the desirable professional characteristics of the learners, including attitudes, learning styles, and beliefs and values. Attributes are sometimes considered as those characteristics that allow someone to be competent in a variety of settings.

It is necessary to consider various tools to measure the identified KSAs. For example, in order to assess knowledge, learners may be asked to demonstrate understanding and identification through a written exam on specific constructs or on a task trainer or anatomical model (e.g., anatomy and anatomical structure). Skills may be assessed by having the learner utilize the anatomical constructs and apply them in a task (e.g., construct a model of a cranial nerve using household items). In this example, the learner uses the foundational elements learned in anatomy to apply in the psychomotor construction of the nerve. This includes identifying the materials, spatial orientation, relationship among constructs, and so on to build a model. The skill requires a higher order of cognition, critical thinking, recall, organization, and application. Therefore, as we discuss competency assessments moving forward, it is imperative to discern the difference between knowledge (real or perceived) and skills. Attributes are more often assessed as part of more advanced SBLEs, such as interprofessional practice.

Competency includes a range of knowledge and behaviors that, collectively, when applied, indicate a level of function commensurate with expected ability to perform professional services across a variety of professional settings. (McAllister, 2006; McGaghie et al., 1978). Within health care professions, one can extend certain professional competencies to include the acceptance and application of a professional role of valuing human life, public health improvement, prevention of illness, as well as the demonstration of leadership in health education and provision of care (McGaghie et al., 1978). That is, competency goes beyond an extensive checklist of demonstrated behaviors. A broader definition of competency recognizes a learner's development of expertise with different client populations, professional settings, and service delivery models. (Harris et al., 1995; Heywood et al., 1992). The reader is referred to Chapter 2 for a full discussion of professional and occupational competency.

Objective Structured Clinical Examination

The most common type of competency-based clinical assessment employed in medicine and nursing education is the OSCE. The OSCE was described in 1979 by Harden and Gleason as a series of timed examinations using simulated patients in stations to assess skills such as history taking and/or conducting a physical exam. Since that time, the description of the OSCE has been expanded to "a versatile multipurpose evaluative tool that can be utilized to evaluate health care professionals in a clinical setting. It assesses competency, based on objective testing through direct observation" (Zayyan, 2011, p. 219). Typically, multiple domains of competency can be assessed, including history taking, physical examination, medical knowledge, interpersonal skills, communication skills, professionalism, data gathering/information collection, evidence-based decision making, patient-centered care, health promotion, and disease prevention (Homer et al., 2020; Zayyan, 2011).

Currently, most OSCEs are conducted using SPs, but given the rapid emergence of computer-based and virtual technologies, this is likely to change. Kachur and colleagues (2013) present a useful 10-step approach to organizing SPs and OSCEs (Figure 3-1). These steps allow the clinical educator to transform what may seem like a major undertaking in creating an OSCE into a manageable process using available resources in an efficient and effective manner. As Kachur and colleagues (2013) point out, much of what is required for a successful OSCE is independent of specialty or profession.

OSCEs employing SPs have been used with both undergraduate and graduate students in CSD. Zraick et al. (2003) were the first to report the use of an OSCE with students in speech-language pathology. Beginning graduate students interacted with SPs portraying a diagnosis of aphasia while enrolled in a class on the diagnosis and management of aphasia. Quigley and Regan (2020) evaluated undergraduate speech-language pathology students' perceptions of the OSCE and whether perceptions differed depending on stage of undergraduate education. In these studies, students reported that OSCE was a fair and meaningful assessment approach (Quigley & Regan, 2020) and should be incorporated into their future clinical coursework (Zraick et al., 2003).

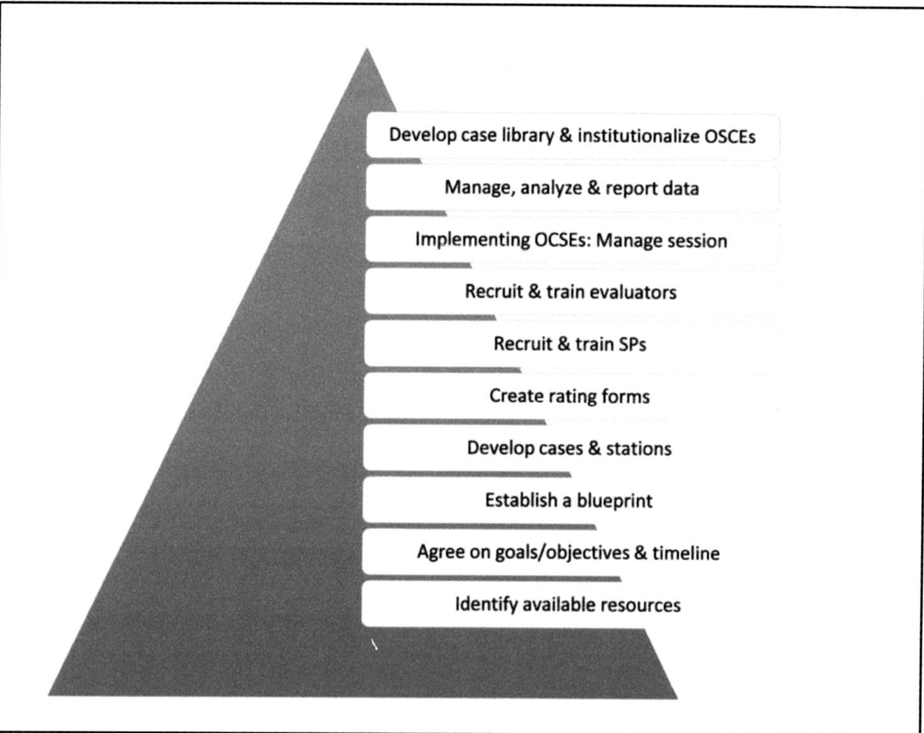

Figure 3-1. Ten-step approach to OSCEs. (Data source: Kachur, E. K., Zabar, S., Hanley, K., Kaler, A., Bruno, J. H., & Gillespie, C.C. [2013]. Organizing OSCEs [and other SP exercises] in 10 steps. In S. Zabar, E. K. Kachur, A. Kalet, & K. Hanley [Eds.], *Objective Structured Clinical Examinations* [pp. 7-35]. Springer.)

Simulation for Student Remediation

As educators, we are aware of the times when learners fail to meet the expected competencies and require additional practice in the form of remediation. Simulation offers the opportunity to structure a learning experience specific to the gaps in KSAs. For example, consider a graduate student in audiology who has not demonstrated the required level of competency in assessing vestibular disorders. As part of the remediation plan, the learner is required to first independently and repeatedly practice the vestibular evoked myogenic potential test using a virtual simulator. This allows for repeated practice in a safe and controlled environment, without risk of harm to patients. Once the learner is confident administrating the procedure, they are again assessed to demonstrate competency in this skill. The experienced clinical educator may well imagine other uses for simulations within the remediation process.

Simulation for Interprofessional Education and Collaborative Practice

Today's management of complex and challenging health care problems is highly dependent on ICP (Barr, 2002; D'Amour & Oandasan, 2005; Gilbert et al., 2010). Studies indicate that ICP improves health care outcomes and patient/provider satisfaction, as well as promotes more effective use of resources (Hammick et al., 2007; Reeves et al., 2012; World Health Organization, 2010). This awareness has led health professions to integrate IPE into the curricula. IPE is defined as "students from two or more professions learning about, from and with each other to enable effective collaboration and improve health outcomes" (World Health Organization, 2010, p. 10). Several studies have shown that students report increased confidence, improved communication skills, improved attitudes toward team care, positive attitudes regarding interprofessional learning, and a deeper understanding of other professions' roles and responsibilities after participating in interprofessional learning experiences (Arenson et al., 2015; Griffin et al., 2016; Nichols et al., 2019; Ruebling et al., 2014; Thomas et al., 2017). Under an IPE framework, students are deliberately exposed to interactive learning opportunities with those outside their professions and learn to collaborate with other professionals to improve education and service provision outcomes.

Over the past decade, IPE and ICP have become required components in many health care professions' accreditation standards, including audiology and speech-language pathology. IPE and ICP are now considered to be critical components in preparing health care professions students to provide safe, high-quality, patient-centered care (Wise et al., 2015). Some of the barriers to IPE are lack of training in conflict resolution (Sexton & Orchard, 2016), hierarchical limitations of teamwork (Dariel & Cristofalo, 2018), or fear of working with teams (Baker-Rush et al., 2021).

SBLEs offer a unique and effective opportunity for integrating IPE/ICP into CSD curricula. This is sometimes referred to as *simulation-enhanced interprofessional education*. Simulation-enhanced interprofessional education offers a method of overcoming these barriers in a safe environment. It also allows for learners to experience the continuum between IPE and ICP. Several researchers have published examples and frameworks integrating IPE and simulation experiences into graduate speech-language pathology training (Hill et al., 2020; Weir-Mayta et al., 2020). Low-stakes and low-fidelity simulation early in health care training may allow for understanding of interprofessional roles and responsibilities, developing confidence and communication skills, and practicing teamwork among professions (Baker-Rush et al., 2021; Mazur & Baker-Rush, 2020). Interestingly, the use of more complex simulation with higher fidelity, prior to establishing foundational knowledge, facilitates interprofessional socialization but does not consistently lead to competency in teamwork (Lockeman et al., 2017). This example further highlights that simulation technologies are a tool and are best used when aligned with learner needs and objectives.

The use of simulation for ICP is another area for consideration. As with IPE initiatives in university programs, training in the workplace faces factors that may promote or limit the opportunity for ICP through simulation. Some of challenges include employer resources (time, money, staff), work culture and environment, return on investment, and the ability to allow staff to step away from patient care to participate in ICP simulation. These challenges provide a unique opportunity for universities and work settings to partner in the provision of IPE/ICP proving that necessity is indeed the mother of invention. For example, practicing nurses who need to demonstrate annual competency on dysphagia screening as part of an annual review process may elect to participate in a simulation for graduate speech-language pathology students being offered at the university. Additional collaborators can be added to this scenario, including pharmacy students. This type of collaboration in IPE/ICP provides all stakeholders (e.g., students, nurses, university, hospital) the opportunity to share resources and overcome some of the barriers described earlier. The opportunity to learn from, with, and about the variety of health care providers—from early learners in low-stakes, low-fidelity simulations to practitioners in high-stakes, high-fidelity simulations—may result in mitigating barriers to ICP when new graduates enter the workforce.

Integrating Simulation Into the Curriculum

In order to be successful, simulation must be implemented across the curriculum, and not simply thought of as an additional assignment. In this section, we will provide some examples of how simulation-based education can be applied within coursework, clinic settings, and a simulation lab (Table 3-2).

Regardless of the physical setting, the considerations remain the same:

- What are the learning objectives?
- How will you know if they achieve the objectives?
- What resources are needed (financial, personnel, time)?
- How was psychological safety ensured?

Simulation in Academic Coursework

Simulation-based education is not the sole domain of one individual or setting. Quality SBLEs can be developed by academics and clinical educators. In fact, the more educators engaged in simulation-based learning the better it is integrated within the curriculum. Educators are encouraged to consider ways to integrate SBLEs into courses as a way of meeting learning objectives. The SBLE can serve a variety of purposes including as a method of instruction (e.g., how to conduct a standardized assessment of a 2-year-old) or assessment tool (e.g., an OSCE demonstrating competency). One group of educators has developed a series of four course-based SBLEs that span the medical speech-language pathology curriculum (Stead et al., 2020). Cases range from mild, moderate, or severe traumatic brain injury, dementia, and Parkinson's disease. Equipment includes full-size manikins, SPs, realistic baby dolls, walkers, feeding utensils, and worksheets. The SBLEs were nongraded in order to reduce anxiety about performance and allow learners to focus on skill development. Learners engaged in repeated practice in which they received formative feedback from experienced educators. This allowed them to develop confidence before a high-stakes summative assessment (e.g., OSCE). Learners who failed to demonstrate clinical competency in the summative assessment were offered remediation until they demonstrated the skill.

TABLE 3-2

Application of Simulation Throughout the Curriculum

SIMULATION MODALITY	GENERALLY DEFINED	LEVEL OF LEARNER	ENGAGEMENT	INTERPROFESSIONAL OPPORTUNITY
Paper case	A written patient health record focal to deciphering, interpreting, navigating, reading, and comprehension	Novice to mid-level learner	Student group learning, faculty-led discussion, independent student self-directed learning	High
Patient management problems or patient-oriented problem solving	A written patient health record focal to a specific skill or task to be addressed or completed; apply basic knowledge to clinical problems and collectively find information necessary to solve problems using sources	Novice to mid-level learner	Student group learning, faculty-led discussion, independent student self-directed learning	High; intended for group-based learning and use of resources
Task trainer	A section or portion of a manikin that simulates a process, system, or anatomical section	Novice to expert	Student group learning, faculty-led discussion, independent student self-directed learning, invasive procedural training	Mid; only a few individuals can be hands on around a task trainer (based on size of task trainer)
Manikin	A lifelike, life-size replica of a being in which procedural skills can be completed (can be high or low fidelity)	Novice to expert	Student group learning, faculty-led discussion, independent student self-directed learning, invasive procedural training	Mid to high
Virtual reality	A four-dimensional experience through the use of combined computer-generated imagery and multisensory components that offer an immersive simulated experience	Novice to expert	Independent student self-directed learning, faculty-directed learning	Low to mid; only one individual may wear the VR system at a time, possibility of more than one learner as the software interface allows
Standardized patient	A professionally trained person who portrays a patient with a health condition or situation	Novice to expert	Student group learning, faculty-led discussion, independent student self-directed learning	Low to high
Hybrid	A combination of two or more simulation modalities (e.g., SP and wearable task trainer)	Novice to expert	Student group learning, faculty-led discussion	Low to high
Computer-based simulation	Computer software created to replicate a real-world process or event	Novice to expert	Student group learning, faculty-led discussion, independent student self-directed learning	Low to mid; based on interactivity capabilities of software

(continued)

TABLE 3-2 (continued)

Application of Simulation Throughout the Curriculum

SIMULATION MODALITY	GENERALLY DEFINED	LEVEL OF LEARNER	ENGAGEMENT	INTERPROFESSIONAL OPPORTUNITY
Game-based simulation	A game in which the focus is to train rather than entertain	Novice to expert	Student group learning, faculty-led discussion	High
Surgical simulator	Can be virtual, hybrid, or realistic and may include a variety or combination of other modalities; can be task/procedural based or scenario based	Mid-level to expert	Faculty-led discussion, independent student self-directed learning Allows deliberate practice of technical procedures	Low to mid
Computer-assisted instruction	A combination of computer or web delivery with an interactive component	Novice to expert	Independent student self-directed learning	Low to mid; based on interactivity capabilities of software
Audio simulation	Sound files of respective health conditions presented in an audio format; can be in isolation or in conjunction with other modalities	Novice to expert	Student group learning, faculty-led discussion, independent student self-directed learning	Low to mid; based on interactivity capabilities of software

Commercially available simulations in CSD, such as Simucase, are attractive to programs invested in the training of future CSD professionals. Simucase is a web-based platform that includes interactive simulations and patient/client videos across multiple settings. "The user can complete observations, screenings and assessments, and provide intervention while interacting with virtual clients, family members, and professionals" (Ondo et al., 2020, p. 5). These simulations offer predefined content, repeated practice, and assessment data that can be used by educators and learners. They save educators time and offer a comparable experience across learners. What these commercially available simulations do not do in themselves is satisfy the necessary components of an SBLE. That is, while these and other types of computer-based simulations have value as a stand-alone course assignment, without a prebrief, feedback, and debrief, these experiences are not to be considered simulation. In order to gain the full benefit of simulation-based education, the educator should follow best practices in simulation-based learning as discussed in the literature and throughout this book.

It is the responsibility of the educator to ensure that the simulation aligns with learning objectives for the course. The educator may choose to begin the process of the simulation design by conducting an analysis to identify the needs of the learners. The next step is the development of learning objectives that include the related KSAs. The learning objectives are intended to move the learners from lower-order thinking skills to higher-order thinking skills as identified by Bloom and Krathwohl (1956). In addition, learning objectives aim to advance cognitive skills along the continuum from factual to conceptual to procedural to metacognitive knowledge (Miller, 1990; Figure 3-2). From this very critical step of developing the learning objectives, all things follow (e.g., development of assessment plan and creating the scenario, select technologies, planning of the prebrief and debrief). (Refer to Chapter 5 for more detail.) Whether the educator continues with the development of the simulation, employs an already developed simulation, or collaborates with an experienced simulation educator to design a simulation, they should be prepared to actively participate in all phases of development and implementation—prebrief, simulation, and debrief—to ensure that the learning objectives are being addressed.

As part of implementation of an SBLE within a course, the educator is reminded to include time for the prebrief and debrief. This is especially important given that the debriefing allows the learner to reflect on their performance, including, but not limited to, psychomotor skills and communication through guided discussion targeting the objectives. The educator can either lead the debriefing process or collaborate with a skilled facilitator until they feel confident in facilitating.

Throughout every step of this process, it is paramount to provide the learners with psychological safety within a safe learning environment. Psychological safety is defined as "a feeling (explicit or implicit) within a simulation-based activity that participants are comfortable participating, speaking up, sharing thoughts, and asking for help as needed without concern for retribution or embarrassment" (Lioce et al., 2020, p. S38). Simulation governing bodies and

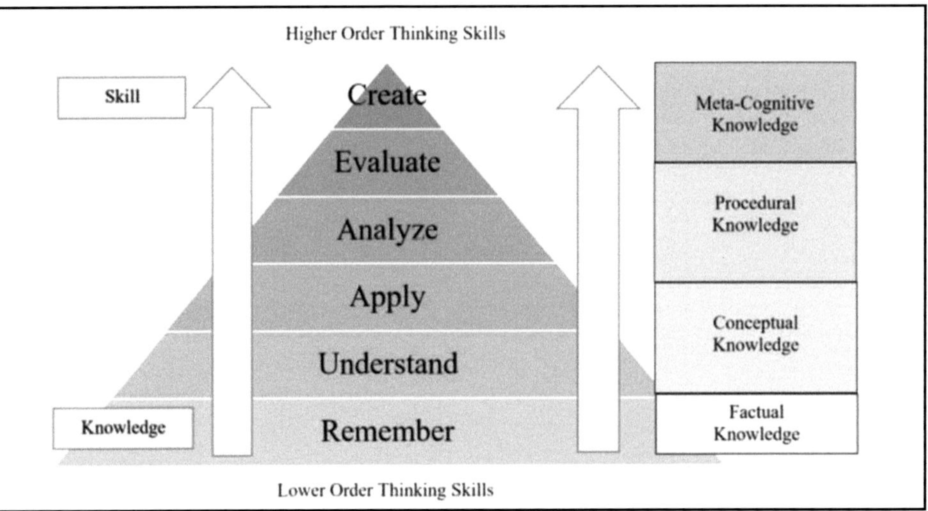

Figure 3-2. Level of learner and cognitive processes. (Image based on the combined works of Krathwohl, D. R., & Anderson, L. W. [Eds.]. [2001]. *A taxonomy for learning, teaching, and assessing: A revision of Bloom's taxonomy of educational objectives.* Allyn & Bacon; Bloom, B. S., & Krathwohl, D. R. [1956]. *Taxonomy of educational objectives: The classification of educational goals, Handbook I: Cognitive domain.* Longmans, Green; Krathwohl, D. [2002]. A revision of Bloom's taxonomy: An overview. *Theory into Practice, 41*[4], 212-218. https://doi.org/10.1207/s15430421tip4104_2; and Miller, G. [1990]. The assessment of clinical skills/competence/performance. *Academic Medicine, 65*[9], S63-S67.)

simulation science report psychological safety as a key tenant (International Nursing Association for Clinical Simulation and Learning [INACSL], 2016c; Society for Simulation in Healthcare [SSH], 2016) and must be considered for learners and all participants involved in the simulation activity. Refer to the Resources for Implementation section of this chapter for in-depth example of how to employ simulation as part of coursework.

Simulations in the University Clinic

Many university programs in CSD house a clinic to serve members of the community. Within these clinics, both graduate and undergraduate students have the opportunity to learn, practice skills, and bolster foundational practice behaviors, including interprofessional competencies, under the direct supervision of a certified and/or licensed professional. There has been an emergence of simulation-based education occurring in these university clinics.

The physical set-up of the clinics (e.g., audiological equipment, treatment rooms, observation monitors) makes them an authentic and realistic space in which to conduct simulations. As is the case for course-based simulation, clinical educators have the option of designing simulations independently/in collaboration with someone experienced in simulation design, or selecting an existing simulation for implementation. Several forms of simulation can be readily integrated into university clinic settings, including the use of task trainers, SPs, computer-based simulations, and VR experiences. Refer to the Resources for Implementation section of this chapter for an example of the use of simulation in the university clinic setting.

Simulations in the Simulation Lab

The simulation lab, or simulation environment, has multiple definitions (Lioce et al., 2020). For clarity and purposes of this discussion, the simulation lab will be defined as a designated space in which simulations may occur. This space may consist of various equipment covering an array of modalities that represents real-world spaces, such as a hospital or a clinic. Within this dedicated simulation lab, it is common to have one-way mirrors, observation booths, and cameras or other observational options. In addition to the physical considerations, a simulation lab provides a supportive atmosphere that is free of humiliation or retributive action.

Perhaps your program does not have access to a simulation lab or high-tech simulation tools and equipment. It is important to explore the resources that may be available to you. Perhaps there is a simulation lab housed in the medical or nursing school at your university or a nearby university that is willing to share resources for a modest fee. A good first step in exploring such a partnership is to ask to observe an upcoming simulation, even if it does not relate to CSD. People like to share what they are passionate about, and those engaged in simulation-based education are passionate about simulation. You may discover that the local hospital houses a simulation lab for their employees. Again, ask to observe and begin to build those networks. The potential benefits go both ways. A partnership between a university program and a local hospital may assist the hospital by way of sharing of expenses and by offering university personnel to assist in the design and implementation of the simulation. It also provides all parties with the opportunity for IPE and ICP. For example, a new graduate speech-language pathology program at a particular university may decide to work collaboratively with a medical college at another university. By working collaboratively, it results in diversifying professions across both universities and creates opportunity for interprofessional simulation that did not previously exist in either university. This would support IPE and ICP practice initiatives at both institutions.

Just as there are best practices and standards for training programs in CSD, there exist practices and standards for simulation labs. The SSH was established in January 2004 to represent educators, researchers, and advocates who utilize simulation methodologies for education, testing, and research in health care. As part of their mission, SSH offers the development of best practice and accreditation standards. Simulation programs and labs accredited through SSH must demonstrate the following seven core standards of practice (SSH, 2016):

1. Mission and governance
2. Program management
3. Resource management
4. Human resources
5. Program improvement
6. Ethics
7. Expanding the field

Readers interested in either establishing a simulation lab or partnering with an existing lab would be well served to be familiar with the standards of best practice for a simulation lab and/or utilize organizations such as SSH to identify simulation labs in your area.

This section provided some considerations and examples of how simulation-based education can be integrated within coursework, clinic, and simulation lab environments. By having knowledge of best practices in simulation, the educator can adjust these examples to meet the needs of their learners—as undergraduate, graduate, or practicing professionals—in a way that utilizes the resources available to the program. The reader is directed to the Resources for Implementation section at the end of this chapter for additional examples and resources.

Impact of a Pandemic on Simulation in Health Care

At the time of this writing, the world continues to be experiencing the COVID-19 (coronavirus disease 2019) pandemic. Maintaining standards in health professions education, keeping clinical learning on track, and minimizing the assessment disruption are unprecedented challenges under pandemic conditions. A key challenge for health profession educators is to simulate clinical encounters during a time with limited access to traditional clinical placements as well as continuing to train learners in the necessary critical thinking skills. The current crisis is stressing the necessity for online learning opportunities and virtual education that allow a learner to be an active participant in the learning regardless of location of the teaching (Nes et al., 2020).

During a time of a pandemic where in-person experiential learning is limited or nonexistent, educators must be mindful, creative, innovative, adaptive, and forward thinking to morph and implement pedagogical teaching designs that continue to build and train critical thinking (Nes et al., 2020). For example, a multimodal approach using videoconferencing (e.g., broadcasting, telecoaching, telesimulation, didactic lecture series) offers a unique and beneficial way to replace the hands-on in-person training that medical surgical residents were lacking (Madani et al., 2021). This creative and multimodal approach provides a new pedagogical teaching design that was not previously used in student training (Madani et al., 2021). This approach aids in critical decision making, application of skills, and assessment of performance (Madani et al., 2021). While it does not allow for the social interaction that in-person training provides, the key aspects of training elements were addressed; however, it is important to note that the social engagement and mentor relationship continue to be a limitation of this approach.

It is projected that the challenges to educators in health care will continue beyond the pandemic and will have a lasting impact on the manner in which we provide clinical education, specifically in the use of simulation. Therefore, educators in CSD will be called upon to utilize creativity, innovation, adaptation, and forward thinking in implementing simulation using strong pedagogical teaching designs that will continue to address learner needs, such as critical thinking, acquisition of knowledge and the application of skills, and authentic assessment. This is a perfect opportunity to develop a set of knowledge and skills to implement high-quality simulation in CSD programs, both in-person and across virtual and remote platforms.

BOX 3-4

INACSL and SSH Joint Position Statement on Use of Virtual Simulation During the Pandemic

In response to the global crisis and in support of the programs struggling to meet the needs of learners, the International Nursing Association of Clinical Simulation and Learning and the Society for Simulation in Healthcare issued a joint statement on the use of virtual simulation during the pandemic (2020).

March 30, 2020

Synopsis

The International Nursing Association of Clinical Simulation and Learning (www.inacsl.org) and the Society for Simulation in Healthcare (www.ssih.org) support the use of virtual simulation as a replacement for clinical hours for students currently enrolled in health sciences professions (i.e., nursing students, medical students) during the current public health crisis caused by COVID-19.

The Problem

The COVID-19 pandemic is currently affecting over 80 countries and has spread throughout every state in the United States. With the pandemic expected to surge in waves and last for months, it is critical that the pipeline of educating healthcare professionals remains intact. Universities across the world have transitioned to continuing education through online or virtual means. In the context of health professions education, many regulatory bodies (such as state boards of nursing) require completion of a set number of hours within the clinical setting.

The Resolution

The professional organizations of INACSL and SSH encompass the world's leading experts in simulation-based education for healthcare providers. We can attest that virtual simulation has been used for over a decade successfully. Further, research has repeatedly demonstrated that use of virtual simulation—simulated healthcare experiences on one's computer—is an effective teaching method that results in improved student learning outcomes. Based on the current and anticipated shortage of healthcare workers, we propose that regulatory bodies and policymakers demonstrate flexibility by allowing the replacement of clinical hours usually completed in a healthcare setting with that of virtually simulated experiences during the pandemic. By supporting this innovative yet effective way of teaching as a solution to address the clinical hour shortage of health professions students, education efforts will continue seamlessly, and we will support timely career progression of healthcare providers needed immediately to battle COVID-19.

Dr. Cynthia Foronda, President, INACSL

Bob Armstrong, President, SSH

Reproduced from International Nursing Association of Clinical Simulation and Learning and Society for Simulation in Healthcare. (2020). COVID-19: *SSH/INACSL position statement on use of virtual simulation during the pandemic.* Society for Simulation in Healthcare. https://www.ssih.org/COVID-19-Updates/ID/2237/COVID-19-SSHINACSL-Position-Statement-on-Use-of-Virtual-Simulation-during-the-Pandemic

Summary

Simulation-based education is a science with methods and best practices supported by learning theory and best practice standards. In this chapter, the authors have provided a brief overview of best practices in simulation. The potential applications of simulation in CSD were considered (e.g., clinical clock hours, guided observation, remediation, competency assessment). Considerations and examples were provided for integrating simulation into the curriculum, and opportunities for IPE and practice.

It is our hope that as you continue learning about and developing simulation in your setting, you will continue to reflect on your growth as a clinical educator. Simulation is not adding to your workload, but rather it is morphing your learning environment into a new and exciting way to teach using scientific principles and educational theory. Not only will you find that the learners will grow in their professional skills, you will, too.

Resources for Implementation

This section includes examples and resources to add to your toolbox of simulation resources and guides. Through these resources, as well as the framework provided within this chapter, we hope that you continue learning and growing in simulation science.

Knowledge Check Simulations

1. What is the purpose of the simulation (e.g., clinical hours, assessment of competency, acquisition of KSAs, remediation, IPE/ICP, student remediation)?
2. What are the learning objectives (i.e., psychomotor, cognitive affective)?
3. What is the method of assessment (i.e., formative or summative assessment)? How do you know?
4. What are the possible settings for this scenario (i.e., coursework, clinic, or simulation lab)?

Coursework Implementation Example

Coursework Scenario

An instructor might employ an SP to demonstrate how to conduct a cognitive screening as part of the classroom experience. The instructor conducts the screening while an SP responds as someone with a communication impairment. The students take note of the instructor's and SP's behaviors. Students might then take turns interacting with the SP, either individually or in small groups. The SP, instructor, and students participate in a debriefing session.

Questions for the Educator

1. What are the learning objectives?
2. How will you know if they achieve the objectives?
3. What resources are needed?
4. How was psychological safety ensured?

Possible Responses

1. Learning objectives
   a. Demonstrate use of a screening measure.
   b. Practice observational skills.
   c. Practice professional communication.
2. Assessment tools (formative): A short checklist focal to the screening tool completed by the faculty member, and a short checklist focal to communication completed by the SP.
3. Resources (SPs): The screening instrument needed to be provided to students in advance. The SPs require training of the case and checklist, case development, and faculty training for checklist and debriefing.
4. Psychological safety: Orientation and expectation of simulation activity and post-encounter debriefing.

Clinic Implementation Example

Clinic Scenario

An SP may portray a parent for history taking and information sharing in a case involving a child with a hearing loss. The students would be provided the results of an audiological exam and child intake form collected by the clinic administrator. The SP would meet with students one-on-one in a clinic room. The students are to collect medical and communication history, review the audiological test results with parent, and provide a verbal summary of results and a plan for follow-up. Faculty will observe and complete a checklist.

Questions

1. What are the learning objectives?
2. How will you know if they achieve the objectives?
3. What resources are needed?
4. How was psychological safety ensured?

Possible Responses

1. Learning objectives
   a. Collect medical and communication history
   b. Explain the audiological test results to the parent
   c. Prepare and produce a verbal summary of results
   d. Formulate a plan for follow-up
2. Assessment (formative): Checklist completed by the faculty member, and a checklist completed by the SP
3. Resources (SPs): Case development, SP training for case and checklist, faculty training for checklist, and development of audiological exam and report findings, cleaning materials, cleaning time, and staff
4. Psychological safety: Orientation and expectation of simulation activity, one-on-one encounters with SP with individual faculty observation; SPs provide immediate feedback on soft skills

Simulation Lab Example

Simulation Lab Scenario

Students are provided information regarding medical equipment typically found in an inpatient hospital space as part of class lecture. Students then report to the simulation lab space equipped as an inpatient hospital room dressed in appropriate health care attire (e.g., lab coat, scrubs). Students are asked to identify and discuss the purpose and function of the medical equipment within the inpatient hospital room. The accompanying faculty leads a hands-on simulation engagement with a stop-start debrief approach. The faculty conducts a comprehensive debrief at the conclusion of the simulation.

Note: This example is an opportunity for IPE. Consider combining two or more professions within the class lecture and during the simulation experience. The debrief would ideally occur with all groups present, but it can occur in professional groups.

Questions

1. What are the learning objectives?
2. How will you know if they achieve the objectives?
3. What resources are needed?
4. How was psychological safety ensured?

Possible Responses

1. Learning Objectives:
   a. Identify medical equipment within an inpatient hospital room
   b. Discuss the purpose of such medical equipment
   c. Discuss function of the medical equipment
2. Assessment: Formative assessment during debrief
3. Resources: Orientation and expectation of simulation activity, various medical equipment, simulation tech support, tech for equipment set-up and tear down, students' attire, cleaning materials, cleaning time, and staff
4. Psychological safety: Ensured by orientation and expectation of simulation activity, facilitated by faculty, small groups

Not All Simulations Are Created Equal

The authors wish to note that not all simulations are created equal and that the use of simulation for obtaining clinical clock hours comes with some considerations. Within the INACSL best practices documents and current literature in nursing, it is noted that a combined approach to high-fidelity simulations and conventional clinical experiences resulted in a higher level of learning, knowledge, and skills (Curl et al., 2016; Haerling, & Prion, 2020; Hayden et al., 2014; INACSL, 2016). Furthermore, it is important to highlight several factors that may impact the learner's ability to translate and apply clinical knowledge and skills into the real clinical environment (e.g., type and volume of simulation, environment, stress, team members, acuity). Thus, it is critical to consider when simulation will and will not suffice when teaching, applying, advancing, or translating clinical skills. Again, guiding documents such as *Best Practices in Clinical Simulation in Speech-Language Pathology and Audiology* (Dudding et al., 2019), the INACSL Standards of Best Practices (INACSL, 2016a-e), *Articles of Influence* (SSH, 2020) and the ASPE Standards of Best Practice (Lewis et al., 2017) offer a guide to decision making and best practices. Furthermore, needs assessments and curricular gaps and needs will help facilitate decisions toward the use and frequency of simulation to aid in clinical clock hours. Refer to Figure 3-3 for a schematic representation of decision points in designing and evaluating simulations.

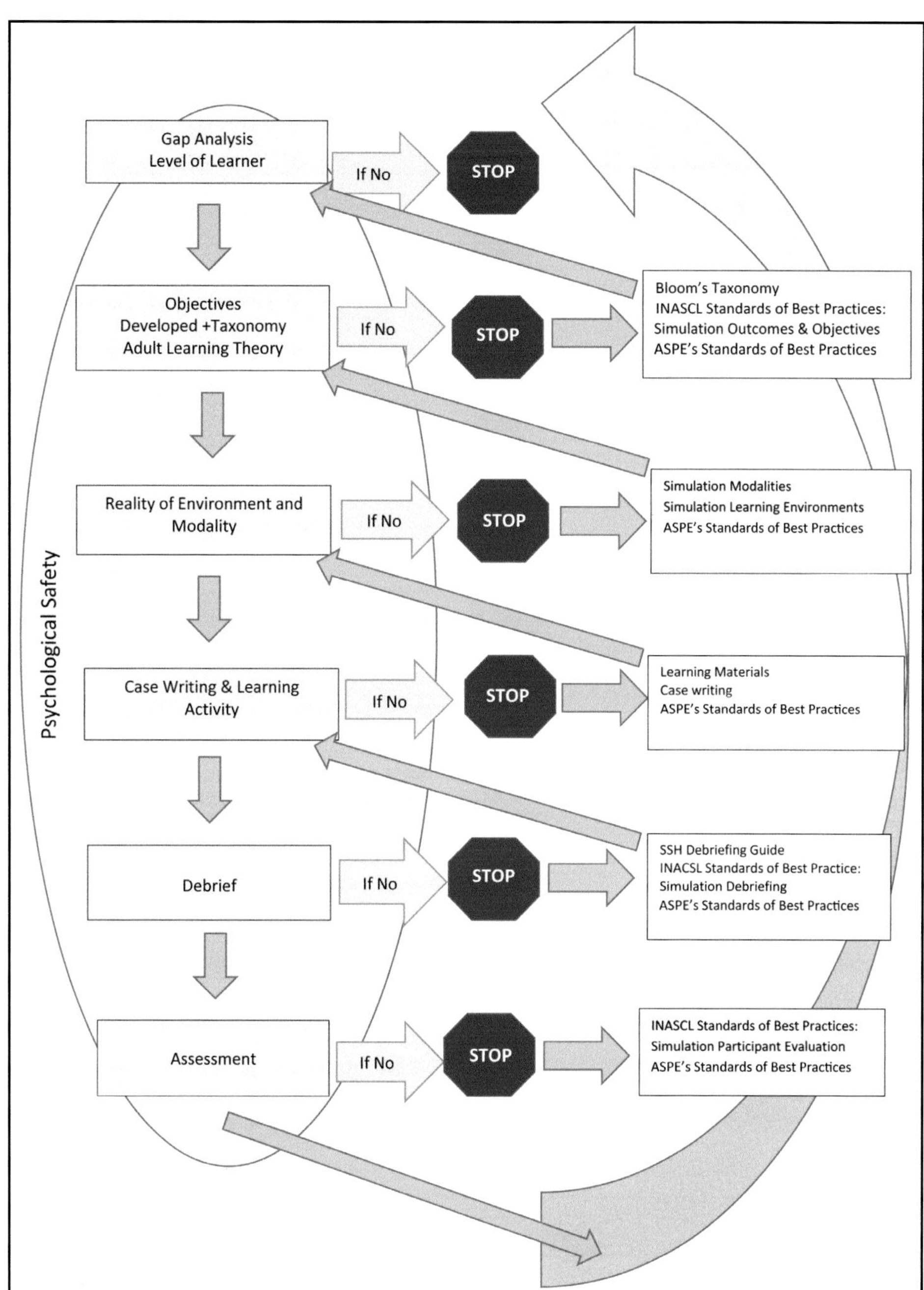

Figure 3-3. Simulation design best practices flow chart.

References

Accreditation Commission for Audiology Education. (2016, March). *Accreditation standards for the doctor of audiology (Au.D.) Program.* https://www.acaeaccred.org/wp-content/uploads/sites/1543/2016/07/ACAE-Standards-5.11NEW-WEB-2.pdf

American Academy of Audiology. (2020). *Academy supports audiology students.* https://www.audiology.org/academy-supports-audiology-students/

American Speech-Language-Hearing Association. (2021). *Certification standards for audiology: Clinical simulation.* https://www.asha.org/Certification/Certification-Standards-for-Aud-Clinical-Simulation/

Anderson, L. W., Krathwohl, D. R., Airasian, P. W., Cruikshank, K.A., Mayer, R. E., Pintrich, P. R., Raths, J. D., & Wittrock, M. C. (Eds.). (2001). *A taxonomy for learning, teaching, and assessing: A revision of Bloom's taxonomy of educational objectives.* Allyn & Bacon.

Anson, W. (2015). Assessment in healthcare simulation. In J. C. Palaganas, J. C. Maxworthy, C. A. Epps, & M. E. Mancini (Eds.), *Defining excellence in simulation programs* (pp. 509-543). Wolters Kluwer.

Arenson, C., Umland, E., Collins, L., Kerns, S. B., Hewston, L. A., Jerpbak, C., Antony, R., Rose, M., & Lyons, K. (2015). The health mentors program: Three years' experience with longitudinal, patient-centered interprofessional education. *Journal of Interprofessional Care, 29*(2), 138-143. https://doi.org/10.3109/13561820.2014.944257

Baker-Rush, M. (2016). *Self-efficacy, perceived skills, and real knowledge of Speech Language Pathologists.* (Publication No.10247267) [Doctoral dissertation, Walden University]. ProQuest Dissertations and Theses Global.

Baker-Rush, M., Mazur, Z., & Friedman, L. (2020, September). *Interprofessional experiential educational programming: PA and DPT students self-reports of growth.* NEXUS Summit 2020 Virtual Conference.

Baker-Rush, M., Pabst, A., Aitchison, R., Anzur, T., & Paschal, N. (2021). Fear in interprofessional simulation: The role of psychology and behaviorism in student participation and learning. *Journal of Interprofessional Education and Practice, 24*, 100432. https://doi.org/10.1016/j.xjep.2021.100432

Barr, H. (2002). *Interprofessional education today, yesterday and tomorrow: A review.* LTSN HS&P.

Bloom, B. S., & Krathwohl, D. R. (1956). *Taxonomy of educational objectives: The classification of educational goals, by a committee of college and university examiners. Handbook I: Cognitive domain.* Longmans, Green.

Council for Clinical Certification in Audiology and Speech-Language Pathology. (2014). Standards for the certificate of clinical competence in speech-language pathology. American Speech-Language-Hearing Association. http://www.asha.org/Certification/2014-Speech-Language-Pathology-Certification-Standards/

Curl, E., Smith, S., Chisholm, L., McGee, L., & Das, K. (2016). Effectiveness of integrated simulation and clinical experiences compared to traditional clinical experiences for nursing students. *Nursing Education Perspectives, 37*(2), 72-77. https://doi.org/10.5480/15-1647

D'Amour, D., & Oandasan, I. (2005). Interprofessionality as the field of interprofessional practice and interprofessional education: An emerging concept. *Journal of Interprofessional Care, 19*(Suppl. 1), 8-20.

Dariel, O., & Cristofalo, P. (2018). A meta-ethnographic review of interprofessional teamwork in hospitals: What it is and why it doesn't happen more often. *Journal of Health Services Research & Policy, 23*(4), 272-279. https://doi.org/10.1177/1355819618788384

Dudding, C. C., Brown, D. K., Estis, J., Szymanski, C., Zraick, R. I., & Mormer, E. (2019). *Best practices in healthcare simulations: Communication sciences and disorders.* Council of Academic Programs in Communication Sciences and Disorders. https://growthzonesites-prod.azureedge.net/wp-content/uploads/sites/1023/2020/03/Best-Practices-in-CSD.pdf

Dudding, C. C., & Nottingham, E. E. (2018). A national survey of simulation use in university programs in communication sciences and disorders. *American Journal of Speech-Language Pathology, 27*(1), 71-81.

Dzulkarnain, A. A. A., Pandi, W. M., Rahmat, S., & Zakaria, N. A. (2015). Simulated learning environment (SLE) in audiology education: A systematic review. *International Journal of Audiology, 54*(12), 881-888.

Gaba, D. M. (2004). The future vision of simulation in health care. *BMJ Quality & Safety, 13*(Suppl. 1), i2-i10.

Gilbert, J. H., Yan, J., & Hoffman, S. J. (2010). A WHO report: Framework for action on interprofessional education and collaborative practice. *Journal of Allied Health, 39*(3), 196-197.

Griffin, D. P., Matte, M. C., Clements, J. M., Palmer, E. A., Bahlke, L. A., Gardon Rose, J. J., & Salvati, L. A. (2016). From introduction to integration: Providing community-engaged structure for interprofessional education. *Journal of Medical Education and Curricular Development*, 3, 139-148.

Haerling, K., & Prion, S. (2020). Questions regarding substitution of simulation for clinical. *Clinical Simulation in Nursing, 50*, 79-80. https://doi.org/10.1016/j.ecns.2020.06.014

Hammick, M., Freeth, D., Koppel, I., Reeves, S., & Barr, H. (2007). A best evidence systematic review of interprofessional education: BEME Guide no. 9. *Medical Teacher, 29*(8), 735-751.

Harden, R. M., & Gleeson, F. A. (1979). Assessment of clinical competence using an Objective Structured Clinical Examination (OSCE). *Medical Education, 13*(1), 39-54.

Harris, R, Guthrie, H., Hobart, B. & Lundberg, D. (1995). *Competency-based education and training: Between a rock and a whirlpool.* Macmillan Education Australia.

Hayden, J., Smiley, R., & Gross, L. (2014). Simulation in nursing education: Current regulations and practices. *Journal on Nursing Regulation* 5(2), 25-30.

Hewat, S., Penman, A., Davidson, B., Baldac, S., Howells, S., Walters, J., Purcell, A., Cardell, E., McCabe, P., Caird, E., Ward, E., & Hill, A. E. (2020). A framework to support the development of quality simulation-based learning programmes in speech-language pathology. *International Journal of Language & Communication Disorders, 55*(2), 287-300.

Heywood, L., Gonczi, A., & Hager, P. (1992). *A guide to development of competency standards for professions.* Canberra.

Hill, A. E., Ward, E., Heard, R., McAllister, S., McCabe, P., Penman, A., Caird, E., Aldridge, D., Baldac, S., Cardell, E., Davenport, R., Davidson, B., Hewat, S., Howells, S., Purcell, A., & Walters, J. (2020). Simulation can replace part of speech-language pathology placement time: A randomised controlled trial. *International Journal of Speech-Language Pathology, 23*(1), 92-102. https://doi.org/10.1080/17549507.2020.1722238

Homer, M., Fuller, R., Hallam, J., & Pell, G. (2020). Shining a spotlight on scoring in the OSCE: Checklists and item weighting. *Medical Teacher, 42*(9), 1037-1042.

INACSL Standards Committee (2016a). INACSL standards of best practice: Simulation Simulation design. *Clinical Simulation in Nursing, 12*(S), S5-S12. http://dx.doi.org/10.1016/j.ecns.2016.09.005.

INACSL Standards Committee (2016b). INACSL standards of best practice: Simulation debriefing. *Clinical Simulation in Nursing, 12*(S), S21-S25. http://dx.doi.org/10.1016/j.ecns.2016.09.008

INACSL Standards Committee (2016c). INACSL standards of best practice: Simulation simulation glossary. *Clinical Simulation in Nursing, 12*(S), S39-S47. http://dx.doi.org/10.1016/j.ecns.2016.09.012.

INACSL Standards Committee (2016d). INACSL standards of best practice: Simulation outcomes and objectives. *Clinical Simulation in Nursing, 12*(S), S13-S15. http://dx.doi.org/10.1016/j.ecns.2016.09.006

INACSL Standards Committee (2016e). INACSL standards of best practice: Simulation participant evaluation. *Clinical Simulation in Nursing, 12*(S), S26-S29. http://dx.doi.org/10.1016/j.ecns.2016.09.009

International Nursing Association of Clinical Simulation and Learning & Society for Simulation in Healthcare. (2020, March 30). *COVID-19: SSH/INACSL position statement on use of virtual simulation during the pandemic.* Society for Simulation in Healthcare. https://www.ssih.org/COVID-19-Updates/ID/2237/COVID-19-SSHINACSL-Position-Statement-on-Use-of-Virtual-Simulation-during-the-Pandemic

Kachur, E. K., Zabar, S., Hanley, K., Kaler, A., Bruno, J. H., & Gillespie, C. C. (2013). Organizing OSCEs (and other SP Exercises) in 10 Steps. In S. Zabar, E. K. Kachur, A. Kalet, & K. Hanley (Eds.), *Objective Structured Clinical Examinations* (pp. 7-35). Springer.

Krathwohl, D. (2002). A revision of Bloom's taxonomy: An overview. *Theory Into Practice, 41*(4), 212-218. https://doi.org/10.1207/s15430421tip4104_2

Lewis, K., Bohnert, C., Gammon, W., Holzer, H., Lyman, L., Smith, C., Thompson, T., Wallace, A., & Gliva-McConvey, G. (2017). The Association of Standardized Patient Educators (ASPE) Standards of Best Practice (SOBP). *Advances in Simulation, 2*(10). https://doi.org/10.1186/s41077-017-0043-4

Lioce, L. (Ed.), Lopreiato, J. (Founding Ed.), Downing, D., Chang, T. P., Robertson, J. M., Anderson, M., Diaz, D. A., Spain, A., (Assoc. Eds.) & the Terminology Concepts Working Group. (2020). *Healthcare Simulation Dictionary* (2nd ed.). Agency for Healthcare Research and Quality. https://doi.org/10.23970/simulationv2

Lockeman, K., Lanning, S., Dow, A., Zorek, J., DiazGranados, D., Ivey, C., & Soper, S. (2017). Outcomes of introducing early learners to interprofessional competencies in a classroom setting. *Teaching and Learning in Medicine, 29*(4), 433-443.

MacBean, N., Theodoros, D., Davidson, B., & Hill, A. E. (2013). Simulated learning environments in speech-language pathology: An Australian response. *International Journal of Speech-Language Pathology, 15*(3), 345-357.

MacKinnon, R. (2011). Editorial: The rise of the collaborative inter-professional simulation education network. *Infant, 7*, 6-8.

Madani, A, Hirpara, D., Chadi, S., Dhar, P., & Okrainec, A. (2021). Leveraging videoconferencing technology to augment surgical training during a pandemic. *Annals of Surgery, 2*(2), e035. https://doi.org/10.1097/AS9.0000000000000035

Mazur, Z., & Baker-Rush, M. (2020, October). *An innovative simulation-based activity to increase early learner's confidence.* Physician Assistant Education Association (PAEA). Austin, Texas [Poster].

McAllister, S., Lincoln, M., Ferguson, A., & McAllister, L. (2006). *COMPASS©: Competency Assessment in Speech Pathology.* Speech Pathology Association of Australia.

McGaghie, W. C., Sajid, A. W., Miller, G. E., Telder, T. V., & Lipson, L. (1978). *Competency-based curriculum development in medical education: An introduction.* World Health Organization. https://apps.who.int/iris/handle/10665/39703

Miller, G. (1990). The assessment of clinical skills/competence/performance. *Academic Medicine, 65*(9), S63-S67.

Mills, B., Hansen, S., Nang, C., McDonald, H., Lyons-Wll, P., Hunt, J., & O'Sullivan, T. (2019). A pilot evaluation of simulation-based interprofessional education for occupational therapy, speech pathology and dietetic students: Improvements in attitudes and confidence. *Journal of Interprofessional Care, 34*(4), 472-480. https://doi.org/10.1080/13561820.2019.1659759

Nes, A. A. G., Steindal, S. A., Zlamal, J., Landfald, Ø., Martini, J. G., Bresolin, P., Riegel, F., & Gjevjon, E. L. R. (2020). Nursing education in the light of the COVID-19 pandemic: Stimulating critical thinking through innovative teaching methods. *International Journal of Sciences and Research, 76*(2), 144-149. https://doi.org/10.21519/j.ponte.2020.12.06

Nichols, A., Wiley, S., Morrell, B. L. M., Jochum, J. E., Moore, E. S., Carmack, J. N., Hetzler, K. E., Toon, J., Hess, J. L., Meer, M., & Moore, S. M. (2019). Interprofessional healthcare students' perceptions of a simulation-based learning experience. *Journal of Allied Health, 48*(3), 159-166.

Ondo, K., Johnson, C., Jansen, L. J., Williams, S. L., & Pantalone, B. (2020). *Simucase user guide 4.0.* Simucase. https://d1e47g7vecbcl4.cloudfront.net/pdf/SC_1117_UserGuide_April_2020.pdf

Owen, H. (2016). *Simulation in healthcare education: An extensive history.* Springer.

Quigley, D., & Regan, J. (2020). Introduction of the Objective Structured Clinical Examination in speech and language therapy education: Student perspectives. *Folia Phoniatrica et Logopaedica, 73*(4), 316-325. https://doi.org/10.1159/000508445

Reeves, S., Tassone, M., Parker, K., Wagner, S. J., & Simmons, B. (2012). Interprofessional education: An overview of key developments in the past three decades. *Work, 41*(3), 233-245.

Ruebling, I., Pole, D., Breitbach, A. P., Frager, A., Kettenbach, G., Westhus, N., Kienstra, K., & Carlson, J. (2014). A comparison of student attitudes and perceptions before and after an introductory interprofessional education experience. *Journal of Interprofessional Care, 28*(1), 23-27.

Scerbo, M. W. (2016). Simulation in healthcare: Growin' up. *Simulation in Healthcare, 11*(4), 232-235.

Sexton, M., & Orchard, C. (2016). Understanding healthcare professionals' self-efficacy to resolve interprofessional conflict. *Journal of Interprofessional Care, 30*(3), 316-323. https://doi.org/10.3109/13561820.2016.1147021

Society for Simulation in Healthcare. (n.d.). Articles of Influence. https://www.ssih.org/SSH-Resources/Articles-of-Influence

Society for Simulation in Healthcare Committee for Accreditation of Healthcare Simulation Programs. (2016, May). CORE standards and measurement criteria. Society for Simulation in Healthcare. https://www.ssih.org/Portals/48/Accreditation/2016%20Standards%20and%20Docs/Core%20Standards%20and%20Criteria.pdf

Stead, A., Lemoncello, R., Fitzgerald, C., Fryer, M., Frost, M., & Palmer, R. (2020). Clinical simulations in academic courses: Four case studies across the medical SLP graduate curriculum. *Teaching and Learning in Communication Sciences & Disorders, 4*(3), Article 6. https://doi.org/10.30707/TLCSD4.3/ACVJ1784

Theodoros, D., Davidson, B., Hill, A., & MacBean, N. (2010). Integration of simulated learning environments into speech pathology clinical education curricula: A national approach. Health Workforce Australia. https://www.academia.edu/6618513/Integration_of_simulated_learning_environments_into_speech_pathology_clinical_education_curricula_A_national_approach

Thomas, E. M., Rybski, M. F., Apke, T. L., Kegelmeyer, D. A., & Kloos, A. D. (2017). An acute interprofessional simulation experience for occupational and physical therapy students: Key findings from a survey study. *Journal of Interprofessional Care, 31*(3), 317-324.

Weir-Mayta, P., Green, S., Abbott, S., & Urbina, D. (2020). Incorporating IPE and simulation experiences into graduate speech-language pathology training (O. Khaiyat, Ed.). *Cogent Medicine, 7*(1). https://doi.org/10.1080/2331205X.2020.1847415

Wise, H. H., Frost, J. S., Resnik, C., Davis, B. P., & Iglarsh, A. Z. (2015). Interprofessional education: An exploration in physical therapist education. *Journal of Physical Therapy Education, 29*(2), 72-83.

World Health Organization (2010). *Framework for action on interprofessional education & collaborative practice.* http://whqlibdoc.who.int/hq/2010/WHO_HRH_HPN_10.3_eng.pdf

Zayyan, M. (2011). Objective Structured Clinical Examination: The assessment of choice. *Oman Medical Journal, 26*(4), 219-222. https://doi.org/10.5001/omj.2011.55

Zraick, R. I. (2020). Standardized patients in communication sciences and disorders: Past, present and future directions. *Teaching and Learning in Communication Sciences & Disorders, 4*(3), 4.

Zraick, R. I., Allen, R. M., & Johnson, S. B. (2003). The use of standardized patients to teach and test interpersonal and communication skills with students in speech-language pathology. *Advances in Health Sciences Education, 8*(3), 237-248.

PART II

Clinical Simulation Learning Experiences

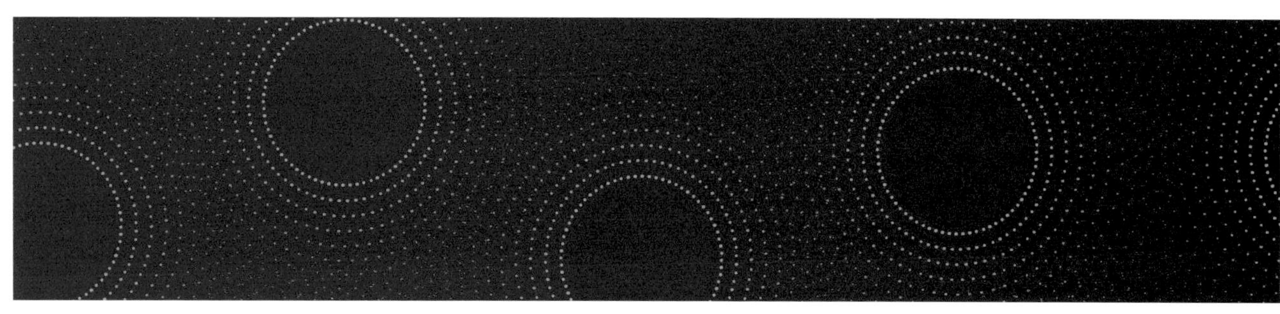

Simulation Technology

David K. Brown, PhD, CCC-A

Tell me and I'll forget, show me and I may remember, involve me and I will understand.
—Confucius (as cited in Dubbs, 1927)

Learning environments that utilize simulation provide standardized learning opportunities in a safe environment for their learners (Kardong-Edgren, 2015). The simulation-based learning experiences (SBLEs) used in these environments go beyond the technologies and are grounded in educational philosophies and learning theories (Gaba, 2004). According to Kneebone (2005), quality SBLEs include four components: (a) deliberate practice in a safe environment, (b) skilled instructors, (c) simulated real-life experiences, and (d) learner-centered experiences. The benefit of simulation is that its use before actual patient experience is cost effective; provides a safe, relatively risk-free context for learning; and improves patient outcomes (Barsuk et al., 2009; McGaghie et al., 2014; Sanko et al., 2012). As such, it is really indispensable as an alternative to hands-on experience with real-life patients (Andersen et al., 2019). This chapter introduces the reader to the simulated real-life experiences component of the SBLE, which includes the key types or modalities of simulation used in the major pedagogies underlying a quality SBLE.

The Technique of Simulation

Simulation is becoming a popular way to both teach and evaluate a learner. It has been depicted in movies such as *Monsters, Inc.* (Docter et al., 2001), where trainees practice scaring simulated children to capture their screams. When things go wrong, the monsters participate in a debriefing session to evaluate their scenario and reflect on the events of the simulation. The monsters (i.e., learners) utilize high-technology manikins to simulate a very dangerous environment (i.e., collecting screams) while performing it in a psychologically safe environment (i.e., simulation). Through this scenario, the monsters are trained in a specific skill or task (i.e., collecting screams), and the educators use an evaluation tool (i.e., skill checklist) to assess clinical competencies. Simulation allows learners to be able to learn a technique and practice it repeatedly until they feel comfortable and are prepared to be assessed on that skill (Barrows, 1993; Ziv et al., 2003). They can practice the same task on various pieces of equipment until they are proficient with that equipment. Manikins do not care how many times you need to repeat a

Dudding, C. C., & Ginsberg, S. M. (Eds.).
Simulation-Based Learning in Communication Sciences and Disorders: Moving From Theory to Practice. (pp. 55-72).

BOX 4-1

Society for Simulation in Healthcare Accreditation Standards

The Society for Simulation in Healthcare (SSH) has developed a set of Core Standards for all programs. This will allow the programs to maintain the basic attributes of simulation in order to provide and sustain quality simulation opportunities for their learners. The seven sections of the Core Standards include:

1. Mission & Governance
2. Program Management
3. Resource Management
4. Human Resources
5. Program Improvement
6. Ethics
7. Expanding the Field

Adapted from Society for Simulation in Healthcare. (2021). Core accreditation standards: 2021 standards revisions. https://www.ssih.org/Portals/48/2021%20SSH%20CORE%20ACCREDITATION%20STANDARDS.pdf

procedure before you feel comfortable performing the test. Working with people trained to portray a patient means that you will not compromise patient care while learners develop communication skills and other clinical techniques. Most training programs do not have ready access to patients with a variety of disorders, but they can gain access through simulation. Simulation will also allow the learner to quantify their clinical skills through both self-assessment and mentored assessment. Learners can be taught a skill or learn it in a self-guided method, practice those skills, monitor their improvement through self-assessment, and finally demonstrate proficiency in a mentored assessment, all before putting hands on a patient.

Simulation Fidelity

Simulation has been used to train health care professionals to perform clinical skills and to work in teams with the goal of improved patient safety. Health care simulations develop a realistic scenario where the learner can experience a representation of a real health care event so that they can learn, practice, and be assessed in order to gain an understanding of the task or the people with whom they are interacting (Lopreiato et al., 2016). In addition to nursing and medicine, health care simulations are used by allied health professionals such as audiologists, occupational therapists, physical therapists, and speech-language pathologists. Health care simulations are often described in levels according to how closely the simulation replicates the real-world experience in terms of physical, environmental, and psychological elements (Lopreiato et al., 2016).

What Is Fidelity?

In the world of simulation, technology is often described by its fidelity. Fidelity is the level of realism that exists in the simulated learning experience—or as Phrampus (2011) defined it, how close something represents reality. This means that fidelity is more of a continuum than an absolute. As shown in Figure 4-1, Leonardo da Vinci's painting of Mona Lisa in the panel on the left is more realistic and more representative of the real Mona Lisa than the drawing on the right. However, fidelity can be described as either functional fidelity or structural fidelity depending on its relationship to either the task/function or how it replicates a part of the body (Hamstra et al., 2014). Functional fidelity is the realism of the simulation scenario relative to its clinical task. Structural fidelity is the physical resemblance of the scenario to a human patient, so it is important for it to appear like what it is representing.

Technology is defined as the materials and devices created or adapted for use in training learners in an SBLE (Lioce et al., 2020). For example, technology could include everything from plastic models or manikins to computer-based virtual-reality (VR) simulators (Cook et al., 2011). Within simulation, we often try to define fidelity by the technology rather than by the ability to reflect a realistic SBLE. For example, a task trainer is often thought to have low fidelity because it costs less or represents only a part of the body, whereas a fully computerized manikin or VR system that comes with a high cost is often thought to be high fidelity (Charnetski, 2019). It is often the case that fidelity is being defined by the amount or cost of the technology; however, it is not the technology that should be defining the fidelity but the SBLE. It has been suggested that the concept of technology should be separated from that of fidelity. In this way, the fidelity or realism is removed from the technology and a high degree of technology does not always mean the simulation is more realistic (Charnetski, 2019; Slone & Lampotang, 2014).

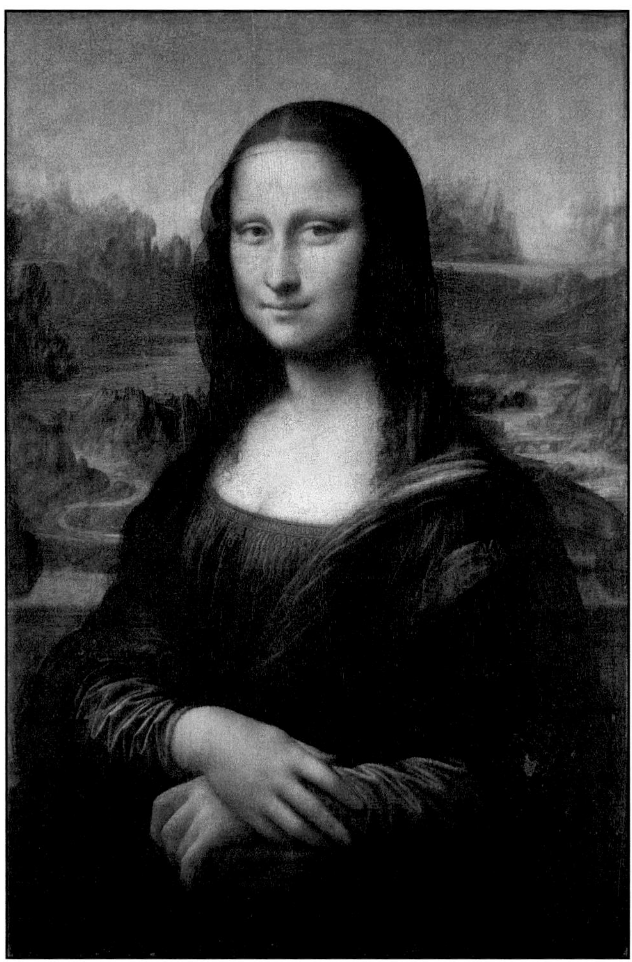

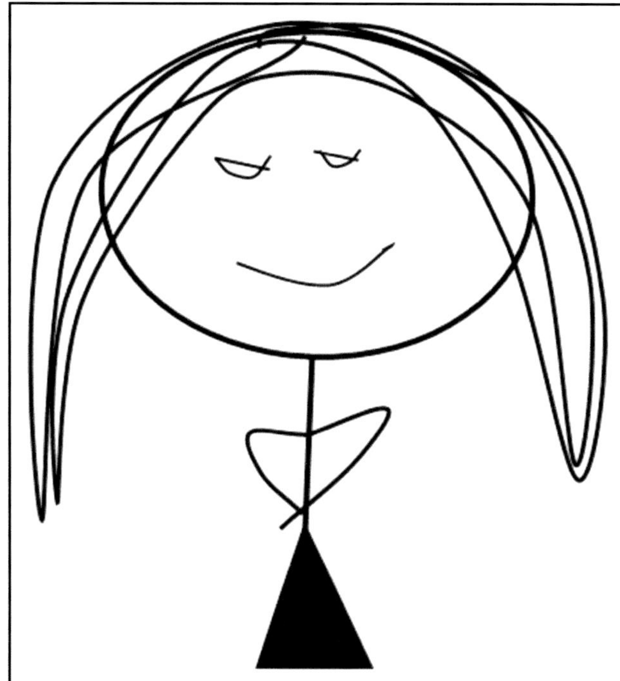

Figure 4-1. Mona Lisa sketch. Leonardo da Vinci's Mona Lisa (left) has greater fidelity than the Mona Lisa sketch above.

Just as fidelity can be described as being low or high, technology can also be described as low or high. For example, a specific task trainer could be designed with either low or high technology. A task trainer that consists of a plastic head and a rubber ear to allow the learner to practice cerumen management may be low technology compared to a rubber ear with a projector at the end of the ear canal to allow the learner to view a picture of the eardrum through an otoscope. But, what about their fidelity? In this example, both could be considered to be high fidelity in that they are both able to provide a very realistic SBLE, yet one clearly incorporates more technology. In this way, higher fidelity is not guaranteed by an increase in technology. However, in certain situations high technology and high fidelity are related, in that fidelity can be increased by including components such as sight, touch, sound, and smell. Thus, a manikin, which is very lifelike, can increase its fidelity by increasing its technology by making it cry or speak.

BOX 4-2

Resusci Anne

The first medical simulator was Resusci Anne; developed in the 1960s, it allowed individuals to practice cardiopulmonary resuscitation prior to seeing critically ill patients. The doll, made of soft plastic, had a collapsible chest so that students could practice chest compressions and open lips so that they could practice mouth-to-mouth resuscitation.

Types of Simulation Technology

Simulation technology includes models, devices, or scenarios that allow the learner to practice a particular skill using a simulator or simulation scenario. Simulators are specialized devices that replicate components of a real-world task and are used as a part of the simulation activity (Lioce et al., 2020). A variety of types of simulation or modalities are available. The modality or type refers to the simulation equipment or technique that constitutes a method of simulation

BOX 4-3

Elements of Fidelity in Simulation Design

The International Nursing Association for Clinical Simulation and Learning (INACSL) has developed a set of Standards of Best Practice™: Simulation (2021). The Standard for Simulation Design requires varying levels of fidelity be employed to create the perception of realism (Criterion 6). Several required forms on fidelity are identified:

Physical (or environmental)—how realistically the physical context of the simulation experience represents the actual environment in real life. Physical fidelity goes beyond technology and considers the appropriate use SPs, equipment, moulage, and related props.

Conceptual fidelity—how well the scenario replicates real-world cases. Cases should be of sufficient detail, reviewed by content experts, and piloted before use with learners.

Psychological fidelity—works with physical and psychological fidelity to create an experience that allows the learner to perceive the experience as real and fully immersed in the experience.

Adapted from INACSL Standards Committee, Watts, P. I., McDermott, D. S., Alinier, G., Charnetski, M., & Nawathe, P. A. (2021). Healthcare Simulation Standards of Best Practice Simulation Design. *Clinical Simulation in Nursing, 58*, 14-21. https://doi.org/10.1016/j.ecns.2021.08.009

(Rutherford-Hemming et al., 2019). Table 4-1 outlines these modalities, which include standardized patients (SPs), task trainers, manikins, computer-based simulators, and VR and shows them across the continuum of technology.

These modalities have been used in a wide array of educational learning activities across the health professions. There is an abundance of research that has studied the various types of simulators; however, studies related to the use of simulations in communication sciences and disorders (CSD) are limited. Research using SPs has shown its worth as a feasible educational strategy in CSD (Alanazi et al., 2017; Hill et al., 2013; Naeve-Velguth et al., 2013; Syder, 1996; Zraick, 2002; Zraick et al., 2003). Other modalities including task trainers (Benadom & Potter, 2011), manikins (Alanazi et al., 2016; Estis et al., 2015; Potter & Allen, 2013; Ward et al., 2015), and computer-based game scenarios (Lieberth & Martin, 2005) have been studied. Positive outcomes with these SBLEs have shown that they are acceptable to learners in CSD programs as training and evaluation tools. Learners have demonstrated an increase in comfort levels with various skills or techniques and gained foundational knowledge for working with a variety of different disorder groups. Table 4-1 describes applications for both audiology and speech-language pathology for the various types of simulation from low to high technology.

Standardized Patients

A widely used type of simulation uses human role players who interact with learners in a wide range of experiential learning and assessment activities. Early on, these human role players were a well-accepted form of simulation as they portrayed patients in various scenarios. In the 1960s, Barrows began referring to the "patients" he used to train medical students as *programmed patients* (Barrows, 1993). Since then, they have been referred to by a variety of names including *patient instructors, professional patients, patient educators, simulated person*, and *scenario role player* (Sanko et al., 2020). More commonly, they are referred to as *simulated patients, standardized patients*, or *simulated participants* (Barrows, 1971). These terms are often used interchangeably, but they have slightly different definitions, (Barrows, 1993).

For purposes of this chapter, we will make a distinction between simulated patients, SPs, and standardized participants. Simulated patient (SiP) is a broad term referring to a person who has been trained to portray a patient with a variety of different clinical conditions (Collins et al., 2011). As Barrows (1993) stated, SiPs should be sufficiently trained as to not be discerned or recognized by an expert clinician. The SiP engages in scenarios that include history taking, physical examination, and communication skills. The learner may encounter difficult personality types and sensitive subject matter through interviews with the SiP (Taylor, 2011; Thacker et al., 2007).

SPs are a type of SiP as they are trained to consistently portray a patient in a specific scripted scenario for the purpose of instructing or assessing health care providers or for letting them practice various skills (Churchouse & McCafferty, 2012; Robinson-Smith et al., 2009). The distinction in these terms is that SPs are consistent in the content of verbal and behavioral responses to a learner or examinee, while the SiP is free to respond according to the needs of the learner. Therefore, an SP encounter is a SiP encounter, but a SiP encounter is not necessarily standardized (Adamo, 2003).

SPs are not volunteers or peers but individuals trained to portray a patient in a realistic and repeatable way, ensuring all learners have similar experiences. Most programs require that their SP have a high school diploma; pass a criminal

TABLE 4-1

Types of Simulation Used in Audiology and Speech-Language Pathology

	TYPE OF SIMULATION	DEFINITION	AUDIOLOGY APPLICATION	SPEECH-LANGUAGE PATHOLOGY APPLICATION
Low Technology	Standardized patients	A person simulates an actual patient in a realistic, standardized, and repeatable way	Delivering bad news, such as identified hearing loss in newborn	Counseling patient regarding risks of aspiration
	Task trainers	A device to train in a specific procedure or skill, represents a part or region of a body, can be worn by an SP	Using an otoscopy trainer to practice insertion and viewing landmarks in the ear	Employing head and neck trainer to practice speaking valve placement
	Hybrid simulations	Using a combination of two or more simulation technologies	Combining the use of a pediatric manikin and a standardized participant to portray the family member observing a newborn hearing assessment.	Utilizing an SP with a wearable task trainer that can simulate chest expansion, lung sounds, and a tracheostomy tube in the care of the patient
	Manikin	A life-size, human-like simulator, vary in fidelity and cost, can include movement, hearing, and voice functioning, controlled by computers and software	Programming a specialized manikin to estimate auditory brainstem response (ABR) thresholds	Using a manikin programmed with oxygen saturation values to teach tracheostomy and speaking valve management
High Technology	Computer-based simulations	A simulation represented on a computer screen, often based on interactive gaming technologies	Allowing learners to practice hearing assessments on a virtual audiometer	Implementing virtual case studies to teach diagnostic skills
	Immersive VR	A computer-based, three-dimensional representation that has the feeling of immersion	Nothing available at this time	Role-playing with use of avatars in an interprofessional environment

Adapted from Dudding, C. C., & Nottingham, E. E. (2018). A national survey of simulation use in university programs in communication sciences and disorders. *American Journal of Speech-Language Pathology, 27*(1), 71-81.

background check, a drug test, and a physical examination; and have current immunizations. They must have a talent for acting and a desire to help train learners to become more effective professionals. Large programs have SP of all ages, ethnicities, socioeconomic statuses, and physical characteristics, including hearing loss and balance issues.

SPs provide a safe and controlled learning and testing environment to prepare learners to see real patients. They provide learners with the same, consistent case each time, and as a result, the faculty can be sure that all learners practice the same skills. With every learner having the chance to both learn and practice a clinical skill with an SP, they can also demonstrate that skill in the same situation, which can assist faculty with assessing clinical skills; thus, making for a fair exam or learning experience for everyone.

SPs are considered a low-technology modality but are a mainstay in the majority of medical fields from medicine to nursing to the allied health fields. Sanko and colleagues (2012) reported finding that low and high technology can have similar effectiveness for achieving learning objectives

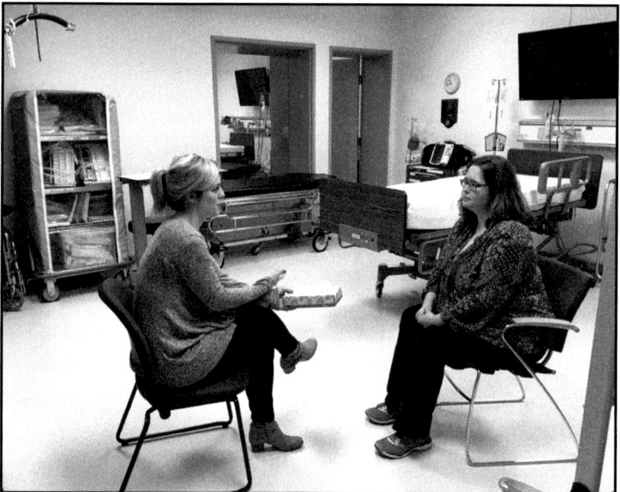

Figure 4-2. A learner presenting bad news to a patient. In this example, they are discussing the results of the hearing evaluation, which indicated that the patient's newborn has a profound hearing loss in both ears. After this "session," the SP will evaluate the learner and provide them with formal feedback about the clinician's behavior and interpersonal skills. (Courtesy of AudProf LLC.)

and for the demonstration of skills, but students preferred interacting with SPs. Figure 4-2 shows a learner interacting with an SP; the interaction between the learner and an unknown "patient" enhances the experience over the use of a peer. The concept of SPs provides clinical education opportunities allowing learners to practice communication skills with patients; practice dealing with difficult patients or difficult situations; review learners' own clinical behavior and terminology when communicating with patients; and receive feedback on the encounter from the SP perspective (see Chapter 6 for further information). The use of SP improves counseling skills, such as case history taking, ability to recognize and empathize with a client's perspective, and general counseling skills, such as breaking bad news (Gilmartin et al., 2010).

Interactions with SPs help a learner gain self-awareness of their own communication and clinical strengths and weaknesses and their reactions to stressful situations (Shemanko & Jones, 2008). Debriefing from these sessions, whether self-assessment or mentor assessment, is a critical component of the use of SPs. One standardized evaluation tool to assess a simulated counseling session or interaction with an SP is the Audiologic Counseling Evaluation (English et al., 2007). Use of this type of tool and a skillful mentor with a positive attitude and constructive criticism can reinforce learning.

As the use of SiPs and SPs continue to expand and develop, the term simulated participant has become popular in use. Simulated participant is a term used to include all role players in any simulation context or activity with varying levels of experience. The simulated participant does not necessarily portray a patient. They may play roles such as clients, family members, and health care professionals. Simulated participants are sometimes referred to as *confederates*.

Simulation participants are selected from different population pools, including faculty, medical students, and children, and portray an expanded scope.

Standardized Patient Examples in Communication Sciences and Disorders

Delivering News

As a part of a pediatric audiology course, graduate-level clinicians are taught to conduct the hearing assessment that will identify hearing loss in young infants. Typically, a newborn receives a threshold ABR test to determine the type and degree of hearing loss. To attain mastery of the use of this assessment tool requires the learner to spend a significant amount of time practicing and learning how to perform the test and to understand the outcome; however, that is only one part of the process of identifying an infant with a hearing loss. It turns out it is just as difficult to learn how to present the news as it is to do the test, yet we spend more time practicing the mechanics of the test and little time learning how to communicate the results to our patients and their families. Most clinicians are not prepared to communicate the news, with all of its emotion and communication complexity; they have fear about the family's reaction and fear of the unknown and untaught, which can lead to their own fears and emotional distress (Monden et al., 2016). Use of an SP to practice delivering news has been shown to increase clinicians' levels of competence in interpersonal and communication skills (Cvengros et al., 2016). The role of an SP is to grade the learner and provide them with feedback on their behaviors and interpersonal skills, not on the content or information they presented.

A Clinical Encounter

A faculty member designs an SBLE as part of their graduate-level adult language disorders course. Learner objectives may focus on any aspect of the clinical encounter—whether informally as part of the interview process, administering a standardized assessment, and/or providing a therapeutic strategy to promote word finding. In this case, the educator decides to focus on the administration of a standardized measure for assessing receptive and expressive language skills in adults (i.e., the Western Aphasia Battery [WAB]). Based on the learning objectives, the educator decides to use an SP recruited from the SP pool at the university. An SP is trained on how to respond as a person with moderate expressive aphasia (e.g., word finding, short sentences, halting speech). Each learner is required to prepare for the SBLE much like they would prepare for an actual evaluation. In this case, the prebrief includes a meeting with the academic educator and learner in which they discuss the case, expectations of performance, and aspects of the simulation (e.g., their role as evaluator, items needed for administration of the WAB, and issues related to safety and confidentiality). The learner enters the SBLE prepared to administer the WAB to an SP. Following best practices in simulation, the student participates in a debrief with the academic educator. The educator engages the learner in a discussion that includes reflection on what went well and what they might do differently. In some cases, as shown in Figure 4-3, an SP will also participate in the debrief. An SP can provide the student with feedback from the perspective of a patient. That is, they can provide the student information about their style of communication, whether they felt rushed, or listened to.

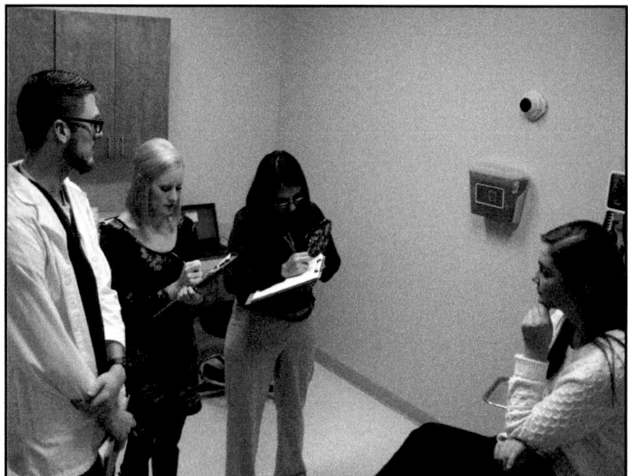

Figure 4-3. SP participates in debrief. (Courtesy of Julie Estis, PhD, Department of Communication Sciences and Disorders, University of Southern Alabama.)

Task Trainers

A type of simulation technology used in training learners in speech-language pathology and audiology are task trainers. They are the simulator of choice when you want to practice a psychomotor skill as they allow the learner to practice repeatedly until a skill is acquired. These devices can be used to teach concepts or as assessment tools. Task trainers can be either lifelike models of different body parts, such as an ear or head/neck region, or nonanatomical devices/mechanical models used to teach function, pathologies, or testing concepts. There have been recent developments in the area of wearable technologies. A wearable technology is a task trainer that can be worn by an SP to increase fidelity. No matter the form, all task trainers have the ability to break down a specific physical task into easily grasped action steps and pieces of information. They lack the provision of feedback or information from the patient, such as vital signs or if you come in contact with a structure or landmark. An example of this technology is an otoscopy trainer, which is a computer-based trainer consisting of an artificial ear and otoscope, through which the student can learn about the anatomy of the tympanic membrane and practice identifying a variety of middle ear pathologies.

Task Trainer Examples in Communication Sciences and Disorders

Ear Mold Impression

An SBLE has been developed to teach and assess learning outcomes in the task of making ear mold impressions (EMIs). Although audiologists perform EMIs as a routine part of their daily practice, it is considered a procedure that has considerable safety concerns. Therefore, patient safety must be paramount in any training procedure and the use of a task trainer when practicing or evaluating EMI is justified. This task uses a low-technology approach, and the EMI can be accomplished with a task trainer, which can be as simple as a styrofoam wig head with the temporal bone cut out to hold a standard rubber ear or a three-dimensional printed life-size bust of a person with detachable ears. These task trainers allow the learner to practice with or without supervision present, as there are no safety concerns with the trainers. Use of this technology divides the task into different components and allows the students to learn and self-assess prior to summative assessment on the activity. Learners receive instruction on making EMIs, including mixing the impression material, placing the otoblock, and the technique of inserting the impression material into the external ear canal and concha of the ear (Brown, 2017). Learners are trained to distinguish between an appropriate EMI and a poor EMI as well as to distinguish between the various problems that can appear when making an EMI. Checklists have been developed for use by learners so they can self-evaluate. Creating a checklist for the learner allows the learner to practice in a safe environment prior to any assessment and before seeking independent status through a skills assessment. As shown in Figure 4-4, learners can practice placing an otoblock in the external ear canal and mixing and inserting the material; the self-assessment tool is then used for evaluating their product. When the learner is comfortable with the methodology and the way they are able to complete the skill, and satisfied with the final product, they can proceed with a mentor assessment and then onto guided mentored assessment on real patients. Not all students are at the same level, and some need additional practice before being assessed on a skill.

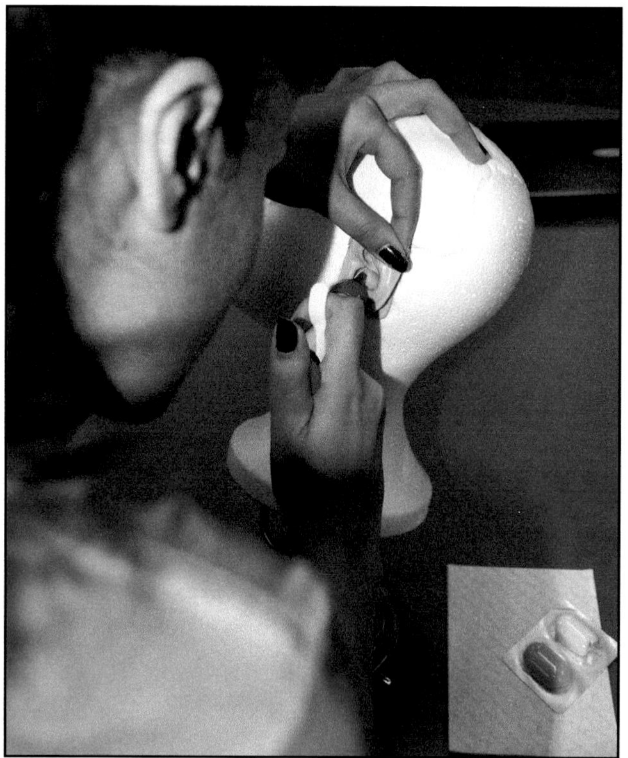

Figure 4-4. Practicing a skill. The low-technology task trainer for developing skills in making EMIs. The task is broken down into different stages, all of which can be portrayed with the task trainer. (Courtesy of AudProf, LLC.)

This technique allows the student to practice as much as is required before they move on to the next level.

Cerumen Management

Figure 4-5 shows a learner practicing cerumen management techniques, which is another example of a low-technology task trainer. Within audiology, cerumen management is one of the most invasive procedures we learn to perform. Therefore, it is paramount that we use simulation to train learners prior to their practice on real patients. With this simulation technology, students can practice unsupervised and become familiar with the different methods, visualization systems (i.e., loupes), and removal tools used in cerumen removal but without needing to be concerned with patient safety. Figure 4-5 shows a learner practicing with the various instruments to remove artificial cerumen from a task trainer. Utilizing artificial cerumen, they can gain experience with different consistencies of cerumen prior to touching a patient. Mentored assessment can be used to determine when they are ready for clinical experience.

Fiberoptic Endoscopic Examination of Swallowing

Task trainers are typically used for the training and assessment of clinical skills that are considered invasive and/or high risk. According to the American Speech-Language-Hearing Association (2001) Scope of Practice, individuals with specialized training and expertise in fiberoptic endoscopy may assess swallow functions of the upper aerodigestive tract using a procedure known as *fiberoptic endoscopic examination of swallowing*. This, and similar procedures, requires that the speech-language pathologist is skilled in passing an endoscope through the nasal passage and upper airway. The risks associated with this procedure on an actual patient is self-evident. A task trainer, as shown in Figure 4-6, that allows a learner to practice insertion of the scope while identifying relevant anatomical structures would be invaluable to expanding the number of clinicians qualified to perform these procedures. Such task trainers have not yet been developed specifically for speech-language pathologists. However, there are task trainers used by our colleagues in medicine that may be adapted for our purposes.

Manikins

Manikins are high-technology simulators that allow students to practice conducting tests or procedures. These life-size human patient simulators are designed to be realistic and are available in a variety of preterm, infant, child, and adult models. High-technology simulators can simulate physiologic functions (e.g., cardiac function, pulse rate, respiratory patterns, pupil dilation, muscle tone, electroencephalogram, cochlear hair cell movement) that may be programmed to respond accordingly to interventions or interactions (Damassa & Sitko, 2010). In order to facilitate this, the manikin needs to have a computer control system to manage the results and program the responses based on the selected outcome, a human–machine interface or program to allow the educator to select the test or practice protocol they would like the learner to use, and a manikin or device that models the real-world human system (Lopreiato et al., 2016). Physiologic parameters are displayed on a simulated patient monitor and/or controlled by a computer. These high-technology simulators or manikins give the learner the opportunity to practice more complex procedures in a safe yet realistic and responsive environment. For example, otoacoustic emissions (OAEs) or ABR testing can be completed on a lifelike infant manikin (Brown, 2017). High-technology preterm manikins have also been used to train clinical and nonclinical students to assess oral feeding skills in preterm infants (Broadfoot,

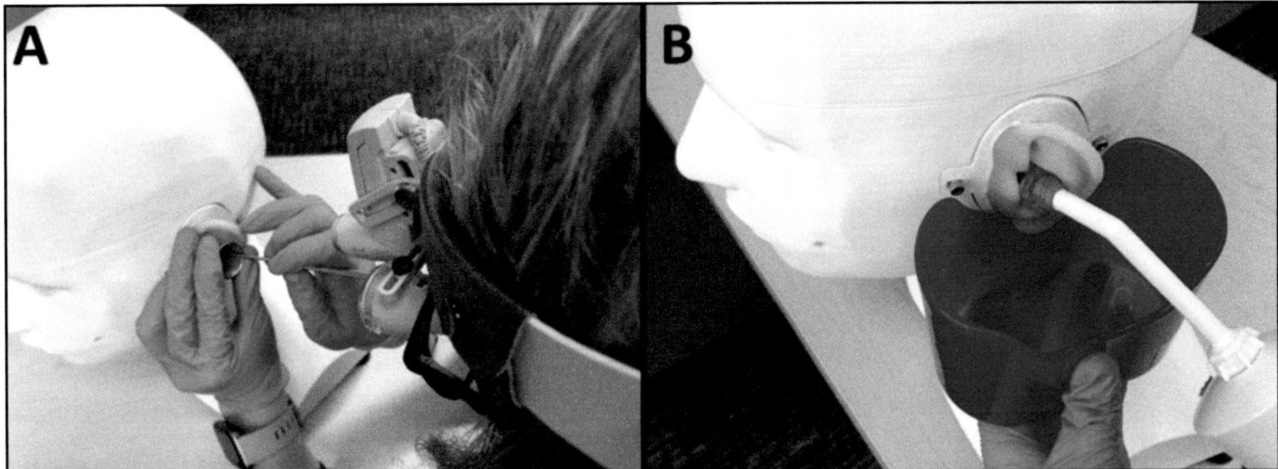

Figure 4-5. Task trainer. This low-technology task trainer allows the learner to practice with the various tools and become comfortable at removing artificial cerumen from the patient's ear canal. (A) The learner practices removal with a curette. (B) The learner uses lavage practice to remove the cerumen. (Courtesy of AudProf, LLC.)

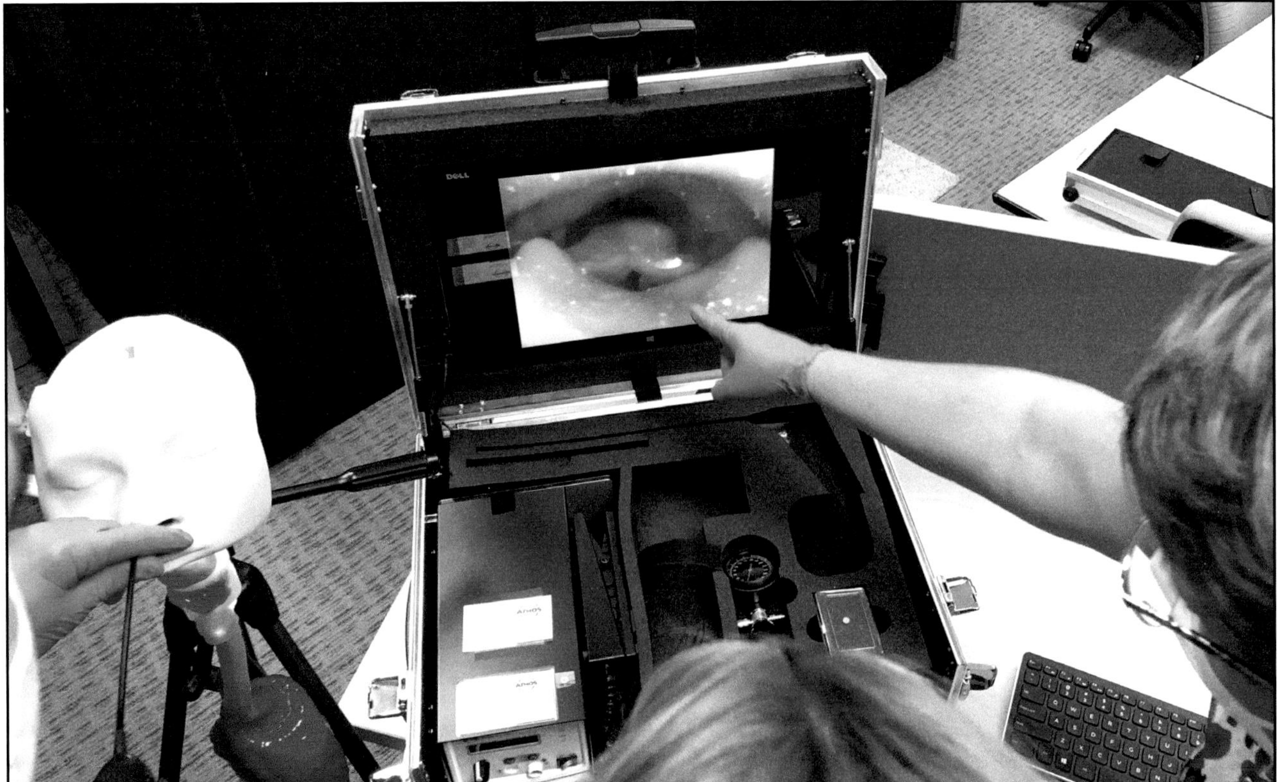

Figure 4-6. Task trainer. Simulator for practicing fiberoptic endoscopic examination of swallowing assessments. (Courtesy of AudProf, LLC.)

2015; Ferguson & Estis, 2018). Often, these manikins are required because parents will not allow you to practice on their newborn until you are competent conducting a threshold ABR. Having multitudes of learners hovering over and spending hours practicing these techniques are not possible with a real infant, but manikins do not complain.

Manikin Examples

Auditory Brainstem Response and Otoacoustic Emissions

High-technology manikin simulators allow learners to conduct both ABR and OAE testing with any manufacturer's diagnostic ABR system. Learners are able to practice making any evoked potential recording from neurodiagnostic testing

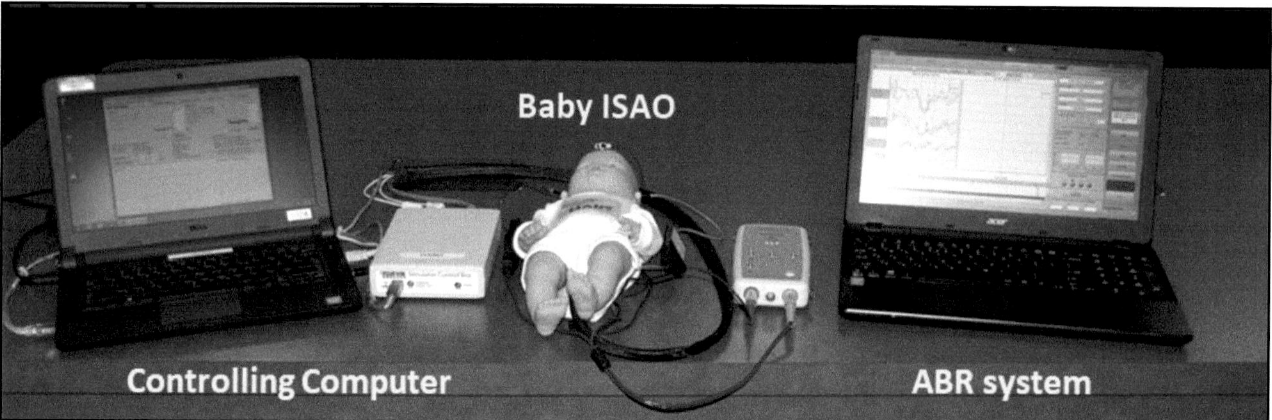

Figure 4-7. Manikin simulator. Baby ISAO, the ABR/OAE manikin simulator simulating a newborn. Any ABR system can be used with this high-technology manikin, so it can be used for learners to practice the procedure or for learning how to use different ABR systems. After attaching electrodes to the forehead and earlobe and the ear is stimulated through the insert earphones, the tone burst or click stimuli is presented to the ear in order to record either a neurodiagnostic or threshold ABR. (Courtesy of AudProf, LLC.)

to threshold estimation. They can practice picking peaks, measuring latencies, and determining the degree of loss using air conducted stimuli. Both transiently evoked otoacoustic emissions and distortion product otoacoustic emissions testing can also be completed with this manikin. Learners can practice each of the tests, receive self-assessment, and prepare for mentored assessment. The controlling computer controls the output of the desired response to the baby. The system can be self-run as a practice platform or as an assessment tool. The mentor has the ability to develop assessment tests that can evaluate any ABR or OAE test. In an assessment, the operator can control the background noise (e.g., electromyography, line noise) and even make the child cry. This high-fidelity, high-technology manikin is used in our clinical proficiency exam for newborn diagnostic hearing testing (see Chapter 6 for an example of our rubric used for this exam). Figure 4-7 shows the manikin and a test result for a neurodiagnostic test.

Infant Oral Feeding

Medically fragile infants, especially those born prematurely, often begin their lives in neonatal intensive care units. It is the role of speech-language pathologists to work as part of an interprofessional team to make decisions about safe oral feeding for these infants. One aspect of that decision is to determine readiness for oral feeding. Educators have used a pediatric manikin, such as Super Tory (Gaumard) or Newborn HAL (Gaumard), to train speech-language pathology students in assessing readiness for oral feeding (Figure 4-8; Clinard, 2018). The high-fidelity manikin allows the educator to manipulate variables such as crying, heart rate, and muscle tone. Graduate students engaged in this type of high-fidelity training with a manikin reported greater confidence in assessing readiness in medically complex infants when compared to students who did not engage in simulation (Clinard, 2018).

Tracheostomy Valves

Training to prepare speech-language pathology, respiratory therapy, and nursing students for interprofessional collaborative practice for patients with Passy Muir valves is effectively conducted with manikins (Estis et al., 2015). Through the computer-controlled manikin, many pathologies or disorders can be replicated, and the student can practice each of the tests or protocols to diagnose or identify them while gaining practice in teamwork and communication.

Hybrid Simulation

Hybrid simulation is the union of two or more modalities of simulation with the aim of providing a more realistic experience for the learner (Lous et al., 2020). In health care simulation, hybrid simulation is most commonly applied to the situation where a task trainer, for example with a chest and tracheostomy model, is realistically attached to an SP. In this way, it allows the learner to interact with an SP and the task trainer for the teaching and assessment of technical and communication skills in an integrated fashion. The use of SP, because of the ability for patient–clinician interaction, increases the realism of the training for the learner, and further engages their feelings and emotions (Dunbar-Reid et al., 2015).

The strength of this type of simulation is that it allows for both procedural and communication skills training simultaneously and adds a sense of realism to the training that may not be attained by using either an SP or simulator alone. An SP elicited more patient interaction, including greater explanation of procedures, the need for reassurance, and

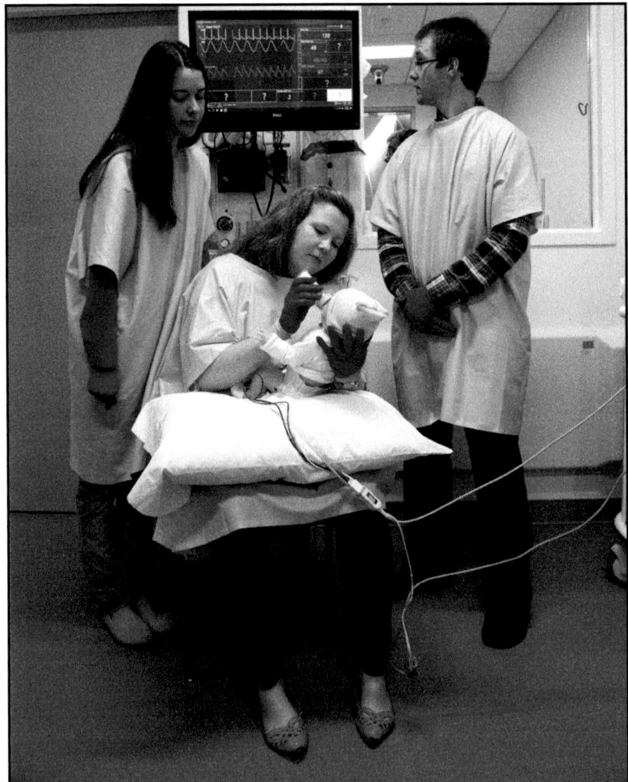

Figure 4-8. Student with Super Tory manikin. (Reproduced with permission from Erin Clinard.)

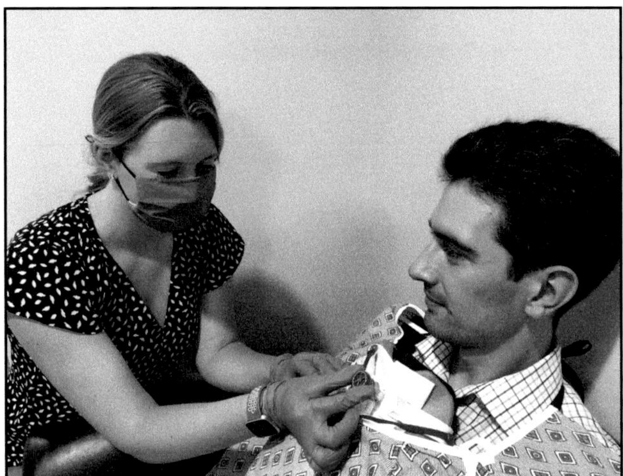

Figure 4-9. SP wears a task trainer. The learner is practicing clearing stoma on this SP that is wearing an Avtrach Wearable Tracheostomy Simulator. This device consists of a chest and a throat with an inserted tracheostomy tube. The learner can listen to various lung sounds and practice suctioning the antimicrobial mucus. Sensors monitor pressure on the trachea and warns the learner if too much pressure is applied. (Courtesy of AudProf, LLC.)

questions for the caregiver (Brown & Tortorella, 2020), all of which are almost nonexistent when high-fidelity simulators are used. It is possible through the use of hybrid simulators to allow learners to realistically experience working with vulnerable groups, such as pregnant people or patients with tracheostomy. Lous and colleagues (2020) reported that hybrid simulation, with its multiple types of simulation giving the appearance that it is more realistic, is associated with better learner satisfaction. The use of two or more simulation modalities in the same simulation activity has been shown to be as efficient as using high-fidelity training (Lous et al., 2020).

Hybrid Simulation Example

Care of the Patient With a Tracheostomy

Task trainers that replicate tracheostomy tubes are helpful in training for medical procedures such as suctioning for feeding assessment and placement of speaking valves. While task trainers are helpful in training the procedural aspects of these high-risk procedures, they do not account for the complexity of the actual human response. As shown in Figure 4-9, this is where combining two or more technologies comes into play. An SP is able to wear a task trainer designed to simulate chest expansion, lung sounds, and a tracheostomy tube. Now imagine the SP coughing and grabbing the hand of the learner during suctioning or valve placement, much like what is likely to occur in the real world. Through this tracheal simulation experience learners will gain both clinical and communication skills. This is an example of enhancing the fidelity of the SBLE by combining types of simulation technologies.

Computer-Based and Web-Based Simulations

Computer-based simulations are "the modeling of real-life processes with inputs and outputs exclusively confined to a computer, usually associated with a monitor and a keyboard or other simple assistive device" (Lopreiato et al., 2016, p. 12). Computer-based simulation can take many forms, including virtual patients, VR task trainers, and immersive VR simulation. Computer-based simulation programs can engage and encourage learners and promote active individual learning of knowledge and skills. As a function of this, the learner will experience what can or will happen as a result of their action, and based on their result, they will be able to repeat a scenario with hopefully a different outcome (Cant & Cooper, 2014; Donovan et al., 2018).

Computer-based simulations tend to originate from a combination of interactive gaming technologies and learning theory. They are designed to present a clinical experience through story or scenario where the learner is forced to make choices to complete the simulation. The learner controls the simulation experience by starting and stopping the simulation at will, they make choices rather than follow a predetermined sequence, and they can restart the experience at any point in the scenario and as often as they want. This type of learning is well suited for promoting skills such as critical thinking, communication, and decision making (Guise et al., 2012).

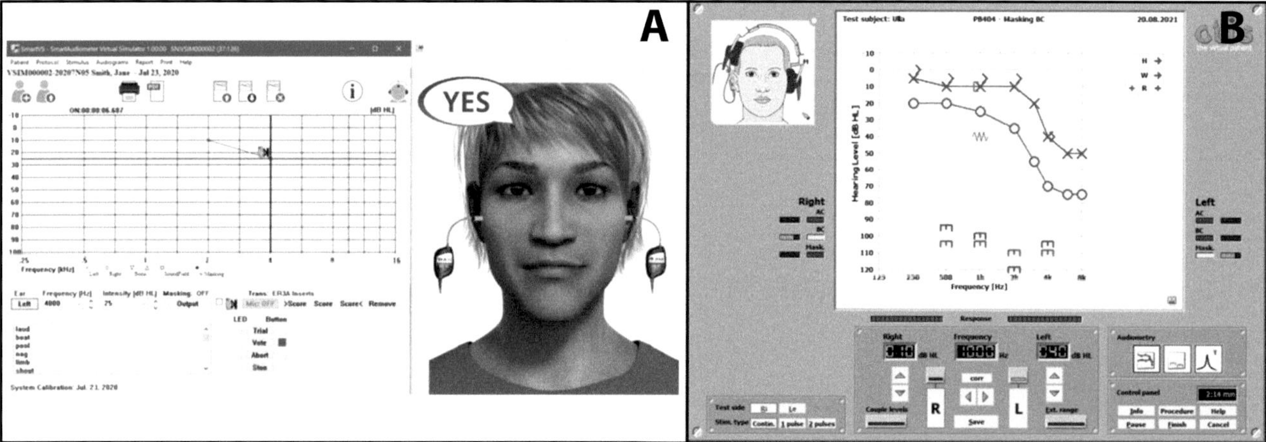

Figure 4-10. Computer-based simulation systems. Examples of two different computer-based simulation systems. There are different systems available including the (A) SmartVS and (B) Otis—the virtual patient. (Courtesy of [A] Intelligent Hearing Systems, [B] INNOFORCE Creative Solutions.)

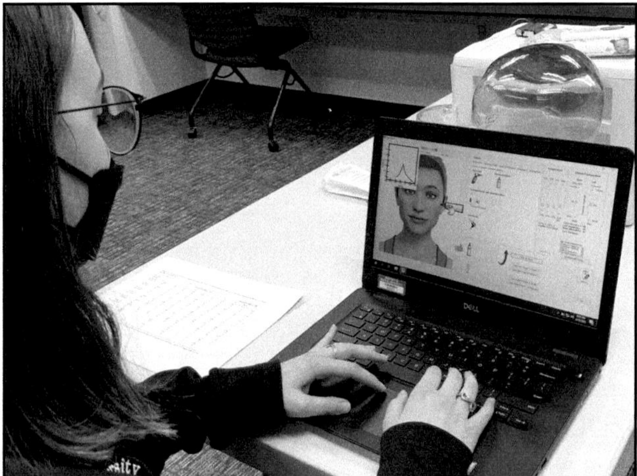

Figure 4-11. Software for testing virtual patients. The learner is practicing various procedures on this patient to be able to determine the type, degree, and configuration of their hearing loss. This assessment can be used by both undergraduates and graduate students. Undergraduates may only look at the basic test battery for their patient, but graduate students could complete the assessment and scrutinize the case history to find additional areas that need to be addressed (e.g., diabetes). (Courtesy of AudProf, LLC.)

Examples of Computer-Based and Web-Based Simulations in Communication Sciences and Disorders

Audiometry

There are existing computer-based simulation technologies that use a virtual patient and a variety of audiology tests from the audiologist's toolbox, such as otoscopy, pure-tone air and bone audiometry, speech audiometry, tympanometry, acoustic reflex thresholds, OAE, and ABR to teach basic audiometric techniques, including masking. These computer-based programs emulate diagnostic test equipment, such as audiometers, tympanometers, OAE, and ABR units and allow the student to perform a variety of tests on a variety of patients (Figure 4-10). Some of the systems are more basic providing only pure-tone audiometry (with or without masking), and some are more comprehensive including advanced diagnostic tests such as OAE and ABR. The virtual patients have a variety of hearing loss patterns with different types and degrees of hearing loss.

The SmartVS (Intelligent Hearing Systems) software has more than 40 cases that include a comprehensive case history. The learner needs to get the patient from the waiting room, and then has the option to review the referral form and case history or begin testing. Patients have their own image, so the learner begins to develop a connection with the patient. After entering the testing room, they have a choice of tests they would like to conduct based on the case history. The learner will have to set up the patient for each test before completing the test and reviewing the results. Figure 4-11 shows the learner conducting various tests on their virtual patient. There are two types of patients, practice and testing. The practice patients provide additional information and guidance on what is happening in real time (e.g., the inserts have been placed on the wrong ears, the electrodes are not attached in the correct location).

For self-assessment, the student can compare their results to the intended results set out by the software. This can also be used to assess a student's ability to conduct an audiometric test, for use by the mentor to evaluate their readiness to test real patients. After completing the various tests, the learner can create a report to submit for grading along with a billing form. Each case includes a debriefing form (Figure 4-12) that asks the learner to reflect on the experience, to identify their own gaps in knowledge and practice, and evaluate methods for improvement.

Debrief Questions?

Testing Patient

1. **Were you satisfied with your ability to test this patient?** (Begin this debrief by gauging how you would rate your performance with the tests/assessments that you performed on this patient.)

Faculty: The student should retrace their steps from the beginning of the case and determine if they were "right" or "wrong."

Reflection

2. **What did you do well and what could have been handled differently in this case?** (Reflect on why you are satisfied with how the case went and what did not go as you expected.)

Faculty: Participants can learn a lot about themselves during this portion of the debrief. In responding to this question, learners reflect on their experience and debate the correct clinical pathway. This can help improve self-awareness and a stronger understanding of the curriculum material.

Learn From the Case

3. **What did you learn from this case?** (As the learner, what is the most important concept that you have taken away from this case?)

Faculty: Because the answers are individualized, one learner may experience an "Aha!" moment and finally grasp a specific diagnostic skill and another learner may develop the confidence to point out a patient diagnosis. Whatever the learner's takeaway is, you can use this to coach them to refine their skills.

Improving the Simulation

4. **How could this simulation experience be improved?** (As the learner, what did you think of the case? Was the simulation realistic enough? Were you adequately prepared? What is the most important concept that you have taken away from this case?)

Faculty: The post-simulation debrief gives you a chance to ask the learner what they think of the teaching method. There is always room to improve a case. Feedback from the learner can improve the case.

Final Remarks

5. **Is there anything else you would like to tell us about this case or your experience with it?**

Faculty: The post-simulation debrief gives the learner a chance to ask the learner what they think of the teaching method. There is always room to improve a case; therefore, the feedback from the learner can assist with making the case better. Improvements can include a number of unexpected and valuable nuggets of information about the case and the learner's experience.

Figure 4-12. Debrief questions. (Courtesy of Intelligent Hearing Systems.)

Case-Based Simulation Technology

Simucase is a computer-based simulation technology that allows learners to observe, assess, diagnose, and provide intervention for virtual patients. Figure 4-13 illustrates the case format from Simucase. As you can see, it provides the learner with information both in the form of a case history and from other family members and professionals. With this information, the learner is to develop a clinical hypothesis and plan for the client. From here the learner moves to the assessment tools (including standardized and non-standardized tests) and evaluates the client. The learner then indicates a diagnosis and completes a recommendation plan for the client. Once this is complete, the learner is provided a competency rating for each of these areas.

Simucase is used in more than 320 CSD programs across the United States and internationally. Between 2019 and 2021, the number of computer-based simulations being submitted by students to receive clinical hours and competencies grew exponentially, increasing from 85,353 simulations completed in 2019 to 176,908 in the first half of 2021 (S. Williams, personal communication, August 5, 2021). This points to the growing acceptance of computer-based simulation to provide access to clinical education opportunities.

Extended Reality Simulation

The VR industry is undergoing rapid expansion and changes even as this chapter is being written. Definitions and classifications are being developed to accommodate these and future technologies. One such change is the use of the term *extended reality* (XR). XR is a term that encompasses several forms of technology, including augmented reality (AR), virtual reality (VR), and mixed reality (MR). Figure 4-14 depicts the relationship of these technologies.

AR refers to when objects and virtual information are overlaid on the real world. You may be familiar with *Pokémon GO*, which overlays digital creatures (Pokémon) onto the real world. Another example of AR would be Snapchat filters that allow users to transform into cats and space aliens. In AR, the real world is central, but it is enhanced by additional digital details. This occurs by layering on new perceptions to supplement your reality or environment. VR is the most common and fully immersive form of XR technologies. Through the use of a head-mounted display, you can experience sights and sounds, and you have the ability to move around and manipulate objects with haptic controllers while being connected to a computer. MR brings together both real-world and digital elements. Through MR technology, you interact with and manipulate both physical and virtual items and environments, using different sensing and imaging technologies. MR allows you to see and immerse yourself in the world around you even as you interact with a virtual environment using your own hands. Mixing these two environments, the real world and a virtual place, allows you to break down basic concepts of real and imaginary and be able to work in this new environment.

Virtual Reality in Simulation

VR typically involves a headset that allows learners to become completely immersed in a three-dimensional virtual world created by computer technologies. Wilson and Wittmann-Price (2019) suggest that the key features to the VR environment are (a) it provides a three-dimensional immersive experience, (b) uses an avatar to interact in the virtual world, (c) provides both visual and auditory feedback, and (d) replicates real-world activities. The benefit of VR is that it can reproduce a problem and allow the learner to work out the best response and/or steps to improve the technique, starting and stopping as frequently as required. Examples of virtual simulations include flight simulators, surgical simulators (e.g., laparoscopic surgery), and vestibular testing.

VR introduces us to the concept of immersion. Immersion or immersive environment means that it tricks your senses into the perception of being physically present in a different nonphysical environment or world (Lui & Slotta, 2014). Like fidelity, immersion and depth of VR occurs on a continuum. Depth of VR experiences begins at the level of learner perception (passive observation) and progresses to simulation (guided experience), followed by interaction (directing the flow of content) and then immersion (active, user-led experience). As with other simulation technology, the reader is directed to select the depth of VR experience that is best suited to the learning objectives. Refer to Figure 4-15 for depths of reality.

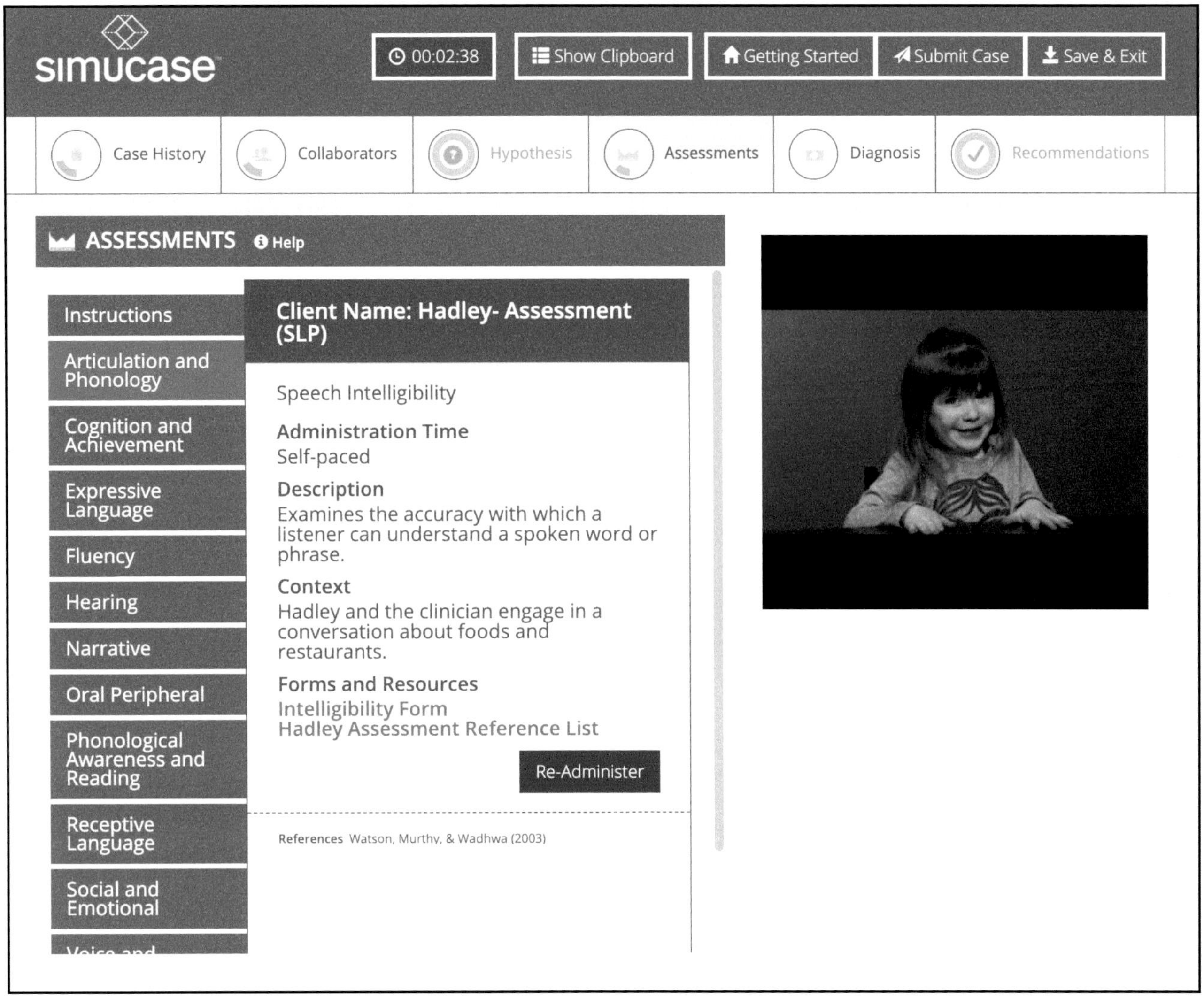

Figure 4-13. Simucase. An example of a Simucase client case format. Through the tabs across the top, the learner has access to the client's case history information, documents from other professionals, assessments, and places to add in the clinical hypothesis, diagnosis, and recommendations. (Reproduced with permission from Simucase.)

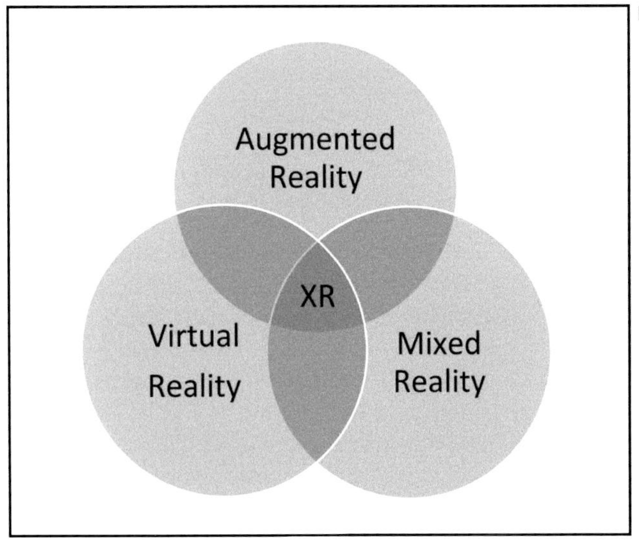

Figure 4-14. Classification of XR technologies.

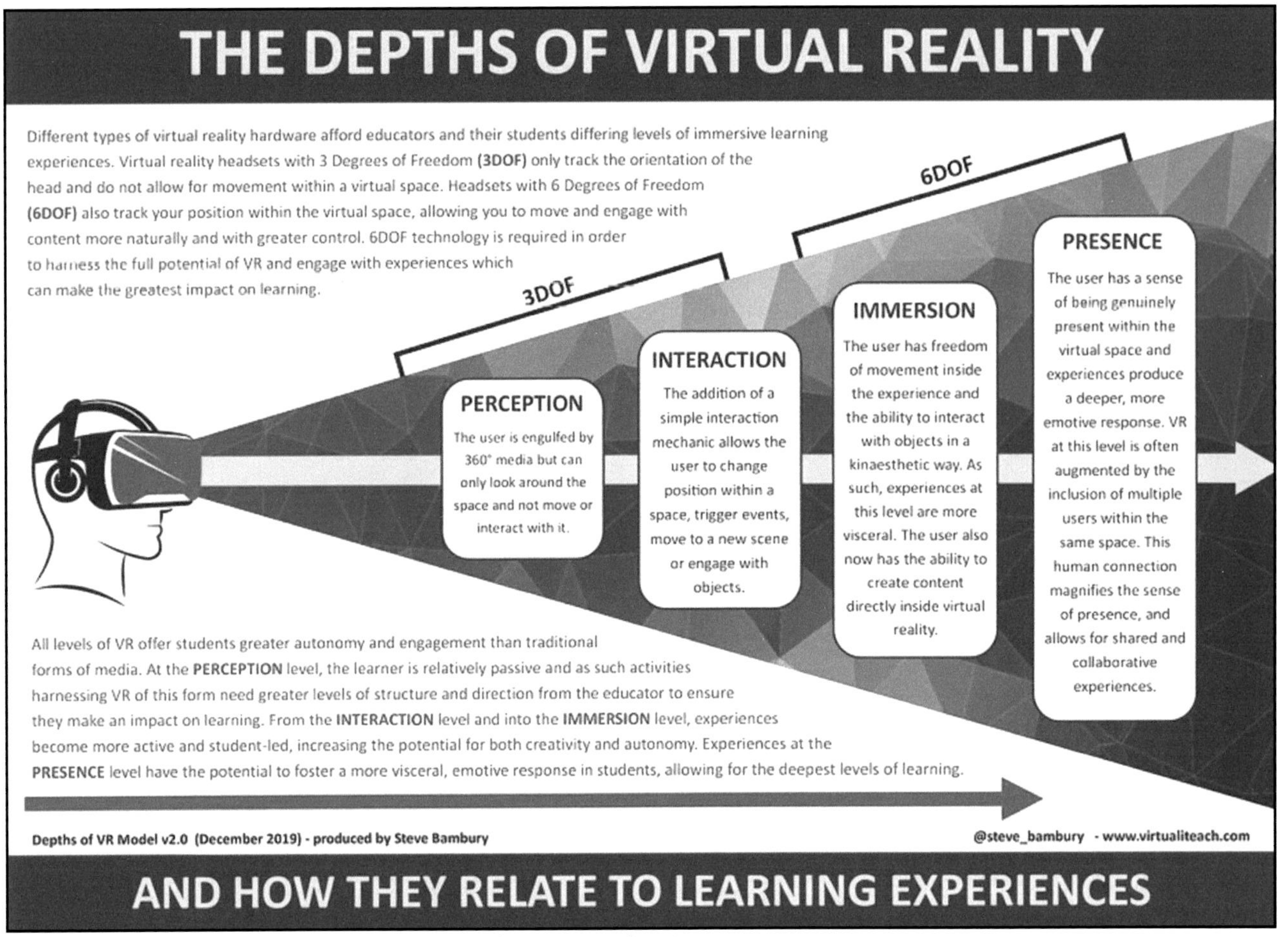

THE DEPTHS OF VIRTUAL REALITY

Different types of virtual reality hardware afford educators and their students differing levels of immersive learning experiences. Virtual reality headsets with 3 Degrees of Freedom **(3DOF)** only track the orientation of the head and do not allow for movement within a virtual space. Headsets with 6 Degrees of Freedom **(6DOF)** also track your position within the virtual space, allowing you to move and engage with content more naturally and with greater control. 6DOF technology is required in order to harness the full potential of VR and engage with experiences which can make the greatest impact on learning.

3DOF

6DOF

PERCEPTION
The user is engulfed by 360° media but can only look around the space and not move or interact with it.

INTERACTION
The addition of a simple interaction mechanic allows the user to change position within a space, trigger events, move to a new scene or engage with objects.

IMMERSION
The user has freedom of movement inside the experience and the ability to interact with objects in a kinaesthetic way. As such, experiences at this level are more visceral. The user also now has the ability to create content directly inside virtual reality.

PRESENCE
The user has a sense of being genuinely present within the virtual space and experiences produce a deeper, more emotive response. VR at this level is often augmented by the inclusion of multiple users within the same space. This human connection magnifies the sense of presence, and allows for shared and collaborative experiences.

All levels of VR offer students greater autonomy and engagement than traditional forms of media. At the **PERCEPTION** level, the learner is relatively passive and as such activities harnessing VR of this form need greater levels of structure and direction from the educator to ensure they make an impact on learning. From the **INTERACTION** level and into the **IMMERSION** level, experiences become more active and student-led, increasing the potential for both creativity and autonomy. Experiences at the **PRESENCE** level have the potential to foster a more visceral, emotive response in students, allowing for the deepest levels of learning.

Depths of VR Model v2.0 (December 2019) - produced by Steve Bambury **@steve_bambury - www.virtualiteach.com**

AND HOW THEY RELATE TO LEARNING EXPERIENCES

Figure 4-15. Depths of VR. (Reproduced with permission from Steve Bambury.)

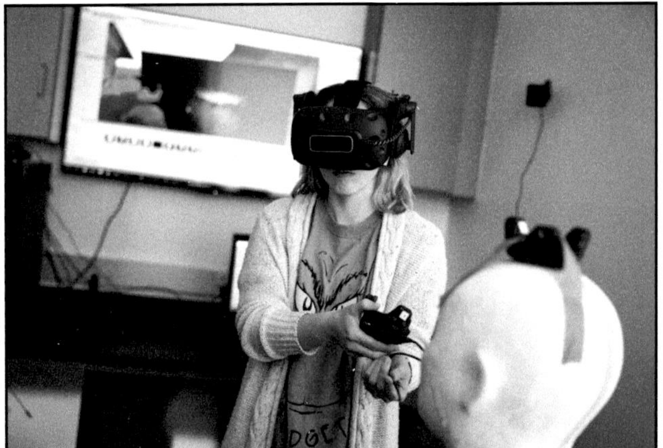

Figure 4-16. Using MR simulation. (Reproduced with permission from James Madison University.)

Example of Mixed Reality in Communication Sciences and Disorders Endoscopic Evaluation

Dudding and colleagues developed an immersive MR experience using a HTC Vive Headset. As shown in Figure 4-16, graduate students put on the headset to get visual feedback while practicing passing an endoscope through a styrofoam head (Long, 2019). This MR experience builds on the mechanical part task simulators that allow only for practice in inserting the scope. By pairing this experience with the virtual environment created by the headset, the students were able to identify anatomical structures as the scope passed through the nasal passage and pharynx. Figure 4-16 depicts the use of MR simulation.

Summary

The goal of simulation is for the learner to incorporate the skills and lessons learned from the simulation experience and assessment/debriefing and apply them to their real-world clinical situations. Using an educational model for training audiologists and speech-language pathologists that includes simulation, future students will be better prepared for clinical practice. The use of simulation serves to heighten the experience, develop and refine clinical skills, and enhance a learner's ability to interact with patients. Self-assessment, feedback from mentors, and the opportunity for remediation will produce better-prepared audiologists.

References

Adamo, G. (2003). Simulated and standardized patients in OSCEs: Achievement and challenges 1993-2003. *Medical Teacher, 25*(3), 262-270. https://doi.org/10.1080/0142159031000100300

Alanazi, A. A., Nicholson, N., Atcherson, S. R., Franklin, C., Anders, M., Nagaraj, N. K., Franklin, J., & Highley, P. (2016). Use of Baby ISAO simulator and standardized parents in hearing screening and parent counseling education. *American Journal of Audiology, 25*, 211-223. https://doi.org/10.1044/2016_AJA-16-0029

Alanazi, A. A., Nicholson, N., Atcherson, S. R., Franklin, C., Nagaraj, N. K., Anders, M., & Smith-Olinde, L. (2017). Audiology students' perception of hybrid simulation experiences: Qualitative evaluation of debriefing sessions. *Journal of Early Hearing Detection and Intervention, 2*(1), 12-28.

American Speech-Language-Hearing Association. (2001). Scope of practice in speech-language pathology. Author.

Andersen, P. A., Downer, T., O'Brien, S., & Cox, K. (2019). Wearable simulated maternity model: Making simulation encounters real in midwifery. *Clinical Simulation in Nursing, 33*, 1-6. https://doi .org /10 .1016/j.ecns.2019.04.007

Barrows, H. S. (1971). *Simulated patients (programmed patients): The development and use of a new technique in medical education.* Charles C. Thomas.

Barrows, H. S. (1993). An overview of the uses of standardized patients for teaching and evaluating clinical skills. *Academic Medicine, 68*(6), 443-453.

Barsuk, J. H., McGaghie, W. C., Cohen, E. R, O'Leary, K. J., & Wayne, D. B. (2009). Simulation-based mastery learning reduces complications during central venous catheter insertion in a medical intensive care unit. *Critical Care Medicine, 37*(10), 2697-2701. http://doi.org/10.1097/00003246-200910000-00003

Benadom, E. M., & Potter, N.L. (2011). The use of simulation in training graduate students to perform transnasal endoscopy. *Dysphagia, 26*, 352-360. http://doi.org/10.1007/s00455-010-9316-y

Broadfoot, C. K. (2015). *Assessing oral feeding skills in preterm infants using a simulation-based approach* (Publication No. 1604551). [Master's Thesis, University of South Alabama]. ProQuest LLC.

Brown, D. K. (2017). Simulation before clinical practice: The educational advantages. *Audiology Today, 29*(5), 16-25.

Brown, W. J., & Tortorella, R. A. W. (2020). Hybrid medical simulation—A systematic literature review. *Smart Learning Environments, 7*(16). https://doi.org/10.1186/s40561-020-00127-6

Cant, R. P., & Cooper, S. J. (2014). Simulation in the internet age: The place of web-based simulation in nursing education. An integrative review. *Nurse Education Today, 34*(12), 1435-1442. https://doi.org/10.1016/j.nedt.2014.08.001

Charnetski, M. D. (2019). Simulation methodologies. In: S. Crawford, L. Baily, & S. M. Monks (Eds.), *Comprehensive healthcare simulation: Operations, technology, and innovative* (pp. 27-45). Comprehensive Healthcare Simulation. Springer. https://doi.org/10.1007/978-3-030-15378-6_3

Churchouse, C., & McCafferty, C. (2012). Standardized patients versus simulated patients: Is there a difference? *Clinical Simulation in Nursing, 8*(8), e363-e365. https://doi.org/10.1016/j.ecns.2011.04.008

Clinard, E. (2018) Effectiveness of high-fidelity human patient simulation in learning to manage medically-complex infants [Doctoral dissertation, James Madison University]. https://commons.lib.jmu.edu/diss201019/196

Collins, L. G., Schrimmer, A., Diamond, J., & Burke, J. (2011). Evaluating verbal and non-verbal communication skills, in an ethnogeriatric OSCE. *Patient Education Counseling, 83*(2), 158-162.

Cook, D. A., Hatala, R., Brydges, R., Szostek, J. H., Wang, A. T., Erwin, P. J., & Hamstra, S. J. (2011). Technology enhanced simulation for health progressions education: A systematic review and meta-analysis. *Journal of the American Medical Association, 306*(9), 978-988.

Cvengros, J. A., Behel, J. M., Finley, E., Kravitz, R., Grichanik, M., & Dedhia, R. (2016). Breaking bad news: A small-group learning module and simulated patient case for preclerkship students. *MedEdPORTAL, 12*, 10505. https://doi.org/10.15766/mep_2374-8265.10505

Damassa, D. A., & Sitko, T. (2010). *Simulation technologies in higher education: uses, trends, and implications.* EDUCAUSE Center for Applied Research. https://library.educause.edu/-/media/files/library/2010/2/erb1003-pdf.pdf

Docter, P., Silverman, D., & Unkrich, L. (Directors). (2001) *Monsters, Inc.* [Film]. Pixar Animation Studios; Walt Disney Pictures.

Donovan, L. M., Argenbright, C. A., Mullen, L. K., & Humbert, J. L. (2018). Computer-based simulation: Effective tool or hindrance for undergraduate nursing students? *Nurse Education Today, 69*, 122-127. https://doi.org/10.1016/j.nedt.2018.07.007

Dubs, H.H., tr. (1927). *The Works of Hsüntze. Book 8: The Merit of the Confucian. Probsthain's Oriental Series 16.*

Dunbar-Reid, K., Sinclair, P. M., & Hudson, D. (2015). Advancing renal education: Hybrid simulation, using simulated patients to enhance realism in haemodialysis education. *Journal of Renal Care, 41*(2), 134-139. https://doi.org/10.1111/jorc.12112

English, K., Naeve-Velguth, S., Rall, E., Uyehara-Osono, J., & Pittman, A. (2007). Development of an instrument to evaluate audiologic counseling skills. *Journal of the American Academy of Audiology, 18*(8), 675-687. https://doi.org/10.3766/jaaa.18.8.5

Estis, J. M., Rudd, A. B., Pruitt, B., & Wright, T. (2015). Interprofessional simulation-based education enhances student knowledge of health professional roles and care of patients with tracheostomies and Passy-Muir valves. *Journal of Nursing Education and Practice, 5*(6), 123.

Ferguson, N. F., & Estis, J. M. (2018). Training students to evaluate preterm infant feeding safety using a video-recorded patient simulation approach. *American Journal of Speech-Language Pathology, 27*(2), 1-8. http://dx.doi.org/10.1044/2017_AJSLP-16-0107

Gaba, D. M. (2004). The future vision of simulation in health care. *BMJ Quality & Safety, 13*(Suppl. 1), i2-i110.

Gilmartin, J., Brooke, R., & Killan, T. (2010). The use of simulated clients to enhance counselling skills of audiologists. *British Academy of Audiology Magazine, 17*, 13-15.

Guise, V., Chambers, M., Conradi, E., Kavia, S., & Valimaki. M. (2012). Development, implementation and initial evaluation of narrative virtual patients for use in vocational mental health nurse training. *Nurse Education Today, 32*(6), 683-689. https://doi.org/10.1016/j.nedt.2011.09.004

Hamstra, S. J., Brydges, R., Hatala, R., Zendejas, B., & Cook, D. A. (2014). Reconsidering fidelity in simulation-based training. *Academic Medicine: Journal of the Association of American Medical Colleges, 89*(3), 387-392. https://doi.org/10.1097/ACM.0000000000000130.

Hill, A. E., Davidson, B. J., & Theodoros, D. G. (2013). The performance of standardized patients in portraying clinical scenarios in speech-language therapy. *International Journal of Language and Communication Disorders, 48*(6), 613-624. http://doi.org/10.1111/1460-6984.12034

INACSL Standards Committee. (2021). Healthcare Simulation Standards of Best Practice. *Clinical Simulation in Nursing, 58*, 66. https://doi.org/10.1016/j.ecns.2021.08.018

INACSL Standards Committee, Watts, P. I., McDermott, D. S., Alinier, G., Charnetski, M., & Nawathe, P. A. (2021). Healthcare Simulation Standards of Best Practice Simulation Design. *Clinical Simulation in Nursing*, *58*, 14-21. https://doi.org/10.1016/j.ecns.2021.08.009

Kardong-Edgren, S. (2015). Initial thoughts after the NCSBN National Simulation Study. *Clinical Simulation in Nursing, 11*(4), 201-202.

Kneebone, R. (2005). Evaluating clinical simulations for learning procedural skills: A theory-based approach. *Academic Medicine, 80*(6), 549-553.

Lieberth, A. K., & Martin, D. R. (2005). The instructional effectiveness of a web-based audiometry simulator. *Journal of the American Academy of Audiology, 16*(2), 79-84. https://doi.org/10.3766/jaaa.16.2.3

Lioce, L. (Ed.), Lopreiato, J. (Founding Ed.), Downing, D., Chang, T. P., Robertson, J. M., Anderson, M., Diaz, D. A., Spain, A. E. (Assoc. Eds.), & the Terminology and Concepts Working Group. (2020). *Healthcare simulation dictionary* (2nd ed.). Agency for Healthcare Research and Quality. https://doi.org/10.23970/simulationv2.

Long, H. (2019, January). Scope of practice. *Madison Magazine*. https://www.jmu.edu/news/2019/01/30-mm-virtual-reality.shtml

Lopreiato, J. O. (Ed.), Downing, D., Gammon, W., Lioce, L., Sittner, B., Slot, V., Spain, A. E. (Associate Eds.), & the Terminology & Concepts Working Group. (2016). *Healthcare Simulation Dictionary.* Agency for Healthcare Research and Quality. http://www.ssih.org/dictionary.

Lous, M. L., Simon, O., Lassel, L., Lavoue, V., & Jannin, P. (2020). Hybrid simulation for obstetrics training: A systematic review. *European Journal of Obstetrics & Gynecology and Reproductive Biology, 246*, 23-28. https://doi.org/10.1016/j.ejogrb.2019.12.024

Lui, M., & Slotta, J. D. (2014). Immersive simulations for smart classrooms: Exploring evolutionary concepts in secondary science. *Technology, Pedagogy and Education, 23*(1), 57-80. https://doi.org/10.1080/1475939X.2013.838452

McGaghie, W. C., Issenberg, S. B., Barsuk, J. H., & Wayne, D. B. (2014). A critical review of simulation-based mastery learning with translational outcomes. *Medical Education, 48*(4), 375-385. https://doi.org/10.1111/medu.12391

Monden, K. R., Gentry, L., & Cox, T. R. (2016). Delivering bad news to patients. *Baylor University Medical Center Proceedings, 29*(1), 101-102. https://doi.org/10.1080/08998280.2016.11929380

Naeve-Velguth, S., Christensen, S. A., & Woods, S. (2013). Simulated patients in audiology education: Student reports. *Journal of the American Academy of Audiology, 24*(8), 740-746.

Potter, N. L., & Allen, M. (2013). Clinical swallow exam for dysphagia: A speech pathology and nursing simulation experience. *Clinical Simulation in Nursing, 9*(10), e461-e464. http://doi.org/10.1016/j.ecns.2012.08.001

Phrampus, P. (2011). *Ft. Sam 91 Whiskey combat medic medical simulation training quantitative integration enhancement program.* University of Pittsburgh Medical Center. https://apps.dtic.mil/sti/pdfs/ADA553926.pdf

Robinson-Smith, G., Bradley, P. K., & Meakim, C. (2009). Evaluating the use of standardized patients in undergraduate psychiatric nursing experiences. *Clinical Simulation in Nursing, 5*(6), e203-e211. https://doi.org/10.1016/j.ecns.2009.07.001

Rutherford-Hemming, T., Alfes, C. M., & Breymier, T. L. (2019). A systematic review of the use of standardized patients as a simulation modality in nursing education. *Nursing Education Perspectives, 40*(2), 84-90.

Sanko, J. S., Schneidereith, T., Cowperthwait, A., & Onello, R. (2020). Findings from a human roles terminology survey: Consensus or chaos? *BMJ Simulation and Technology Enhanced Learning, 6*, 158-163. http://dx.doi.org/10.1136/bmjstel-2018-000378

Sanko, J., Shekhter, I., Rosen, L., Arheart, K., & Birnbach, D. (2012). Man versus machine: The preferred modality. *The Clinical Teacher, 9*(6), 387-391. https://doi.org/10.1111/j.1743-498X.2012.00593.x

Shemanko, G., & Jones, L. (2008). To simulate or not to simulate: That is the question. In R. Kyle & W. Murray (Eds.), *Clinical simulation: Operations, engineering and management* (pp. 77-84). Elsevier.

Slone, F., & Lampotang, S. (2014). Mannequins: Terminology, selection, and usage. In J. C. Palaganas, J. C. Maxworthy, C. A. Epps, & M. E. Mancini (Eds.), *Defining excellence in simulation programs* (pp. 183-198). Lippincott Williams & Wilkins.

Syder, D. (1996). The use of simulated clients to develop the clinical skills of speech and language therapy students. *European Journal of Disorders of Communication, 31*, 181-192.

Taylor, J. S. (2011). The moral aesthetics of simulated suffering in standardized patient performances. *Culture, Medicine and Psychiatry, 35*(2), 134-162.

Thacker, A., Crabb, N., Perez, W., Raji, O., & Hollins, S. (2007). How (and why) to employ simulated patients with intellectual disabilities. *The Clinical Teacher, 4*(1), 15-20.

Ward, E. C., Hill, A. E., Nund, R. L., Rumbach, A. F., Walker-Smith, K., Wright, S. E., Kelly, K., & Dodrill, P. (2015). Developing clinical skills in paediatric dysphagia management using human patient simulation (HPS). *International Journal of Speech-Language Pathology, 17*(3), 230-240. https://doi.org/10.3109/17549507.2015.1025846

Wilson, L., & Wittmann, R. A. (2019). *Review manual for the Certified Healthcare Simulation Educator (CHSETM) exam* (2nd ed.) Springer.

Ziv, A., Wolpe, P. R., Small, S. D., & Glick, S. (2003). Simulation-based medical education: An ethical imperative. *Academic Medicine, 78*(8), 783-788.

Zraick, R. (2002). The use of standardized patients in speech-language pathology. *Perspectives on Issues in Higher Education*, 5, 14-16. http://doi.org/10.1044/ihe5.1.14

Zraick, R., Allen, R., & Johnson, S. (2003). The use of standardized patients to teach and test interpersonal and communication skills with students in speech-language pathology. *Advances in Health Sciences Education, 8*, 237-248.

Simulation Design and Facilitation

Erin S. Clinard, PhD, CCC-SLP, CHSE

Learning in Simulation

To some, it may be tempting to jump into using simulation as part of an individual course or across an entire program. To others, figuring out where to begin and how to get started feels overwhelming. It is not simple to do simulation well without preparation, training, and experience, but it also is not so difficult that those interested should be afraid to try. Either way, this chapter provides educators with a foundation of how and where to begin implementing a simulation-based learning experience (SBLE) in communication sciences and disorders (CSD). Regardless of your starting point, it is essential to recognize simulation as a teaching methodology that requires planning and adherence to best practice guidelines in order to ensure design and implementation of evidence-based simulation. Simulation takes knowledge and planning in order to be successful.

Simulation is an educational process that has been used for many years in the training of health professionals but is still relatively new in CSD. An SBLE is defined as "an array of structured activities that represent actual or potential situations in education and practice" in order for learners to develop knowledge, skills, and attributes (KSAs; e.g., confidence; Lioce et al., 2020). SBLEs in CSD, like other health professions, are crafted to achieve clinical learning in authentic and engaging scenarios through the use of appropriate technologies designed to support learning.

Simulation is a natural fit for CSD programs because of its documented advantages in clinical training. These advantages include deliberate and repeated practice, risk-free learning, practical application of knowledge, experiential learning and reflective practice, support of critical learning, and providing a comprehensive learning experience for students (Jansen, 2015). Further, well-designed simulation enhances the transferability of skills learned during an SBLE to real-life experiences, as well as the ability to standardize learning in simulation for the purposes of consistency across iterations or for assessment of learning.

Often discussions about simulation revolve around technology, but technology is only one component of an SBLE. The technology is a tool that should be strategically selected to maximize learning and outcomes (Gaba, 2004). SBLEs do not have to employ fancy or expensive technology in order to provide rich learning. There are many modalities of simulation (see Chapter 4), including the use of task trainers, standardized patients (SPs), computer-based simulations, and high-fidelity human patient simulators (manikins). Modalities can also be combined to create hybrid simulations.

Dudding, C. C., & Ginsberg, S. M. (Eds.).
Simulation-Based Learning in Communication Sciences and Disorders: Moving From Theory to Practice. (pp. 73-90).

Learning can occur with any level of simulation fidelity. Fidelity refers to how authentic a simulation is to real-life clinical environments and circumstances. SBLEs may be designed with different levels of fidelity based on what is appropriate to meet the learning objectives. For example, while a low-fidelity simulation with a task trainer may be the most appropriate to develop the psychomotor skill of passing an endoscope for a fiberoptic endoscopic examination of swallowing assessment, a high-fidelity simulation may be more appropriate for an interprofessional scenario in which learners are conducting a feeding readiness assessment with an infant and their caregiver. Fidelity can also be achieved by combining modalities and technology; for example, an SBLE in which the objectives are that a learner will be able to pass an endoscope while also explaining and discussing what they are seeing with a patient may benefit from a hybrid simulation utilizing an SP with a wearable task trainer. In this way, simulation modalities are able to increase fidelity in order to meet this additional objective of communicating with the patient.

Simulation is not a one-size-fits-all answer to clinical teaching. Every element of a simulation is designed to meet specific learning needs while engaging learners in an immersive and authentic experience. Therefore, the key to designing any successful SBLE is strategically selecting the modality, technology, and level of simulation fidelity that will maximize desired outcomes (Wang, 2011). So, regardless of the type of simulation modality or fidelity, educators must determine *why* they are planning the SBLE in the first place. What do they expect learners to be able to do at the end of the simulation? What would be considered success for the experience? This is not dissimilar to the process of designing any educational experience or activity. Simulation, particularly high-fidelity simulation, takes time and experienced personnel as well as specialized equipment. To be good stewards of program resources and educational costs, consideration of the return on investment must be a consideration in the design process, as well as when selecting the appropriate modality for each SBLE.

Simulation scenarios must also integrate evidence-based clinical practice and uphold expectations of quality clinical intervention because the SBLE will reinforce clinical behaviors. By grounding the scenario in evidence-based practice (EBP) educators can support clinical skill development among learners that will later be transferred to the clinical environment (Waxman, 2010). This chapter will focus on the process of designing and facilitating quality SBLEs regardless of the technology or level of fidelity. For more information about simulation design from a curriculum level, see Chapter 2.

Simulation Framework

Perhaps the most commonly referenced framework in simulation-based education is the National League of Nursing (NLN) Jeffries framework that was designed in 2005, revised in 2007, and revised again 2012 (Rizzolo et al., 2016). This framework provides simulation educators with a guide to designing and facilitating quality, effective scenarios that support learning. In 2015, the framework was reconceptualized as the NLN Jeffries Simulation Theory. This was the result of rigorous evaluation and a thorough systematic review of the literature that clarified the constructs and identified relationships among the framework's components (Adamson & Rodgers, 2016; Jeffries et al., 2015). The NLN Jeffries Simulation Theory, depicted in Figure 5-1, outlines essential principles and practices of simulation that guide design, facilitation, and evaluation of SBLEs (Cowperthwait, 2020; Jeffries et al., 2015).

The original framework identified five major core constructs essential for design, implementation, and evaluation of simulation-based education. The five original constructs were simulation design characteristics, facilitator characteristics, participant characteristics, educational practices, and outcomes. The revised theory retained these key constructs and grounds all of these components in context. Contextual factors, such as the environment/setting and circumstances, influence the entire SBLE and guide the simulation purpose. Additionally, the theory added a sixth construct of background, which encompasses essential factors that influence simulation design, such as specific learning objectives (SLOs), how the SBLE fits within the larger curriculum, and required resource allocation (Jeffries et al., 2015). Design, in this theory, specifically refers to the task of developing the SBLE from developing appropriate and SLOs to designing a scenario with the right content and complexity to achieve those objectives. Design decisions also include fidelity decisions, such as factors that influence physical fidelity (realism of all aspects of the environment), conceptual fidelity (all aspects of simulation relate in a way that is realistic), and psychological fidelity (perceived realism such that it evokes learners' beliefs, emotions, and self-awareness as it would in a real-world setting; Jeffries et al., 2015; Lioce et al., 2020).

The NLN Jeffries Simulation Theory recognizes that there is a dynamic relationship between the facilitators and the participants that is influenced by the characteristics each individual brings to the interaction. Participants bring their age, gender, experience, knowledge, and biases, as well as anxiety and self-confidence. Facilitators bring many attributes that influence the simulation experience, including their skill and experience as well as the educational strategies (i.e., feedback, cues) they employ during the SBLE (Jeffries et al., 2015).

The final key construct in the theory is outcomes. A change from the original framework is the organization of outcomes into participant-, patient-, and system-level outcomes. While the assessment of outcomes is beyond the scope of this chapter, designing an individual SBLE must include, at a minimum, clear expectations for desired learning outcomes at the participant level. Learning outcomes should be an extension of the learning objectives and clearly state

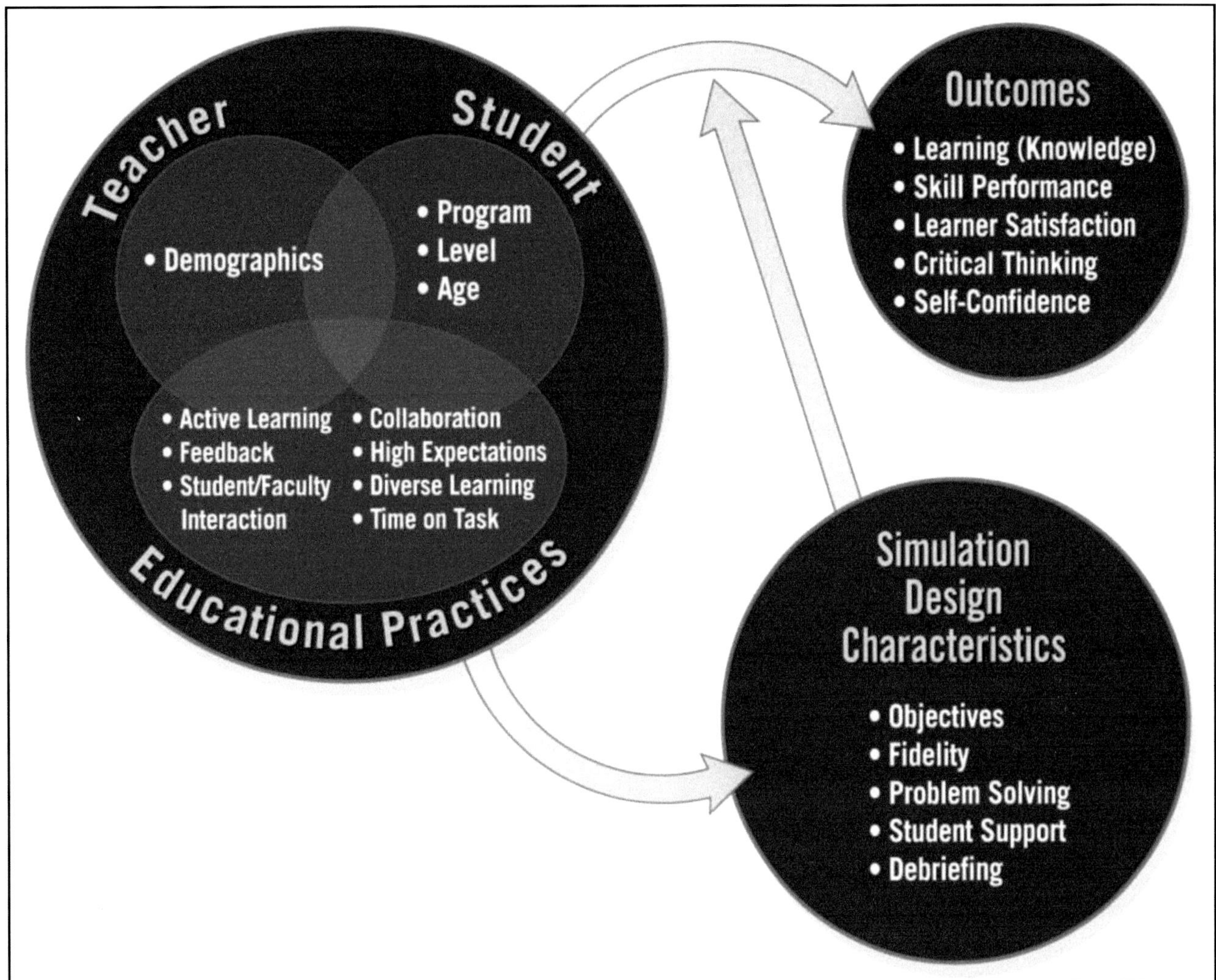

Figure 5-1. NLN/Jeffries Simulation Theory. (Reproduced with permission from Jeffries, P. R. [Ed.]. [2020]. *Simulation in nursing education: From conceptualization to evaluation* [3rd ed.]. National League for Nursing.)

what we hope the learners to be able to do as a result of the simulation experience. However, as educators and clinicians, most individuals in CSD designing SBLEs are also considering the potential for the learning experience to result in improved outcomes at the patient and system levels as well.

Best Practice Guidelines

Best practices in simulation in CSD are guided by the evidence from other health professions, primarily nursing and medicine, with extensive bodies of evidence and guidelines. The International Nursing Association for Clinical Simulation and Learning (INACSL) published evidence-based guidelines in 2016 of best practice for implementation and use of simulation in nursing. These comprehensive guidelines are living documents that outline all aspects of a simulation from design to facilitation to evaluation. The purpose of the INACSL Standards is to ensure that educators designing and implementing SBLEs are doing so in a way that is grounded in the evidence of what makes the methodology effective for learning. As stated on their website, "The International Nursing Association for Clinical Simulation and Learning (INACSL) has developed the INACSL Standards of Best Practice™: Simulation to advance the science of simulation, share best practices, and provide evidence-based guidelines for implementation and training" (INACSL, n.d., para. 1). These guidelines, while written for nursing, apply to simulation-based education in CSD and other health professions as well.

The information presented in this chapter, and throughout this text, aligns with the INACSL Standards. This chapter specifically references the standards of Simulation Design, Outcomes and Objectives, Facilitation, and Debriefing. Any educator interested in implementing simulation must familiarize themselves with all of the best practice guidelines because the methodology is only as effective as the quality of its implementation.

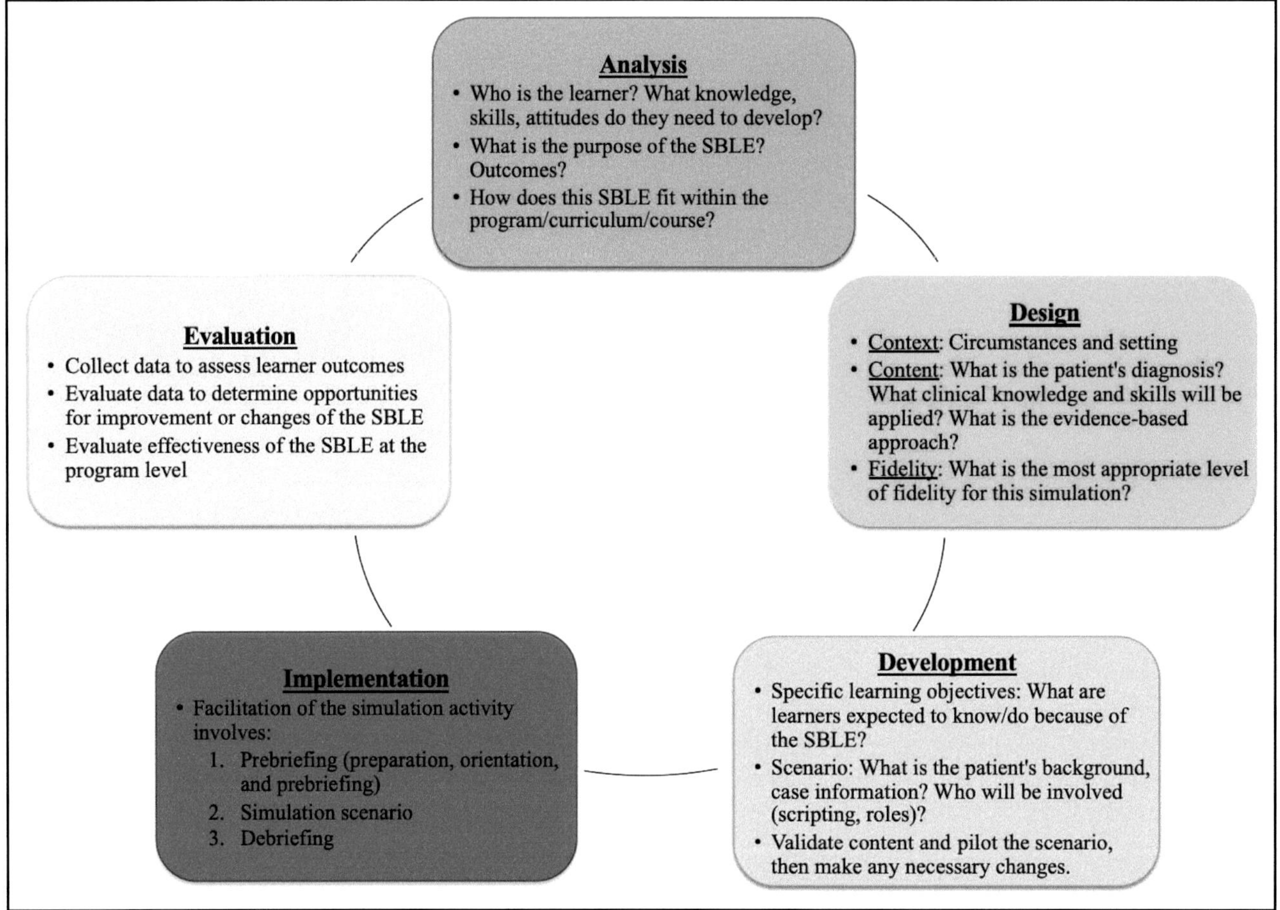

Figure 5-2. ADDIE model and SBLE design. (Adapted from Kurt, S. [2017]. ADDIE model: Instructional design. Educational Technology. https://educationaltechnology.net/the-addie-model-instructional-design/)

Instructional Design Model

In instructional design, there is a commonly used model for designing learning experiences known as the *ADDIE model* (Kurt, 2017; Wang & Hsu, 2009). ADDIE is a simple and flexible design model made up of five phases: analysis, design, development, implementation, and evaluation. Figure 5-2 illustrates how the ADDIE model is useful for developing SBLEs because it provides a systematic process for approaching design focused on developing effective learning experiences that achieve targeted outcomes (Kurt, 2017; Robinson & Dearmon, 2013). The phases are not discrete and will overlap as the process unfolds, but it is important that it is iterative and that as the educator gathers information or makes decisions about the design, they consider the whole picture to be sure everything aligns to achieve the purpose of the SBLE. ADDIE is one of several instructional design models that are applicable to designing SBLEs (see Chapter 2). Regardless of the instructional design model, educators must first consider the SLOs (e.g., what will the learner be able to do at the end of the SBLE?) and design a quality SBLE to achieve those desired learning objectives.

Analyze

The first phase of the ADDIE model is to analyze. Prior to designing and developing an SBLE, it is critical to first analyze the need for the SBLE. This phase is similar to conducting a needs assessment. This process will help to identify the learners and define the overarching purpose by asking who the learners are and what they need to know? It is also important to understand who the learners are by looking at their curriculum and analyzing their knowledge, skills, and experience at this point in their program. Understanding these factors will guide decisions made regarding the complexity of the SBLE based on the learners' knowledge and skills.

Design and Development

Design, guided by the completed analysis, involves situating the SBLE within the curriculum and considering the desired outcomes. Designing an SBLE that is too complex or with learning objectives that are not appropriate for the learners' level will set the learners up for failure and frustration. Ideally, SBLEs are designed to create a supportive learning experience through identifying the right simulated context for the objectives that challenge learners to meet achievable expectations (Robinson & Dearmon, 2013). It is in this design phase that the educator begins to determine what setting or circumstances would be appropriate, what content needs to be incorporated, and what technology or level of fidelity would be necessary to achieve the overall purpose of the simulation. When designing SBLEs at the course and event level, focus must be on selecting the appropriate mode to achieve the desired outcomes. By selecting the appropriate technology and context the educator sets the learners up for success (Robinson & Dearmon, 2013).

The design and development phases often overlap, and there is often much evaluation and revision as the SBLE begins to take shape. An acronym that Robinson and Dearmon (2013) suggest may be helpful for new educators as they begin the design and development phases of the process is I-CARE. This acronym can help you to remember key elements to include in the SBLE design and development. I-CARE stands for:

- **I**nstructional design: Linking the learning objectives to teaching strategies and activities that are appropriate for the learners' level of knowledge and skills.
- **C**ontext: Context, such as situating the SBLE in the clinical environment, makes the SBLE meaningful for the learners and increases engagement in the learning process.
- **A**ttention: Selecting the appropriate mode of delivery based on the learning objectives, complexity, and fidelity will serve to hold learner's attention in the SBLE.
- **R**elevance: Connects with context to make the learning meaningful to the learner, which enhances the value of the activity and learner motivation.
- **E**valuation: In this stage of design and development, a systematic plan to evaluate learners should be formulated.

Implementation

The implementation phase includes requisite training for all personnel involved in the SBLE, clear communication, and explicit directions and expectations so that everyone is operating toward the same goal. During this stage, all aspects of the plan and details must be attended to while maintaining focus on the learning objectives. This attention to detail is critical to ensuring learners have the opportunity to engage and practice skills without cognitive disconnect resulting from errors in the environment.

Evaluation

The final key element of quality instructional design, as outlined by the ADDIE model, is the evaluation. Evaluation of simulation happens both at the curricular and individual event level and serves to inform and guide educators toward quality design of future SBLEs. Evaluation is a critical part of the design process. It is essential that educators also design *how* objectives will be measured and *how* learning will be evidenced when developing learning objectives and considering expected outcomes. Specific assessment and evaluation considerations are beyond the scope of this chapter but are discussed further in Chapter 6.

Design and Development

Whether you are new to simulation or have lots of experience, the ADDIE model and the NLN Jeffries framework (Jeffries, 2007) are a great place to start when designing and developing SBLEs. Thinking through the instructional design elements, including the evaluation plan, will support the development of high-quality learning experiences. "It is evident that without clear simulation design, the outcomes of learning, critical thinking, self-confidence, performance, or satisfaction cannot be achieved" (Waxman, 2010, p. 30).

Templates and checklists are available for designing simulations, which are particularly useful for educators new to designing and planning SBLEs (Alinier, 2011; NLN, 2019; Waxman, 2010). One such example is presented in Waxman (2010) and was designed by a California collaborative of simulation programs in an effort to support faculty in writing evidence-based scenarios. These guidelines, like those designed by others, walk developers through developing evidence-based learning objectives, planning assessment measures and instruments, identifying presimulation activities, and a debriefing plan. These guidelines for clinical simulation development include additional elements consistent with best practice guidelines, including validation of the scenario through peer review, testing or piloting of the scenario, and making needed adjustments before it is time to facilitate the SBLE with learners (Table 5-1).

The benefit of such templates is to provide a structure to the simulation plan and ensure that all of the key details are considered. Another example of a template that is helpful to use and aligns directly with the INACSL best practice standards for simulation was designed by a Certified Healthcare Simulation Educator (CHSE) at James Madison University in Harrisonburg, Virginia (Mullen, 2020). It is available in the Resources for Practice section at the end of this chapter. This template walks educators through the process of designing an SBLE by prompting for responses to each critical component of design. This ensures that the educator has considered all necessary components for a quality SBLE and has clearly outlined the simulation activity so that it can be run successfully and, ideally, replicated at a later time with more learners. It also ensures that all of the information that each member of the team (e.g., facilitator, operator, SP) has the information that they need to do their part to contribute to the success of the SBLE.

When designing an SBLE, educators must first consider the context for the simulation. What is the purpose of the simulation? Is it a formative or instructional experience? Is it

TABLE 5-1

Evidence-Based Guidelines for Clinical Simulation Scenario Development

CRITICAL ELEMENT	RATIONALE
Ensure that the learning objectives are defined. Develop clear, concise learning objectives.	Need a tool that guides learning. Objectives should be broad based. Should be based on the level of the student. Should reflect intended outcome of the experience. Should ask "what competencies are being trained?" Should allow student to integrate and use the theory they were taught in class. After simulation, objectives should be referenced in the debriefing.
Identify the level of fidelity (the extent to which a simulation mimics reality). There are three levels of sophistication (Seropian et al., 2004): high, moderate, and low.	If the purpose of the simulation is task training (e.g., intramuscular injection, nasogastric tube insertion), then a low-fidelity simulation should suffice. If the purpose of the simulation is to enhance critical thinking, communication, and certain skills, then high fidelity should be used.
Define level of complexity (problem solving).	Scenario needs to be appropriate to the experience level of the learner. Should be based on the knowledge and skill level of the learner. Try not to overload the scenario. Should this scenario be multidisciplinary?
Use evidence-based references.	Evidence drives practice. List all key references that serve as the theoretical foundation for the learning objectives. Scenarios should be peer reviewed.
Incorporate instructor prompts and cues.	Instructor should know when support and assistance should be provided by the facilitator. Assistance should be in the form of cues or prompts and guide learners to the path of discovery.
Allow adequate time for debriefing or guided reflection.	Needs to occur immediately after the scenario is completed. Try not to break sense of realism; timing and location are important. Adequate time needs to be allocated and should be at least as long as the scenario, if not twice as long. Session should be guided by an educator skilled in facilitation.

Reproduced with permission from Waxman K. T. (2010). The development of evidence-based clinical simulation scenarios: Guidelines for nurse educators. *Journal of Nursing Education*, *49*(1), 29-35. https://doi.org/10.3928/01484834-20090916-07

for the purpose of evaluating learners? How does this SBLE fit within the program or curriculum as well as an individual course or clinical placement? What setting or circumstances will be the foundation of the SBLE? Once the general purpose and outcomes have been determined, then the instructor must begin designing the specifics of the SBLE. The factors that must be considered in the design of an SBLE include the SLOs, content and complexity of the scenario, fidelity (physical, conceptual, psychological), and prebriefing and debriefing strategies (Jeffries et al., 2015; Lioce et al., 2020).

Learning Objectives

Once the overarching purpose or goal of the SBLE is established, context identified, and level of complexity determined, the next and arguably most critical step is to identify the SLOs. Up to this point, the focus has been on the broad goal and general purpose of the SBLE, so now it is time to detail what specific KSAs are expected to be learned and demonstrated during the SBLE. Developing clear and explicit learning objectives will define the desired outcome and, thereby, must guide all aspects of design. Typically, there are three to four learning objectives for an SBLE, but the exact number depends on the length and complexity of the scenario. The learning objectives should be appropriate for the learners' level and should connect with the purpose of the simulation. Bloom's taxonomy is the more commonly used framework in education for developing learning objectives. Bloom identifies three main learning domains: cognitive (critical thinking and problem solving), psychomotor (technical skills), and affective (behaviors) domains (Anderson et al., 2008). All three of these domains can be targeted during simulation learning.

When we have clear expectations of what successful learning looks like, based on clearly written objectives, then it is easier to develop an SBLE that will allow learners the opportunity to practice and refine clinical skills (Chatterjee & Corral, 2017; INACSL, 2016a). As clinicians and educators, many are familiar with the mnemonic SMART (specific, measurable, attainable, relevant, and time bound) when learning objectives or goals. Just as would be written for any educational and/or clinical activity, SMART objectives should be developed for SBLEs as well. It is also helpful to align the SBLE objectives with the course learning objectives and even with professional standards, which for CSD professionals in the United States would be the American Speech-Language-Hearing Association Standards for the Certificate of Clinical Competence in Audiology or Speech-Language Pathology (Council for Clinical Certification in Audiology and Speech-Language Pathology, 2018a, 2018b).

Content

Now that there is context for the SBLE and SLOs are written, it is time to develop the content for the SBLE. The content of an SBLE is driven by the SLOs and is situated in the context of the curriculum and course in which it is embedded. Typically, the content is presented as part of a scenario or case. The content should be relevant and appropriate for the learners and should be grounded in evidence of best practice in the field in order to ensure that quality intervention is reinforced through the SBLE that will later be translated to the clinical environments (Alinier, 2011). Further, the content of the SBLE should be authentic to ensure that learners are able to fully engage in the simulation without cognitive disconnect. As outlined in the ADDIE design model in Figure 5-2, this requires selecting appropriate technologies and designing an SBLE with an appropriate level of fidelity to support the learner through the SBLE. It is essential that content-matter experts be involved in designing the SBLE and review the scenario to verify accuracy.

When writing the scenario, first start by creating the patient: who is this person and what is their relevant background? It can be helpful to draw from real patients to maintain a level of authenticity, but it is important to adapt details as necessary to meet the appropriate level of complexity for the learners. Who is the patient that will be seen and why are the learners being asked to see this patient (circumstances)? What is their backstory, including all aspects of relevant information (physical, social, emotional)? One strategy to reduce the burden of designing lots of cases for learners of different levels might be to develop one really rich case that can then be adapted or pulled from to meet different learning objectives. For example, you can create one patient that may have a scenario that is appropriate for an acute care visit but also have additional information about that patient post discharge that could be for learners working on follow-up care. Planning with the type of scaffolding and flexibility in mind may be challenging for those new to designing SBLEs but is a worthwhile endeavor as you gain experience.

The scenario should also include details such as writing out what will happen in the scenario and what will unfold (e.g., patient responses to questions asked, changes in status requiring the learners to react), as well as what the expected actions are of the learners. This is sometimes referred to as *scripting* as it is similar to planning out the script of a performance. It is important that the expected actions (what the learners should do in response to the patient's situation) fit with the scenario developed and align with EBP guidelines in order to reinforce good clinical skills. A key step when developing the content of the scenario is to have content experts review the case to validate the content and verify that expectations align with EBP (Alinier, 2011; INACSL, 2016a) to confirm the validity of the case and establish conceptual fidelity.

Logistics

Along with developing the content, it is also essential at this stage to make decisions about details such as the technologies that will be used, personnel required, moulage (use of makeup to enhance realism), allocation of resources, consumable materials needed, time and space requirements, scheduling, and so on. Focusing on every detail during the design and development stages will reduce unanticipated issues during implementation of the SBLE.

Once the overarching purpose and SLOs are determined, it is time to make decisions about the specific details of the SBLE that will meet those objectives. The decisions made during design and development should be guided by the SLOs and seek to create an authentic experience (fidelity) that will support students achieving those objectives.

First, it is critical to consider the space and resources available to you. Not everyone has access to high-fidelity human patient simulators, but that does not mean that you cannot design a rich, immersive learning experience. It is also not necessary to use high-tech simulators for every SBLE, so critical analysis of the most appropriate technology to meet the learning objectives is important. Just because the technology is cool or fancy does not mean that it is necessary. As designers of learning experiences, it is important to create SBLEs that are effective in meeting stated objectives while being good stewards of available resources.

Another key decision when considering logistics is what configuration the SBLE will take. For example, will it take place virtually or face to face? Will it be episodic (one case that will be completed from start to finish during one SBLE), unfolding (a case that will evolve over time, potentially multiple encounters, with new situations that arise for the learners to respond to), or concurrent (one SBLE in a series of related SBLEs)? It is also important that all essential personnel are identified. A qualified facilitator who is knowledgeable of both the content and simulation (including how to prebrief and debrief effectively) must be identified. If the technology being employed requires operation, then a qualified simulation operator is needed. Any additional personnel, such as an SP, must also be identified and trained appropriately. The preparation and training of SPs is beyond the scope of this chapter, but the literature is rich with resources to assist those interested in planning an SBLE with an SP. The Association of Standardized Patient Educators (https://www.aspeducators.org/) offers standards of best practice related to SPs.

Pilot

At this point, the analysis, design, and development phases of the ADDIE design model have been completed. The SBLE context, content, and fidelity have all been determined. But before deploying the SBLE with a group of learners, it is important—and essential according to INACSL Standards (INACSL, 2016a)—that the new SBLE be piloted. During this pilot, which is much like a dress rehearsal, the scenario would be run from beginning to end. The purpose of this step prior to implementing the SBLE with learners is to take an opportunity to evaluate and revise any details that would enhance the learners' experience. Some things to consider when piloting the SBLE may include:

- Did everyone involved in running the SBLE (facilitator, SPs, operator) know and perform their role effectively? Is additional training needed?
- Were the learners provided with ample opportunity to practice skills, apply knowledge, and achieve the learning objectives?
- Is the environment and physical fidelity appropriate for the context of the SBLE?
- Are there risks to psychological safety that need to be examined?
- Does the sequence of events make sense?

Implementation and Facilitation

Simulation is a process comprising three essential components that do not exist independent of one another. The three components of every SBLE are (a) a prebriefing that sets the stage and orients participants to the purpose, equipment, roles, and objectives of the simulation; (b) the simulation scenario, which has been designed according to best practices and integrates EBP with clear learning objectives; and (c) a reflective debriefing that follows the SBLE during which a trained facilitator engages participants in learning through reflection. The facilitator conducts the prebriefing, observes the entire scenario, intervenes as necessary, and guides the debriefing session. According to INACSL (2016b), the facilitator of an SBLE must have knowledge and skills in simulation pedagogy to competently support learners through these three phases at a level that is appropriate given the learner's level of experience. The facilitator is integral to the success of the SBLE and should be trained in simulation and according to whichever debriefing model is being used (INACSL, 2016b). Often the facilitator is an instructor or faculty who is likely a content expert in the areas relevant to the SBLE and has specific knowledge and skills in simulation. For facilitators who are new to simulation and/or debriefing, collaborating with a CHSE or other experienced simulationist can provide excellent mentoring to support the facilitator's learning. Further, INACSL (2016b) recommends formal coursework/training, as well as continuing education to develop and maintain skills to support learning in simulation.

A Three-Phase Model of Prebriefing

Learning how to facilitate a prebriefing in a way that is effective in supporting learner outcomes can be a challenge for educators who are preparing to facilitate SBLEs. One reason for this challenge is that there is a paucity of research about prebriefing methods, and even terminology in the literature lacks consistency (e.g., the prebriefing may also be called a briefing, introduction, or orientation; Chamberlain, 2015; McDermott, 2016; Page-Cutrara, 2015). Despite the fact that the prebriefing has received much less attention in the literature than other phases of simulation and simulation development, the prebriefing is supported as an essential component that establishes an orientation and sets out the expectations for the learners according to best practice guidelines (Chamberlain, 2015; Fanning & Gaba, 2007; INACSL, 2016b; Page-Cutrara, 2015).

Rudolph et al. (2014) suggest that the prebriefing should establish an environment in which learners experience a "deep level of connection to their motivations, each other, and the instructors" (p. 339) before the simulation begins. The facilitator has an ethical duty to establish a safe and confidential learning environment, one in which learners feel valued and respected (Fanning & Gaba, 2007). This can be achieved through a thorough prebriefing of the SBLE and the facilitator taking time during the prebriefing to observe the learners and begin to get to know them as individuals and as a group (Fanning & Gaba, 2007).

According to INACSL (2016b), the prebriefing should include preparatory activities before the SBLE and several components meant to prepare learners for the scenario while establishing trust between the instructor and learners and among the group of learners themselves. While there is not a set protocol or procedures for a prebriefing, Criterion 3 of the INACSL (2016b) Facilitation Standard outlines essential components. The checklist in Figure 5-3 includes these components.

A recent concept analysis of the prebriefing literature suggests the need for a structured prebriefing model that includes all necessary components required to prepare learners for the simulation activity and is also grounded in learning theory and the work of others (Ludlow, 2020; McDermott, 2016). These three phases (preparatory, orientation, and prebriefing) incorporate all of the essential prebriefing components according to INACSL guidelines in a manner that supports success (Ludlow, 2020).

The first phase of prebriefing is the preparatory phase. This phase addresses the cognitive domain and is where learners will prepare for the SBLE. It may take place just prior to, or even days before, the SBLE. Facilitators should provide learners with any necessary readings, videos, lectures, or other materials that may be necessary or helpful as learners prepare for the simulation activity. This information is not intended to give them the answers or tell them what to expect in the simulation, but rather to ensure all learners come into the SBLE with the same foundation upon which they can build their learning (INACSL, 2016b; Ludlow, 2020).

The orientation phase involves the hands-on (psychomotor domain) orientation to the simulation space and equipment in an effort to reduce additional distractions or stress during the simulation activity. For learners new to simulation, providing a video about what the simulation is and what to expect when they arrive at the simulation laboratory is also helpful as a preorientation. During the orientation phase, learners may also practice skills, explore the environment, and familiarize themselves with any technology or equipment in the space allowing them to focus their energy and attention during the scenario on problem solving and making decisions rather than on managing the environment (INACSL, 2016b; Ludlow, 2020).

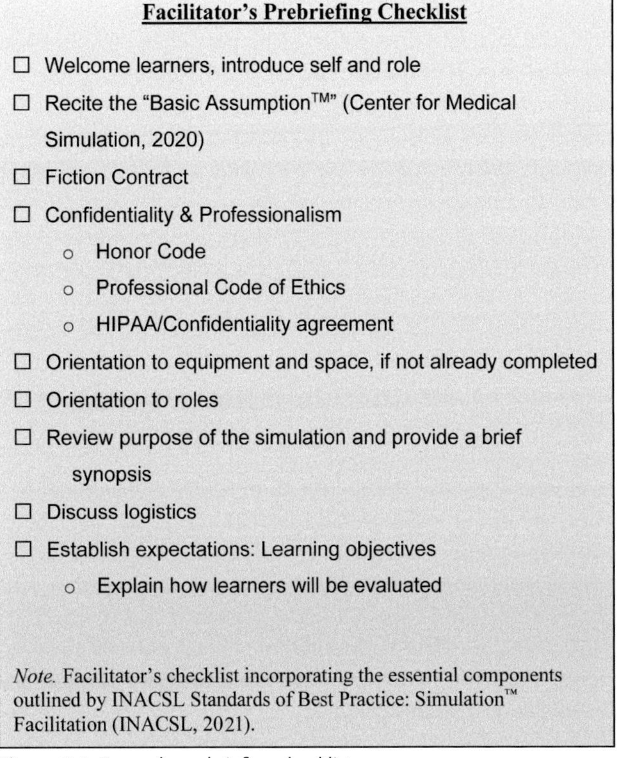
Facilitator's Prebriefing Checklist

- ☐ Welcome learners, introduce self and role
- ☐ Recite the "Basic Assumption™" (Center for Medical Simulation, 2020)
- ☐ Fiction Contract
- ☐ Confidentiality & Professionalism
  - Honor Code
  - Professional Code of Ethics
  - HIPAA/Confidentiality agreement
- ☐ Orientation to equipment and space, if not already completed
- ☐ Orientation to roles
- ☐ Review purpose of the simulation and provide a brief synopsis
- ☐ Discuss logistics
- ☐ Establish expectations: Learning objectives
  - Explain how learners will be evaluated

Note. Facilitator's checklist incorporating the essential components outlined by INACSL Standards of Best Practice: Simulation™ Facilitation (INACSL, 2021).

Figure 5-3. Example prebriefing checklist.

The final phase of prebriefing is where the affective domain is addressed and where facilitators work to establish a safe learning environment. The role of the prebriefing process is to protect psychological safety and trust and establish an agreement to suspend disbelief while engaging professionally in the SBLE as if it were a real visit with a real patient (Center for Medical Simulation, 2020; INACSL, 2016b). This involves establishing expectations, reviewing essential components of the prebriefing plan, and introducing the case information. This final phase is critical for creating an environment in which learners feel safe to learn and can help reduce their anxiety (Alinier, 2011; INACSL, 2016b; Ludlow, 2020).

Discussing ground rules, establishing a noncompetitive environment, and acknowledging that mistakes will happen in the SBLE and be discussed in the debriefing will all contribute to creating the safe learning environment learners need to feel secure enough to take risks in the scenario. Another required element of the prebriefing phase is the fiction contract, which acknowledges that the environment is simulated and, so, while the best efforts are made to make the experience as authentic as possible, there may still be differences in the simulation environment (i.e., a manikin cannot swallow). This agreement among the learners, facilitator, and all involved in the simulation is a commitment everyone makes to suspend disbelief and accept the simulation as real. In order to create a psychologically safe environment, the Center for Medical Simulation (2020) at Harvard recommends that learners agree on a core value known as the *Basic Assumption* that states, "We believe that everyone participating in activities at [insert your institution here] is intelligent, capable, cares about doing their best, and wants to improve" (para. 1). To reinforce the importance of professionalism throughout the simulation activity and treating the situation as real, it is helpful to review the Health Insurance Portability and Accountability Act and even have learners sign a confidentiality agreement that aligns with Health Insurance Portability and Accountability Act, professional organization standards, and any other relevant honor codes (i.e., university integrity policy).

Once trust has been established, the facilitator should then, at a minimum, review necessary background information and SLOs and address any questions the learners may have, including ways they may meet the objectives in the scenario. Learners should be assigned roles in the SBLE. Assigning roles and sharing clear descriptions of each of those roles supports learners in focusing during the scenario on the tasks within their role. Logistics are also covered in the prebriefing (e.g., how to contact others if needed during the scenario, time to prepare before beginning the simulation, how the learners will be informed that the scenario has ended).

This process of prebriefing should also establish psychological safety, allowing learners to feel confident in taking risks during the scenario. When learners feel secure and willing to take risks in the scenario, they are able to reflect on their decisions and actions, correct and repeat behaviors while learning from their mistakes, and be comfortable with uncertainty and not knowing the answers (Rudolph et al., 2014).

Simulation Scenario

The simulation scenario is the part of the SBLE where learners engage in the simulation activity following the case and content that was designed and developed to meet the stated learning objectives. Following the prebriefing, the facilitator will provide the learners with clear instructions to begin the scenario. During the simulation scenario the facilitator needs to attend to the learners' actions in order to be able to provide cues, which may have been anticipated in the design of the simulation (e.g., the nurse entering the room with additional information) or unplanned (e.g., the facilitator notices the learners are way off track and calls into the room as the nurse to provide information to redirect their efforts). The facilitator must have enough skills and knowledge in simulation pedagogy, as well as background of the simulation content, to be able to provide the feedback and cues needed in order to help learners meet the objectives. This time spent by the facilitator observing the scenario also provides necessary observations and information to be able to effectively guide the debriefing session (Dieckmann et al., 2010; INACSL, 2016b). Simulation scenarios usually last between 20 and 30 minutes, or less, long enough to address the developed learning objectives.

Debriefing

The debriefing has long since been held as the most important part of simulation. This assertion is in large part because debriefing engages learners in active reflection about an experiential learning situation, which aligns with methods and preferences for adult learners (Fanning & Gaba, 2007; Gardner, 2013; INACSL, 2016c; Sawyer et al., 2016; Wang, 2011). Shinnick et al. (2011) suggest that "learning does not occur primarily or exclusively in the hands-on portion of the HFS [high-fidelity simulation] experience, and the debriefing component is the most valuable in producing gains in knowledge" (p. e109). In debriefing, learners are tasked with reflecting on the simulation experience. Learners should not only be challenged with what went well and what could be improved but also consider how the simulation scenario might apply to other clinical situations or settings (Fanning & Gaba, 2007; INACSL, 2016c; Shinnick et al., 2011; Voyer & Hatala, 2015). This time spent reflecting on the simulation experience and integrating what they learned with other knowledge and experiences supports the development of clinical reasoning and critical thinking (Dreifuerst et al., 2014; Shinnick et al., 2011).

Role of the Facilitator in the Debriefing

The benefit of a facilitated debriefing in simulation is that the facilitator guides learners through this process to use their reflection and discussion in order to achieve meaningful learning. By having a trained facilitator guiding the debriefing, learners are able to describe and react to experience, identify any emotions involved by exploring how they felt during the scenario, and then consider differences among each member of the group. This process aids them in achieving learning by being able to reflect on their own and others' perspectives and apply those to real-life clinical situations, which is ultimately the goal of simulation-based learning (Fanning & Gaba, 2007).

The facilitator sets the stage and establishes expectations for the debriefing. These expectations are aligned with the ground rules established during the prebriefing (Fanning & Gaba, 2007). This means that the facilitator must uphold the commitment made during the prebriefing to maintain a safe and open learning environment. The facilitator should remind the learners of their role in the debriefing process, introduce the debriefing framework that will be utilized, and share how the session will proceed. Skilled facilitators will encourage learners to share their honest, genuine thoughts and feelings about the performance within the scenario. The facilitator's role is to structure and guide the debriefing so that learners have an opportunity to vent their feelings and provide feedback about the scenario experience. A well-trained facilitator allows learners enough time to express themselves while keeping the discussion focused on the learning objectives and outcomes (Sawyer et al., 2016).

Time and Place of the Debriefing

Criterion 2 of the INACSL (2016c) Debriefing standard requires that the debriefing occur in an "environment that is conducive to learning and supports confidentiality, trust, open communication, self-analysis, feedback, and reflection" (p. s22). Typically, the debriefing takes place immediately following the scenario and in a space, such as a conference room, that is separate from where the simulation scenario occurred. Debriefing right after the end of the scenario is best because the experience is fresh in the learners' minds and they are best able to recall and reflect on their actions in the simulation. The purpose of removing the learners from the simulation environment for the debriefing is to allow them a private, confidential space to diffuse tensions and emotions from the scenario while creating an environment conducive to reflection (Dreifuerst et al., 2014; Fanning & Gaba, 2007).

There are some simulation activities where debriefing may be conducted in situ (in the environment and within the event, rather than post-event) such as for situations focused on teaching a technical skill or if immediate feedback regarding team communication or performance is required (Fanning & Gaba, 2007). In situ debriefing may also be beneficial if there are significant concerns about the progression of the scenario and a time-out is needed to help get the learners back on track (Sawyer et al., 2016). There may also be situations in which a debriefing immediately after the scenario is not possible, such as with some self-paced computer-based simulations; however, debriefing remains an essential component. In the cases when debriefing is not immediate, learners will typically receive feedback during the simulated experience that provides formative feedback to guide their learning. Additionally, having learners complete their own individual written or recorded reflections allows them to reflect on the simulated experience and report their immediate impressions. This may then be followed at a later time by an in-person, structured, reflective debriefing facilitated by a simulation educator. Recent literature also indicates that additional possibilities for effectively debriefing computer-based or virtual simulated experiences, other than immediate face-to-face debriefings, include synchronous virtual debriefings, asynchronous debriefings, computer debriefing, and self-debriefing (Atthill et al., 2021; Luctkar-Flude et al., 2021; Verkuyl, Atack, et al., 2018; Verkuyl, Lapum, et al., 2018).

Components of the Debriefing

According to Lederman (1992) there are seven elements of the debriefing process: (a) the debriefer/facilitator, (b) the participants/learners, (c) the simulation scenario, (d) the impact of the scenario on the learners, (e) learners' recollections, (f) mechanisms for learners to report about the scenario (e.g., written, verbal), and (g) time. All of these elements are integral to the debriefing process and the learner experience. Participants in the debriefing process must include, at a minimum, the facilitator and the learners. Literature has shown that the time between finishing the scenario and participating in the debriefing affects how learners perceive and report about the scenario (Anderson et al., 2008; Jeffries, 2007; Waxman, 2010). Debriefing often takes place immediately after the scenario, but there may be situations where it is necessary for more time to lapse before the debriefing (Gardner, 2013). Elements four, five, and six all align with phases that occur during the debriefing discussion; most debriefing models have at least three phases (names of these phases vary widely) of the debriefing session (Fanning & Gaba, 2007; Gardner, 2013; Sawyer et al., 2016):

1. Reaction/decompression (the impact of the scenario)
2. Reflection/self-assessment (recollection)
3. Summarizing (reporting)

The debriefing process often allows learners an opportunity to emotionally decompress/react following the simulation scenario. They are invited to express any feelings or emotional responses to the simulation without judgment. It is important to realize that simulation is a stressful experience for many learners, especially those new to simulation or if the scenario is particularly challenging or emotionally charged. It is essential to allow learners a safe place to acknowledge and release those feelings and emotions so that they may more effectively engage in the reflection. This is a critical stage of the debriefing, but it is the facilitator's job to ensure that learners do not become so stuck in the venting of their own individual emotional reactions that they are unable to move on to participating effectively in self-reflection.

Most simulation debriefings include a time where learners and the facilitator collaborate in analyzing the scenario and decisions made during the simulation. This reflection stage is learner centered and focuses on what the learners did during the simulation and why they made specific decisions based on the situation and patient condition (Sawyer et al., 2016). The goal is to identify the learners' thought processes by having focused discussion of specific actions during the scenario. This can be an opportunity to reinforce quality clinical judgment when a learner's actions fit with the patient's needs. Or it can reveal a misalignment of a learner's actions in response to cues within the scenario indicating that their frame (thought process) needs to be refined. One example of how a facilitator can do this is by using what is referred to as the *action inquiry approach*. This approach is used in the Debriefing with Good Judgment model (Rudolph et al., 2007) and employs specific observations of actions taken during the scenario and asks an open-ended question about the learners' actions in order to reveal the learners' frames of thought during that moment in the simulation.

Debriefing Methods

There are many debriefing methods in the literature, but no consensus on which method is the most effective, as all have been shown to benefit learning (Sawyer et al., 2016). There are commonalities between the methods as they evolve from what Fanning and Gaba (2007) refer to as the "natural order of human processing: to experience an event, to reflect on it, to discuss it with others, and learn and modify behaviors based on the experience" (p. 117).

Table 5-2 provides a list of some commonly used models of debriefing. Educators interested in facilitating SBLEs are referred to the cited sources for more details and are encouraged to seek training for how to debrief effectively. Some associations and resources for training in debriefing are listed in the section Resources for Practice.

Summary of Learning

Regardless of what model of debriefing is being used, it is important for the facilitator to wrap up the debriefing session by helping learners to make connections between the simulation experience and real-life clinical practice. The ultimate goal of simulation-based education and SBLEs is to improve critical thinking and clinical judgment so that learners transfer the learned KSAs to practice. It should not be assumed that learners will do this naturally or intuitively; instructors must be explicit in helping learners to make connections between the SBLE and other authentic, clinical contexts. Taking a final opportunity to have learners state their takeaways and summarizing the debriefing points will aid learners in transferring the learning, and tie together their learning in the SBLE and future practice in a clinical environment.

TABLE 5-2

Examples of Commonly Used Debriefing Models

DEBRIEFING MODELS	PHASES
• 3D Model (Zigmont et al., 2011)	Defusing, Discovering, Deepening
• Debriefing for Meaningful Learning (Dreifuerst, 2015)	Engage, Explore, Explain, Elaborate, Evaluate, Extend
• Debriefing with Good Judgment (Rudolph et al., 2007)	Reactions, Analysis, Summary
• GAS (Phrampus & O'Donnell, 2013)	Gather, Analyze, Summarize
• Promoting Excellence and Reflective Learning in Simulation (PEARLS) (Eppich & Cheng, 2015)	Reactions, Description, Analysis, Summary
• Plus Delta (Gardner, 2013)	(+) strengths, what went well (-) weaknesses, opportunities for improvement

BOX 5-1

Resources for Training in Debriefing

- Center for Medical Simulation at Harvard: https://harvardmedsim.org/
- George Washington University Massive Open Online Course entitled "Essentials in Clinical Simulation Across the Health Professions" on Coursera: https://www.coursera.org/learn/clinicalsimulations
- HealthySimulation.com courses and webinars: https://learn.healthysimulation.com/
- International Nursing Association for Clinical Simulation and Learning (INACSL): https://www.inacsl.org/
- Mayo Clinic College of Medicine and Science, Multidisciplinary Simulation Centers: https://college.mayo.edu/academics/simulation-centers/courses/
- Society for Simulation in Healthcare: https://www.ssih.org/
- Stanford Medical Center for Immersive and Simulation-based Learning: https://med.stanford.edu/
- WISER Education and Simulation Improving Healthcare at University of Pittsburgh: https://www.wiser.pitt.edu

Summary

Like all quality teaching and learning, SBLEs require careful planning, design, and facilitation in order to consistently meet the learning objectives. SBLEs can be expensive and require resources (e.g., personnel, consumables, facilities), and therefore careful consideration of the most efficient and effective way to meet those learning objectives should be considered from the start. Not all learning requires simulation, and not all simulation needs to be high fidelity to be effective. By adopting a systematic approach to design, such as the ADDIE model and the NLN Jeffries Simulation Theory, as well as any of the design templates mentioned in this chapter, instructors can be confident in their ability to create effective SBLEs. Planning evaluation from the start will ensure that there is a clear plan to demonstrate outcomes and will also provide data to support improvements and enhancement of the SBLE.

Beyond a systematically designed simulation plan, successful SBLEs require skilled facilitation throughout the entire process, including the prebriefing, scenario, and debriefing. Faculty serving as facilitators should seek mentorship and training, such as those included in this chapter, in simulation and debriefing to develop the requisite skills to support student learning. Partnering with other skilled personnel (e.g., CHSE), SPs, and simulation operators will support the design and deployment of quality SBLEs through which students can develop critical thinking and clinical skills.

Resources for Practice

Designing a Simulation-Based Learning Experience for a Graduate Course

This section provides the reader with an in-depth example of integrating simulation into graduate coursework. It follows evidence-based best practices, including the development of SLOs, design of the SBLE, and the facilitation and debriefing processes. Refer to Clinard (2022) for a full description of the SBLE described in this section. The information is organized according to the ADDIE and SBLE design model depicted in Figure 5-2.

Analysis

Analyze, the first phase of the ADDIE model, requires the educator to consider the learners, their existing knowledge and skills, and identify the KSAs they are expected to require. The identified learners are students in the first year of a 2-year graduate program in speech-language pathology. The students are enrolled in a pediatric dysphagia course required in their curriculum. Students report a lack of confidence in working with pediatric patients with feeding and swallowing difficulties, particularly those who are medically complex. The SBLE addresses a gap in student knowledge and skills in working with infants in a medical setting such as a neonatal intensive care unit. The purpose of the SBLE is to increase learner confidence and skills in assessing a child's swallowing in a medical environment (Box 5-2).

The educator developed SLOs as the next step in the process. The SLOs developed for this SBLE are provided in Box 5-2. Note that the SLOs align with the cognitive, psychomotor, and affective learning domains. They are observable and directly related to the needs of the learners. Careful consideration must be given to this step because the learning objectives are critical in guiding all aspects of the simulation experience.

Design and Development

The design and development of the SBLE takes into consideration where it is situated within the curriculum (i.e., a graduate course on pediatric dysphagia) as well as the existing knowledge of the learners (i.e., anatomy and physiology of normal and abnormal swallow). Once the overarching purpose and SLOs are determined, it is time to make decisions about the specific details of the SBLE that will meet those objectives. The goal of this SBLE is for learners to gain confidence and skills assessing pediatric feeding and swallowing in a medical environment; therefore, it is important to create a simulated setting (i.e., hospital room, clinic room) that would immerse them in that environment. Selecting space with authentic sights, sounds, and equipment will help create physical/environmental fidelity to support learners in achieving the SLOs. Another objective of the SBLE is that learners will be able to communicate education to the parent/caregiver. To provide learners an opportunity to achieve this objective, an experienced nurse was utilized as an embedded participant, serving as the caregiver in this scenario.

The SBLE was designed as a hybrid simulation employing the use of a high-fidelity manikin and an embedded (standardized) patient. A high-fidelity manikin, Super Tory (Gaumard Scientific, 2017), was determined to be the most appropriate level of technology given the need for the learners to monitor and assess behavioral markers, such as color change, tone and activity, and sucking. The manikin was positioned in a hospital crib with blanket rolls to support positioning. Leads attached the manikin to a simulated telemetry unit so students could monitor and measure physiological markers, such as heart rate, respiratory rate, and oxygen saturation. Additional moulage that added to the physical fidelity included an IV in the manikin's hand, pulse oximeter, and a nasogastric tube in place.

A case scenario included sufficient detail to provide the learners with a plausible scenario that would allow them to meet the objectives of the SBLE. The simulation design template (Figure 5-4), was developed by a CHSE in the James Madison University School of Nursing (Mullen, 2020). This is aligned with best practice standards established by the INACSL and served as a guide for every aspect of the SBLE. This scenario presented the case of an infant born at 36 weeks' 5 days' gestation, who is now 2 weeks old and status-post gastroschisis repair. Medical background, birth history, and reason for referral were developed as part of the scenario. The role of the bedside nurse was carefully scripted to guide the student's learning. As specified in the INACSL best practice standards, the scenario was piloted by three experienced clinicians before full implementation. Changes were made to the case scenario based on feedback from the pilot.

Implementation

The students participated in a prebriefing, simulation scenario, and a reflective debriefing in accordance with best practices established by INACSL (2021).

Orientation and Prebrief

The day before the simulation, all learners participated in an orientation that included a brief video introduction to the simulation laboratory and the simulation process. Students were placed into groups of three and provided a hands-on orientation in the space where the simulation was to occur. Immediately prior to the simulation experience, each group of students participated in a prebriefing session. During the prebriefing, the groups were provided basic information about the case that included name, diagnosis, age, and reason for referral. Each member of the group was

BOX 5-2
Specific Learning Objectives

Overarching goal: Increase learner confidence and skills in assessing a child's swallowing in a medical environment.

Specific learning objectives: Through participating in this SBLE, learners will:

- Identify signs of distress in an infant during a bottle feeding (cognitive).
- Demonstrate the ability to adjust feeding interventions to support infant stability while eating from a bottle (psychomotor).
- Educate parents/caregivers about signs of distress and provide recommendations for safe feeding (affective, cognitive).

assigned a primary role within the simulation scenario (e.g., assessor, feeder, communicator) and engaged in a discussion about the expectations for each role.

Simulation Scenario

Students entered the simulation environment and were greeted by an embedded participant (SP) assuming the role of the bedside nurse. The nurse provided a report of the infant's case and status to the students, and indicated where they could locate items, such as bottles for feeding, in the room. Students had the opportunity to ask questions about the infant before the embedded participant exited the room. The students then collaborated in their primary roles to assess the infant's feeding readiness and complete the simulation scenario. At the end of the simulation scenario the embedded participant returned as the bedside nurse and the students communicated their findings and recommendations based on their assessment. The simulation scenario was concluded in under 20 minutes. The entire experience was recorded for later viewing.

Debrief

The debriefing occurred immediately following the simulation scenario. As indicated throughout this book, the debriefing process is a critical component of SBLEs precipitating student learning. The educator elected to use an action-inquiry approach to debriefing for this SBLE, specifically the Debriefing with Good Judgment model (Clinard, 2022; Rudolph et al., 2006, 2007). The debriefing session consisted of three phases: (a) the reaction, or decompression, phase allowed students to express their initial thoughts, feeling, and reactions following the simulation scenario; (b) the reflection phase engaged students in discussion using action-inquiry statements based on the scenario and their observed performance in an attempt to address any knowledge and performance gaps; and (c) the summary phase reviewed and summarized the learning objectives, addressed any final questions that the learners had, and discussed any additional knowledge or performance gaps. At the end of the summary phase, students were encouraged to reflect on the scenario and their performance to answer the question "If you could go back, what is one thing you would do differently?" For specific examples from the debriefing, refer to Box 5-3.

Evaluation

Student learners were evaluated at the start of their pediatric dysphagia course and also following completion of the SBLE. Knowledge of infant feeding readiness and assessment was assessed using a researcher-developed instrument. Students also completed confidence surveys that measured their self-efficacy assessing and managing infant oral feeding readiness. Confidence was measured at three time points: before coursework, following coursework but before the SBLE, and after the SBLE. Additionally, students completed an assessment measuring the effectiveness of the SBLE and their experience in simulation. These evaluation data were collected in alignment with best practices and as part of a larger study for publication (Clinard, 2022).

This example highlights aspects of the development, design, and facilitation of an SBLE as discussed throughout this chapter. High-quality simulation learning requires systematic planning, intention, and adherence to best practices. Use of templates and resources to guide the design and facilitation will ensure that alignment and support learners in achieving the SLOs.

Simulation Design Template

JMU School of Nursing

Simulation Foci	What is the topic or course focus?
Modality/Pilot (Standard: Design, criterion 11)	What simulation modalities are available (manikin-based, SP, hybrid, telesimulation)? *Consider course objectives, learning outcomes, academic level, and alignment with curriculum. *ALL new simulations are piloted with representative groups prior to implementation. Select modality/technology and make a plan to pilot new SBLE
Cohort (Standard: Design, criterion 2)	Identify the learner level/cohort characteristics
Interprofessional (Standard: Sim Enhanced-IPE)	Indicate if the experience is interprofessional/interdisciplinary and list competencies being addressed.
Professional Integrity (Standard: Professional Integrity)	We stand against injustice and systemic racism in all its forms. We have a responsibility to act with empathy and inclusiveness to reduce inequities. We pledge to respond against discrimination, violence, and racism with advocacy and collective action. Simulation templates undergo an equity-minded review of content to ensure we are upholding this commitment. ☑
Purpose (Standard: Design, criterion 2)	☐ Promote readiness for clinical practice ☐ Address competencies ☐ Improve quality of care and patient safety ☐ Enhance curriculum in the classroom and/or clinical areas ☐ Provide opportunities for standardized clinical experiences
Fidelity (Standard: Design, criterion 6)	**<u>Physical Fidelity</u>:** Degree to which simulation looks, sounds, & feels like the actual task. *high-fidelity manikin, acute care equipment and supplies, simulated EHR, information technology, diagnostic equipment* **<u>Conceptual Fidelity:</u>** Ensures that all elements of the scenario relate to each other in a realistic way so that the case makes sense, as a whole, to the learner(s) *designed by CHSE, reviewed by content expert, case and moulage aligns with clinical situation.* **<u>Psychological Fidelity</u>:** Extent to which the simulated environment evokes the underlying psychological processes necessary in the real-world setting. *clinical judgment, time pressure, competing priorities, documentation*
Needs Assessment: (Standard: Design, criterion 2)	Spheres of care, concepts, domains, competencies, subcompetencies addressed
Outcomes, Objectives, Competencies (Standard: Design, criterion 3) (Standard: Outcomes and Objectives)	<u>Simulation Outcomes/Objectives:</u> • Develop 3-4 specific, measurable learning objectives o What do you expect learners will gain by participating in this SBLE? o Use active verbs o Address learning domains (cognitive, psychomotor; affective) <u>Course Specific Objectives:</u> • How does this SBLE align with the course or program objectives? • Align with course objectives and/or professional standards
SBLE Structure (Standard: Design, criterion 4)	Prebrief ___minutes ➡ Scenario ___minutes ➡ Group debrief ___ minutes **Schedule**: as above **Space**: ☐ Virtual ☐ FTF **Structure:** ☐ Episodic ☐ Unfolding ☐ Concurrent ☐ Telesimulation

Mullen, L. (2023). Simulation Design Template. JMU School of Nursing

Figure 5-4. Sample simulation design template. (EHR=electronic health record.) (Adapted and reproduced with permission from Mullen, L. [2023]. Simulation design template [unpublished template], School of Nursing, James Madison University.) *(continued)*

JMU School of Nursing

Simulation Design Template

SBLE Preparation (Standard: Design, criterion 8)	How are students prepared for the SBLE experience?
Prebrief (Standard: Prebriefing) **Debrief** (Standard: Design, criterion 9) (Standard: The Debriefing Process)	**Prebrief:** Information or orientation session held prior to start of the SBLE; instructions of preparatory activities provided to learners (SSH Dictionary). Follow INACSL Healthcare Simulation Standards of Best Practice™ (HSSOBP™). Prebriefing to include purpose, objectives, expectations, role, and evaluation methods. **Debrief:** Collaborative session after the SBLE during which clinical judgment and critical thinking are fostered and the simulation experience is re-examined for the purpose of assimilating learning to future situations (SSH Dictionary). • What framework/model of debriefing will be applied? • Who will facilitate the debriefing and what qualifications do they have? • When will the group debriefing take place? Facilitators possess the necessary professional development according to the INACSL HSSOBP™ Professional Development

Evaluation
(Standard: Design, criterion 10)
(Standard: Evaluation of Learning and Performance)
	Learners:
	• How will learners be evaluated?
	  o Evaluation of meeting simulation objectives? Course objectives?
	  o Checklist of performance/actions in response to cues in the scenario?
	  o Formative v. summative feedback?
	• How will students be "graded" (Pass/Fail, narrative feedback only, grade)?
	
	SBLE:
	• SBLE Evaluation is used to strengthen the simulation experience, identify areas for faculty/facilitator professional development, and to assess the application of INACSL HSSOBP™. Should be conducted following the group debriefing.

Facilitation (Standard: Design, criterion 1/7) (Standard: Facilitation) (Standard: Professional Development)	**CHSE** • simulation design • simulation resources, support, & evaluation • embedded participant **Faculty** • prebrief/debrief • logistics • student evaluation **SPs (if applicable)** • patient • family member or caregiver
Orientation to the Simulated Environment (Standard: Design, criterion 8)	How will learners be oriented to the simulated environment (including simulator, equipment, location of supplies, and how to communicate if assistance is needed)?
Clinical Judgment Actions (Standard: Design, criterion 4/5)	Protocols for the facilitator and standardized participant, if applicable, outlining clinical judgment cues and learner expected clinical decisions. • What is the expected action of the learner based on the cues provided?
Faculty/Facilitator Role (Standard: Facilitation)	Developing a "Faculty Guidance" document can assist faculty in preparing for simulation. Role defined by institution based on available resources, expertise, and learning outcomes. For example • Review and provide preparation modules/resources/guidance documents • Perform group prebrief and debrief; serve as facilitator for the duration of the scenario • Assess simulation assignments, if applicable • Assign performance roles • Ensure completion of evaluation measures • Review logistics, capabilities/limitations of simulator, other institution-specific protocols
References *Include any professional standards that guide SBLE design & any relevant references for replication	Dickison, P., Haerling, K. & Lasater, K. (2019). Integrating the National Council State Boards of Nursing-Clinical Judgment Model (NCSBN-CJM) into Nursing Educational Frameworks. *Journal of Nursing Education, 58*(2), 72-78. INACSL Standards Committee. (2021). Healthcare Simulation Standards of Best Practice™. *Clinical Simulation in Nursing,* https://www.inacsl.org/healthcare-simulation-standards

Mullen, L. (2023). Simulation Design Template. JMU School of Nursing

Figure 5-4 (continued). Sample simulation design template. (Adapted and reproduced with permission from Mullen, L. [2023]. Simulation design template [unpublished template], School of Nursing, James Madison University.)

BOX 5-3

Examples From an Action Inquiry Debriefing

Action observed by the facilitator: "I noticed when the baby's respiratory rate increased from 54 to 72 breaths per minute, the team discussed what to do and decided to stop the feeding."

Inquiry: "Were there other options that you discussed that may have supported continued successful feeding?"

Reframe: "Yes, you're correct that repositioning the baby and even taking a break to burp the baby would have been great options to reestablish physiologic stability before continuing the feeding."

Action observed by the facilitator: "When you were talking to the parent about your recommendations, I noticed that she didn't respond to much that you said. She seemed disengaged."

Inquiry: "What do you think she was feeling?"

Reframe: "I agree that she may have felt overwhelmed. It is a stressful time and a lot of information to process. I wonder how you could engage her in learning the strategies to successfully feed her baby?"

References

Adamson, K. A., & Rodgers, B. (2016). Systematic review of the literature for the NLN Jeffries simulation framework: Discussion, summary, and research findings. In P. R. Jeffries (Ed.) *The NLN Jeffries simulation theory* (pp. 9-37). Wolters Kluwer.

Alinier, G. (2011). Developing high-fidelity health care simulation scenarios: A guide for educators and professionals. *Simulation and Gaming, 42*(1), 9-26. https://doi.org/10.1177/1046878109355683

Anderson, J. M., Aylor, M. E., & Leonard, D. T. (2008). Instructional design dogma: Creating planned learning experiences in simulation. *Journal of Critical Care, 23*(4), 595-602. https://doi.org/10.1016/j.jcrc.2008.03.003

Association of Standardized Patient Educators. (n.d.) Home. https://www.aspeducators.org/

Atthill, S., Witmer, D., Luctkar-Flude, M., & Tyerman, J. (2021). Exploring the impact of a virtual asynchronous debriefing method after a virtual simulation game to support clinical-decision making. *Clinical Simulation in Nursing, 50,* 10-18. https://doi.org/10.1016/j.ecns.2020.06.008

Chamberlain, J. (2015). Prebriefing in nursing simulation: A concept analysis using Rodger's methodology. *Clinical Simulation in Nursing, 11*(7), 318-322. http://dx.doi.org/10.1016/j.ecns.2015.05.003

Chatterjee, D., & Corral, J. (2017). How to write well-defined learning objectives. *Journal of Education in Perioperative Medicine, 19*(4), 1-4.

Center for Medical Simulation. (2020). The basic assumption. https://harvardmedsim.org/resources/the-basic-assumption/

Clinard, E. S. (2022). Increasing student confidence with medically-complex infants through simulation: A mixed methods investigation. *American Journal of Speech-Language Pathology, 31*(2), 942-958. https://doi.org/ 10.1044/2021_AJSLP-21-00234

Council for Clinical Certification in Audiology and Speech-Language Pathology. (2018a). 2020 Standards for the Certificate of Clinical Competence in Audiology. American Speech-Language-Hearing Association. www.asha.org/certification/2020-Audiology-Certification-Standards/

Council for Clinical Certification in Audiology and Speech-Language Pathology. (2018b). 2020 Standards for the Certificate of Clinical Competence in Speech-Language Pathology. American Speech-Language-Hearing Association www.asha.org/certification/2020-SLP-Certification-Standards/

Cowperthwait, A. (2020). NLN/Jeffries Simulation Framework for simulated participant methodology. *Clinical Simulation in Nursing, 42*(C), 12-21. https://doi.org/10.1016/j.ecns.2019.12.009

Dieckmann, P., Lippert, A., Glavin, R., & Rall, M. (2010). When things do not go as expected: Scenario life savers. *Simulation in Healthcare, 5*(4), 219-225. https://doi.org/10.1097/SIH.0b013e3181e77f74

Dreifuerst, K. T., Horton-Deutsch, S. L., & Henao, H. (2014). Meaningful debriefing and other approaches. In P. R. Jeffries (Ed.) *Clinical simulations in nursing education: Advanced concepts, trends, and opportunities* (pp. 44-57). Wolters Kluwer.

Fanning, R. M., & Gaba, D. M. (2007). The role of debriefing in simulation-based learning. *Simulation in Healthcare, 2*(2), 115-125. https://doi.org/10.1097/SIH.0b013e3180315539

Gaba, D. M. (2004). The future vision of simulation in health care. *BMJ Quality & Safety, 13*(Suppl 1), i2-i10. https://doi.org/10.1136/qhc.13.suppl_1.i2

Gardner, R. (2013). Introduction to debriefing. *Seminars in Perinatology, 37*(3), 166-174. https://doi.org/10.1053/j.semperi.2013.02.008

Gaumard Scientific (2017). Super Tory S2220 [Newborn Simulator].

INACSL Standards Committee (2016a). INACSL standards of best practice: Simulation Simulation design. *Clinical Simulation in Nursing, 12,* S5-S50. https://doi.org/10.1016/j.ecns.2016.09.009

INACSL Standards Committee (2016b). INACSL standards of best practice: Simulation facilitation. *Clinical Simulation in Nursing, 12*(S), S16-S20. http://dx.doi.org/10.1016/ j.ecns.2016.09.007

INACSL Standards Committee (2016c). INACSL standards of best practice: Simulation debriefing. *Clinical Simulation in Nursing, 12*(S), S21-S25. http://dx.doi.org/10.1016/ j.ecns.2016.09.008

INACSL Standards Committee, Watts, P.I., McDermott, D.S., Alinier, G., Charnetski, M., & Nawathe, P.A. (2021, September). Healthcare Simulation Standards of Best Practice. *Simulation Design. Clinical Simulation in Nursing,* 58, 14-21. https://doi.org/10.1016/j.ecns.2021.08.009

International Nursing Association for Clinical Simulation and Learning. (n.d.). Healthcare Simulation Standards of Best Practice. https://www.inacsl.org/healthcare-simulation standards-of-best-practice/

Jansen, L. J. (2015). The benefits of simulation-based education. *SIG 10 Perspectives on Issues in Higher Education, 18*(1), 32-42. https://doi.org/10.1044/ihe18.1.32

Jeffries, P. R., Rodgers, B., & Adamson, K. (2015). NLN Jeffries Simulation Theory: Brief narrative description. In P. R. Jeffries (Ed.), *The NLN Jeffries simulation theory* (pp. 39-42). Wolters Kluwer.

Jeffries, P. R. (Ed.). (2007). *Simulation in nursing education: From conceptualization to evaluation.* National League for Nursing.

Kurt, S. (2017). ADDIE model: Instructional design. Educational Technology. https://educationaltechnology.net/the-addie-model-instructional-design/

Lederman, L. C. (1992). Debriefing: Toward a systematic assessment of theory and practice. *Simulation and Gaming 23*(2), 145-160. https://doi.org/10.1177/1046878192232003

Lioce, L., Lopreiato, J., Downing, D., Chang, T. P., Robertson, J. M., Anderson, M., Diaz, D. A., & Spain, A. E. (Eds.), & the Terminology and Concepts Working Group. (2020). *Healthcare simulation dictionary* (2nd ed.). Agency for Healthcare Research and Quality. https://doi.org/10.23970/simulationv2

Luctkar-Flude, M., Tyerman, J., Verkuyl, M., Goldsworthy, S., Harder, N, Wilson-Keates, B., Kruizinga, J., & Gumapac, N. (2021). Effectiveness of debriefing methods for virtual simulation: A systematic review. *Clinical Simulation in Nursing, 57*, 1-13. https://doi.org/10.1016/j.ecns.2021.04.009

Ludlow, J. (2020). Prebriefing: A principle-based concept analysis. *Clinical Simulation in Nursing. 56*, 22-28. https://doi.org/10.1016/j.ecns.2020.11.003

McDermott, D. S. (2016). The prebriefing concept: A Delphi study of CHSE experts. *Clinical Simulation in Nursing, 12*(6), 219-227. https://doi.org/10.1016/j.ecns.2016.02.001

Mullen, L. (2020). *Simulation design template* [Unpublished template]. School of Nursing, James Madison University.

National League of Nursing. (2019). Simulation design template. http://www.nln.org/sirc/sirc-resources/sirc-tools-and-tips

Page-Cutrara, K. (2015). Prebriefing in nursing simulation: A concept analysis. *Clinical Simulation in Nursing, 11*(7), 335-340.

Rizzolo, M. A., Durham, C. F., Ravert, P. K., & Jeffries, P. R. (2016). History and evolution of the NLN Jeffries simulation theory. In P. R. Jeffries (Ed.), *The NLN Jeffries simulation theory* (pp. 1-7). Wolters Kluwer.

Robinson, B. K., & Dearmon, V. (2013). Evidence-based nursing education: Effective use of instructional design and simulated learning environments to enhance knowledge transfer in undergraduate nursing students. *Journal of Professional Nursing, 29*(4), 203-209. https://doi.org/10.1016/j.profnurs.2012.04.022

Rudolph, J. W., Raemer, D. B., & Simon, R. (2014). Establishing a safe container for learning in simulation: The role of the presimulation briefing. *Simulation in Healthcare, 9*(6), 339-349. https://doi.org/10.1097/SIH.0000000000000047

Rudolph, J. W., Simon, R., Rivard, P., Dufresne, R. L., & Raemer, D. B. (2007). Debriefing with good judgment: Combining rigorous feedback with genuine inquiry. *Anesthesiology Clinics, 25*(2), 361-376. https://doi.org/10.1016/j.anclin.2007.03.007

Sawyer, T., Eppich, W., Brett-Fleegler, M., Grant, V., & Cheng, A. (2016). More than one way to debrief: A critical review of healthcare simulation debriefing methods. *Simulation in Healthcare, 11*(3), 209-217. https://doi.org/10.1097/SIH.0000000000000148

Shinnick, M. A., Woo, M., Horwich, T. B., & Steadman, R. (2011). Debriefing: The most important component in simulation? *Clinical Simulation in Nursing, 7*(3), e105-e111. https://doi.org/10.1016/j.ecns.2010.11.005

Voyer, S., & Hatala, R. (2015). Debriefing and feedback: Two sides of the same coin? *Simulation in Healthcare, 10*(2), 67-68. https://doi.org/10.1097/SIH.0000000000000075

Verkuyl, M., Atack, L., McCulloch, T., Liu, L., Betts, L., Lapum, J. L., Hughes, M., Mastrilli, P., & Romaniuk, D. (2018). Comparison of debriefing methods after a virtual simulation: An experiment. *Clinical Simulation in Nursing, 19*, 1-7 https://doi.org/10.1016/j.ecns.2018.03.002

Verkuyl, M., Lapum, J. L., Hughes, M., McCulloch, T., Liu, L., Mastrilli, P., Romaniuk, D., & Betts, L. (2018). Virtual gaming simulation: Exploring self-debriefing, virtual debriefing, and in-person debriefing. *Clinical Simulation in Nursing, 20*, 7-14. https://doi.org/10.1016/j.ecns.2018.04.006

Wang, E. E. (2011). Simulation and adult learning. *Disease-a-Month, 57*(11), 664-678. https://doi.org/10.1016/j.disamonth.2011.08.017

Wang, S.-K., & Hsu, H.-Y. (2009). Using ADDIE model to design second life activities for online learners. *Tech Trends, 53*, 76-81. https://doi.org/10.1007/s11528-009-0347-x

Waxman, K. T. (2010). The development of evidence-based clinical simulation scenarios: Guidelines for nurse educators. *Journal of Nursing Education, 49*(1), 29-35. https://doi.org/10.3928/01484834-20090916-07

Simulation Assessment and Evaluation

Julie M. Estis, PhD, CCC-SLP and David K. Brown, PhD, CCC-A

Simulation is a technique—not a technology—to replace or amplify real experiences with guided experiences that evoke or replicate substantial aspects of the real world in a fully interactive manner.
—Gaba (2004, p. i2)

As communication sciences and disorders (CSD) programs begin to design and implement simulation, the initial focus is often on the clinical scenario, patient disorder, or clinical skill that will be addressed. We plan what we are going to do and what the students are going to do, but it is critical that we also explore both the impact of the experience on the student and their perceptions of the simulation. By incorporating assessment and evaluation in simulation-based learning experiences (SBLEs) for speech-language pathology and audiology students, we are able to determine the level of performance achieved, provide meaningful feedback to the learner, and improve the quality of the learning experience.

Defining Assessment and Evaluation in Simulation-Based Learning Experiences

Though the terms *assessment* and *evaluation* are often used interchangeably, assessment focuses on gathering, analyzing, and interpreting evidence to determine how well student learning outcomes are met (Suskie, 2018). Evaluation adds a layer of judgment. That is, through the evaluation process, assessment evidence is interpreted and assessment results are used. For example, a checklist may be used to assess a learner's performance on a case history interview with a standardized patient (SP). The instructor may use that assessment checklist to evaluate the learner's performance and assign a course grade based on their achievement of the associated learning outcomes.

Dudding, C. C., & Ginsberg, S. M. (Eds.).
Simulation-Based Learning in Communication Sciences and Disorders: Moving From Theory to Practice. (pp. 91-102).

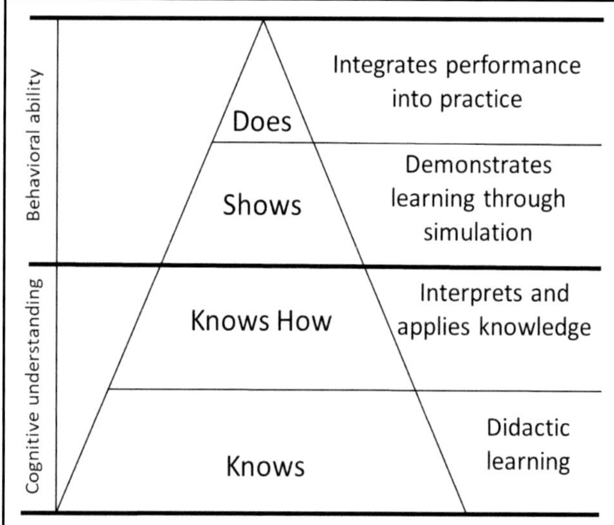

Figure 6-1. Miller's pyramid of competence shows the four levels of competency as they move up the pyramid from cognition to behavior. This pyramid shows the performance across abilities, skills, and knowledge. (Adapted from Miller, G. E. [1990]. The assessment of clinical skills/competence/performance. *Academic Medicine, 65*[9], S63-S67.)

Based on principles of learning assessment in general, there are several reasons assessment is important in this context (Suskie, 2018). Assessment provides insights on the quality of the SBLE and answers the question "Are we giving students the best possible education through this experience?" Through assessment, stewardship of resources may be improved as the utilization of resources to achieve the desired impact is explored. Also, accountability is a benefit of assessment as successes gained from the SBLE are determined and areas for improvement are identified. Meaningful assessment of SBLEs is carefully aligned with learning goals and competencies. It is based on research and best practices, and when conducted effectively, assessment leads to improved teaching, learning, and student success. It also provides evidence that learning has occurred and that evidence of competency has been observed (McGaghie et al., 1978; Scalese & Issenberg, 2008).

Assessment and evaluation are key components of simulation-based education frameworks and instructional design frameworks. Outcomes is a core construct of the National League of Nursing (NLN) Jeffries Simulation Theory (Jeffries et al., 2015) and includes the process of defining and measuring outcomes at the participant, patient, and system levels. The reader is referred to Figure 5-1 for the visual model of this theory. Evidence-based guidelines for simulation in nursing by the International Nursing Association for Clinical Simulation and Learning (INACSL Standards Committee et al., 2021) include participant evaluation as a key component. INACSL Standards require alignment of learning outcomes or intent of the simulation with the planned evaluation and elaborate three types of evaluation: formative, summative, and high stakes. The ADDIE model of instructional design described in Chapter 5 also emphasizes the importance of planning evaluation in the design process. As educators plan simulation activities that are linked to specific learning outcomes, defining how outcomes will be measured is essential.

Determining What Will Be Assessed by Defining Learner Outcomes

Throughout this book, we highlighted the importance of well-developed learning objectives to guide the development of the simulation experience. Learner objectives establish the aim or purpose of what we hope to do. Learner outcomes specify what learners will be able to do as a result of participating in the SBLE. Effective evaluation of SBLE participants hinges on clearly defining the intended learning outcomes for the experience and determining what evidence will be used to show if students met those intended outcomes. As elaborated in the following section, taxonomies are useful in defining learning outcomes of the SBLE that will be assessed.

Bloom's taxonomy was developed to evaluate learning in the domains of knowledge, skills, and attributes (KSAs). It was first described in the late 1950s but was subsequently revised 20 years ago (Anderson et al., 2001). The revised list includes a hierarchy of six levels: remembering, understanding, applying, analyzing, evaluating, and creating. As one moves up from the lower-order thinking skills (remembering) to the higher-order thinking skills and cognitive skills (evaluating and creating), they transition from knowledge acquisition to the synthesis of new ideas, such as generating hypotheses or planning a project (Novotny & Griffin, 2006; Thomas, 2016). These levels are often used to develop goals and objectives that can then be framed as learning outcomes. The outcomes can be reflected in the evaluation of the learning session. Simulation can be used as an evaluation tool since it uses both a controlled environment and experience with each learner (Wittmann-Price & Price, 2019).

Assessment occurs after a learner has had both didactic exposure and experience with a concept. The assessment allows the learner to demonstrate their level of competence in a particular area. This follows Miller's pyramid of competence (1990), where the learner works through the four levels or stages of the pyramid from knows to does. He suggested that there was not a single method of assessment that could provide all of the data required for assessing the entire delivery of health care services. As illustrated in Figure 6-1, Miller proposed a hierarchical structure with four levels, each having their own method of assessment. The lower two levels test a learner's knowledge or cognitive understanding but do not assess how they would behave in a real-life scenario (Miller, 1990). *Knows* and *knows how* are the foundational knowledge that can be assessed by written exams or multiple-choice questions. The top two levels look at the behavioral ability or competency. *Shows* and *does* is the clinical performance, where they look at methods of assessing the analysis, interpretation, synthesis, and application of knowledge. The third level, shows, refers to the learner's ability to demonstrate through performance that they can use their knowledge while being supervised and observed (Cruess et al., 2016). This level is the clinical skills competency level, which can be assessed through the use of simulation, including the use of SPs or manikins (Witheridge et al., 2019). Finally, the does level is the final measure of the behavioral ability of clinical competency, where the assessment is completed by direct observation in a real clinical setting.

Education implies the process of facilitating learning in the acquisition of KSAs. Evaluation is a tool that can provide insight as to the level of performance that a student has achieved in an individual topic, course, or with any simulation activity. Data can be collected during or at the end of a course or objective, thus monitoring their progress as they proceed in meeting the objectives of the course or activity (Kulasegaram & Rangachari, 2018). In simulation, assessments can be used to demonstrate that learning has occurred and that learning occurred in a situation that is as close to the real world as possible. Through these evaluations, both the instructor and the learner share the responsibility for having a successful outcome. The instructor is responsible for the design and implementation of the learning experience, but it is the learner who is responsible for the learning within that environment; therefore, learning and assessment are connected (Black & Wiliam, 2009; Kulasegaram & Rangachari, 2018).

Distinguishing Types of Learning Assessments

Formative and Summative Assessments

Learning assessments are often described as being summative or formative. *Summative assessments* are the most common, or primary, assessment of learning (Kibble, 2017). This type of assessment includes final exams or grades and is used to rank, approve a student's skills, or determine if they have achieved their learning goals or demonstrated competencies (Sadler, 1998). *Formative assessments* are assessments that provide feedback during the learning process and allow students to improve their own learning and achievement (Sadler, 1998). This type of assessment can be used by instructors to identify a student's ability to understand the information and guide and support their progress (National Research Council, 2012), therefore reinforcing and enhancing learning. It is the purpose of the assessment and not necessarily the form that it takes that makes an assessment summative or formative.

SBLEs can be designed to incorporate one or both forms of assessment. The use of simulation can allow learners the repeated practice that allows them to monitor incremental improvement in a clinical skill or procedure (formative assessment). The same SBLE can be used by educators to assess if the learner has achieved clinical proficiency/competency in that skill (summative assessment). In the case of demonstrated competency, the learner moves on to the next course. In the event that competency is not met, the learner may engage in remediation until the desired level of proficiency is achieved. An example of this model is the use of an otoscopy trainer, which uses a self-guided method to enhance the student's knowledge of a variety of conditions found in the ear canal and tympanic membrane. It provides information that the student can study to learn about the problem and then allows them to visualize it through an otoscope in an ear simulator. It then provides them with a self-assessment tool to determine if they are understanding the material. Once they have completed those tasks, the otoscopy trainer can be utilized as part of a more comprehensive skills check or proficiency exam in combination with an SP as a part of a mentored assessment.

High-Stakes Evaluation

When assessment results or outcomes of a simulation experience have a major consequence, they are referred to as *high-stakes evaluation* (Bensfield et al., 2012). For example, major grades or program progression could be linked to learner performance in an SBLE. While formative and summative assessment occur throughout the learning cycle, high-stakes evaluations are often conducted at the end of the learning process. Simulation assessment, particularly high-stakes evaluation, requires careful planning and effective design. The SBLE components are standardized, with the learner as the only variable in the situation and all other aspects remaining the same (Rizzolo et al., 2015). Reliability and validity of assessment tools is particularly important for high-stakes evaluations using simulation. While many examples are available for medicine and nursing, scenarios and assessments for high-stakes evaluations in CSD are not yet widely available. Zraick (2012) reviewed the use of SPs in Objective Structured Clinical Examinations for training and evaluating speech-language pathology students, describing examples and calling for additional research. He described the use of checklists to evaluate student performance, completed by trained judges and SPs. Student questionnaires are used to evaluate the SBLE, and student review meetings with judges or SPs provide additional opportunities for self-evaluation and reflection. Opportunities for practice in advance of the high-stakes evaluation and for remediation to improve skills and demonstrate competencies after high-stakes evaluation are recommended (Bensfield et al., 2012).

Evaluating the Simulation Experience

In addition to evaluating learner outcomes, SBLEs benefit from evaluation of the simulation experience. By obtaining impressions from learners and from facilitators, the SBLE can be continuously improved. A survey of simulation in CSD showed that 42% ($n = 29$) of the programs that reported use of simulations asked learners to rate the SBLE (Dudding & Nottingham, 2018). As simulation in CSD programs is emerging, many SBLEs are novel developments. Learner input allows the SBLE designers and facilitators to plan and implement new SBLEs, then revise and improve the SBLEs for future learners. Likert scales or open-ended questions are often utilized. Published simulation scales include the Simulation Effectiveness Tool (Leighton et al., 2015), the Simulation Design Scale (Jeffries, 2005; Jeffries & Rizzolo, 2006), the Educational Practices Questionnaire (NLN, 2005a), and the Student Satisfaction and Self-Confidence in Learning Scale (Jeffries & Rizzolo, 2006; NLN, 2005b).

Qualitative data on student impressions may be obtained through open-ended survey questions, focus groups, or individual interviews. After qualitative data are collected, it can be analyzed using content analysis or thematic analysis (Miles et al., 2020). Content analysis involves coding data for words or content, identifying patterns, and interpreting meanings. Then, data are sorted based on the coding and patterns are determined. Thematic analysis involves grouping the data into predetermined themes or themes that emerged naturally from the experience. Either of these approaches may be used to analyze and summarize impressions of the SBLE. A mixed methods approach incorporating scaled questionnaires and open-ended responses provides valuable information to support continuous improvement of the SBLE (Estis et al., 2015; VandeWaa et al., 2019).

Educator impressions provide additional insights on the effectiveness and areas for improvement of SBLEs. Impressions may be collected informally, but it is beneficial to plan assessment of the simulation by the educators involved in planning and implementing the SBLE. Written reflections, focus groups, or interviews may be used. For example, each member of the educational team responds to a survey with questions about the experience. They complete a survey with questions such as these: What went well with the SBLE? What actions can be taken to improve the debriefing? Which component of the SBLE needs the most improvement? Another way of obtaining feedback about the process is to conduct a focus group with an interprofessional group of educators. The quantitative and qualitative methods provided for student impressions may also be used to describe educator impressions. For more insights regarding the collection of data related to SBLE implementation, see Chapter 8.

Assessment and Evaluation in Simulation-Based Learning

Assessment is a key component of every stage of an SBLE. During the preparing stage, SBLE planning is driven by the objectives you hope to achieve with consideration of the participants' knowledge or level of experience. It is critical that the preparing stage includes planning for assessment of the expected outcomes. Planned assessments can include the participants, the facilitators, the overall experience, or other identified outcomes of interest. During the prebrief stage, it is beneficial for the facilitators to share with the learners the objectives that will be targeted and assessment measures that will be used. During the simulation phase, participants practice skills and apply knowledge in a safe environment that is representative of a real health care context or event. Unlike the unpredictable nature of clinical settings, SBLEs allow for systematic assessment of targeted interactions and clinical skills in a controlled context. During the debrief, assessment may be used to provide feedback to the participants. Through feedback and reflection, the facilitator enhances critical thinking and fosters clinical skill development.

Using Backward Design to Align Objectives, Activities, and Assessments in Simulation

The backward design process (Wiggins & McTighe, 2011) is a helpful framework for developing, implementing, and assessing SBLEs. Simply stated, backward design is beginning with the end in mind. The first step is to identify and articulate the desired results. The next step is to determine acceptable evidence to demonstrate to what extent the desired result was achieved. From there, the SBLE is planned and implemented. Figure 6-2 presents a model for SBLEs.

After student learning outcomes have been identified for the SBLE, a variety of assessment methods may be utilized. Wiggins and McTighe (2011) present a continuum of assessment methods that range from informal checks for understanding, to observations, to tests, to academic prompts, to performance tasks. Each of these methods may be applied to simulation. For example, the facilitator may informally ask a learner, "Explain your rationale for the order of your case history questions with the standardized patient." For a performance task assessment, a checklist may be used to determine competency for a clinical skill like tracheostomy care. As with other learning contexts, when planning assessments for SBLEs, consider what evidence is needed to show that students understand the concepts or effectively perform the tasks (Wiggins & McTighe, 2005). Also, consider if other

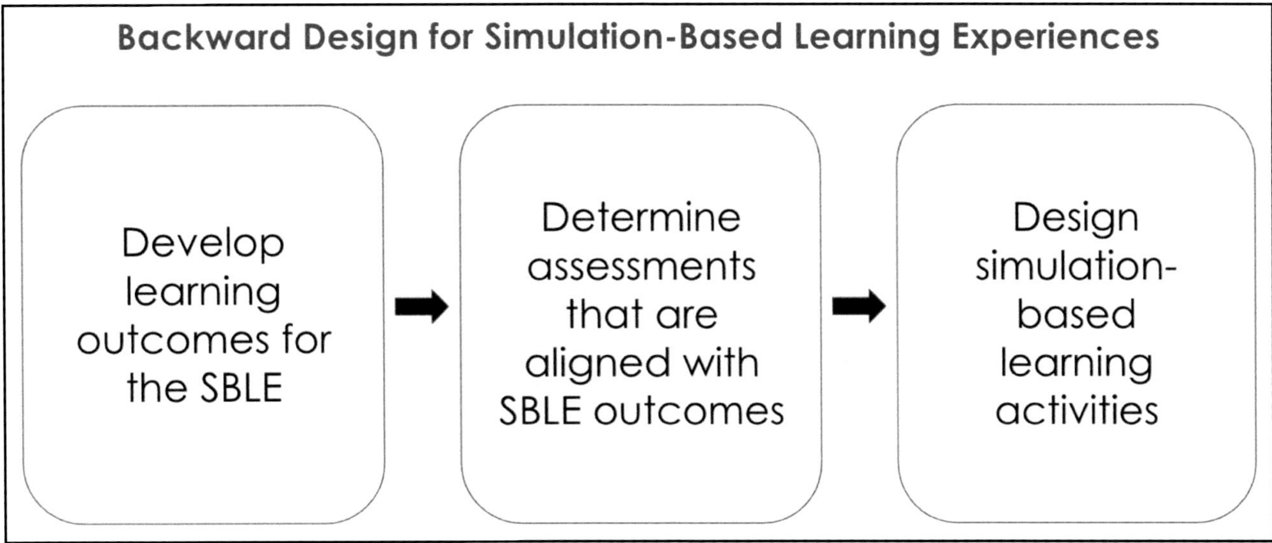

Figure 6-2. Backward design for SBLEs. (Adapted from Wiggins, G., & McTighe, J. [2011]. *The understanding by design guide to creating high-quality units.* Association for Supervision and Curriculum Development.)

BOX 6-1

Participant Evaluation Criteria

When designing SBLEs, it is helpful to use the INACSL Standards of Best Practice in Simulation: Participant Evaluation (2016) criteria:

1. "Determine the method of participant evaluation before the simulation-based experience.
2. Simulation-based experiences may be selected for formative evaluation.
3. Simulation-based experiences may be selected for summative evaluation.
4. Simulation-based experiences may be selected for high-stakes evaluation."

evidence is needed given the desired results. Ask, "How will I determine that the competency has been met or that the goal has been achieved?" After selecting assessment methods that are aligned with the learning objectives, review the quality of your assessments in terms of fairness, validity, and reliability, as well as alignment with learning outcomes and simulation activities. Though there may be a tendency to begin SBLE planning with the activities, the last step in the backward design process is developing learning activities that are linked with the learning outcomes and assessment methods. By designing the activities after articulating the learning outcomes and determining the assessment methods, student learning remains the focus of the SBLE and alignment of learning outcomes, assessment methods, and activities is achieved.

Applying Best Practices for Evaluation of Simulation Participants in CSD

Who Is the Evaluator?

In SBLEs, who has the role of the evaluator? There is not a simple answer as there are a number of individuals who can and do provide the learner with feedback, although not usually all at the same time. Evaluating the SBLE can occur at of the level of the learner themselves, or it might be a high-stakes evaluation completed by an expert in their field. Often the learner will conduct a self-evaluation of their experience. It might also be a peer-to-peer evaluation completed by another learner participating in the SBLE. If the learner is involved in an SBLE that is utilizing an SP, the SP may provide input in the form of an observation of the encounter. The learner may also receive feedback through the use of a formative assessment from the educator.

Self-Evaluation

Self-evaluation affords the learner the opportunity to evaluate their own performance. Learners can utilize techniques such as a skills checklist or a self-confidence survey to investigate their abilities. Often, this can provide valuable information to the learner as well as the educator. Skills checklists are useful only if the learner has the knowledge of what is expected so they can make a judgment as to how close they are to the mark. The ability to use a checklist creates a better understanding of what is correct. In this case, the rubric or checklist is key to improving the learner's performance. The checklist needs to be detailed enough so the learner will know when they have successfully completed the task.

The self-confidence survey allows the learner to move the self-evaluation to the next level, beyond the concept of completing a task to a level of evaluating their performance. These surveys are structured to provide the learner with an opportunity to reflect and provide their perception of their performance and is a valuable learning experience for the learner (Cason & Lee, 2019). The survey can also be enhanced by including video recordings of their performance. Self-confidence surveys provide complementary information to the learner's test performance and will give the learner a better understanding of their strengths and weaknesses when performing various tasks.

Peer Evaluation

Peer evaluation, or peer-to-peer evaluation, is a method that allows the participants to evaluate each other and removes the facilitator from the evaluation process. Learners are open to discuss the activity and provide feedback from their perspective to the other participants and through this process both the learner and the peer evaluator benefit. However, the success of this type of evaluation depends on how it is structured. It must be structured to prevent participants from providing erroneous information or allowing their bias and subjectivity to filter in (Rush et al., 2012). An additional benefit of peer evaluation is that it provides learners with experience in giving and receiving feedback, reflecting on the activity, and working with peers in small groups. The learners develop and gain experience making judgments and providing feedback but most importantly, they have the opportunity to both give and receive constructive criticism (Cason & Lee, 2019). Assessment using this type of evaluation has shown it to be valuable in that there is an established link between the peer-assessment process and clinical skills learning (Rush et al., 2012).

Standardized Patient Evaluation

SPs are trained to portray the role of the patient or a family member or other person and consistently provide standard answers and behaviors to a group of learners (Anson, 2015). Use of SPs allows the learner to practice testing, case history taking, communication skills, and other exercises. In addition to being trained to play the role of the patient, the SP is trained to evaluate the learner's skills and provide them with feedback. After the encounter with the learner, the SP will grade the learner on the basis of their observations of the encounter. The feedback includes the SP's opinion on how they felt in response to what the learner said or did during the interview or assessment. The feedback focuses on the learner's behaviors and interpersonal skills, not on the content or results presented. The SP utilizes a checklist and scores the learner on the basis of their observation of the encounter (McLaughlin et al., 2006).

Educator Evaluation

Simulation is a valuable tool in health care education and can be used for determining clinical competency; however, this must be done by an experienced evaluator. The role of the educator is to determine if the learner is competent, which goes beyond self-evaluation, peer evaluation, and SP evaluation. Most often these evaluations are of high stakes and will require an instrument or tool that is both valid and reliable. The educator evaluation collects outcome data that can be used for assessing the individual learner, but it can also be used for assessing the simulation experience to determine if the activity meets the objective for which it was designed.

Tools for Success

There is a need to provide evidence that learning has taken place in an SBLE, which means that we need to implement an evaluation component within each activity. There are three elements that must be considered when conducting an evaluation (Cason & Lee, 2019; Rosen et al., 2008):

1. The intent of the SBLE
2. The identification of a valid and reliable evaluation tool
3. A plan to implement the assessment and interpret the results

For us to understand the usefulness of simulation, we must understand how it is evaluated. That is, we must understand why we should evaluate, what we should evaluate, and how we would evaluate. Evaluation needs to be done so that we can provide feedback to the learners, validate the usefulness of the activity, and provide a mechanism to demonstrate that the SBLE translates into practice.

Learning objectives drive not only the development and design of the SBLE but the evaluation as well. The learning objectives identify the KSAs that serve as the focus for the evaluation. Once the KSAs have been determined, then it becomes the mechanism of how to evaluate. The determination of the tool to use will differ depending on if you are assessing the knowledge or skill (Kardong-Edren et al., 2010).

TABLE 6-1

Tools for Evaluating the Simulation Experience

TOOL	EVALUATION OF SIMULATION EXPERIENCE	EVALUATION OF KNOWLEDGE, SKILLS, AND/OR ATTRIBUTES
Simulation Effectiveness Tool-Modified (SET-M; Leighton et al., 2015)	• Prebriefing • Scenario • Debriefing	
Simulation Design Scale (Jeffries, 2005; Jeffries & Rizzolo, 2006)	• Objectives and information support • Feedback fidelity	• Problem solving
Educational Practices Questionnaire NLN-2 (NLN, 2005a)	• Active learning facilitation • Collaboration • Diverse ways of learning • High expectations	
Student Satisfaction and Self-Confidence in Learning (Jeffries & Rizzolo, 2006; NLN, 2005b)	• Satisfaction with current learning	• Self-confidence in learning
Seattle University Simulation Evaluation Tool (Mikasa et al., 2013)		• Assessment/intervention/evaluation • Critical thinking • Clinical decision making • Direct patient care • Communication • Collaboration • Professional behavior

Selection of the assessment tool is important as it ensures the tool is appropriate, reliable, valid, and fits well with the testing conditions and requirements of the program. Evaluators utilize checklists, behavioral rating scales, reflections, and rubrics in the completion of their task. Table 6-1 lists several tools available for evaluating the simulation experience. Additional resources are available from INACSL at https://www.inacsl.org

Assessment tool development is highly complex but there needs to be continued development if we want to improve the use of simulation (Adamson et al., 2013). We need to continue the development of valid and reliable measures for simulation instruments, especially those used for CSD. Replication studies using existing instruments with new populations and venues will be part of the process to turn tentative belief into accepted knowledge.

Checklists

Checklists and rating scales have long been used in the evaluation of simulation, each with its own advantages and disadvantages (Ilgen et al., 2005). Checklists allow raters to indicate the observation of a specified behavior. The behavior is scored dichotomously and judged to be present or absent (Anson, 2015). A well-developed checklist should include a task-specific description of the behavior. Use of checklists during SBLE activities allows the rater to determine through observation if the learner has accomplished the item. The checklist can be utilized by anyone from the learner to the educator. Checklists are either weighted or not weighted. A weighted checklist is one in which some items on the list are judged to be more critical to a successful procedure and would, therefore, are assigned a higher point value.

Figure 6-3 is an example checklist used for training tracheostomy care and suctioning procedures to speech-language pathology students using an adult nasogastric tube and tracheostomy care manikin trainer. The column on the left shows items that are being evaluated. The "Yes" and "No" columns are used by the educator to indicate if the skills were demonstrated or not. The right column is used for educator comments. This checklist is not weighted, and every component is required to be assessed before the activity is completed. After feedback and additional instruction, the student repeats the SBLE until all skills are demonstrated.

Skill	Yes	No	Comments
Initiates visit with patient correctly by introducing self, verifying order, gathering equipment, checking expiration date on sterile saline, identifying patient using 2 identifiers, assessing allergies on chart, and explaining procedure to patient.			
Positions patient correctly by raising bed to working height, lowering siderail, and adjusting to a semi-Fowler's or high-Fowler's position			
Dons PPE in proper order: gown, mask, goggles, and clean gloves.			
Assesses for signs and symptoms of upper and lower airway obstruction requiring suctioning			
Maintains sterile environment while preparing for tracheostomy care by opening sterile tracheostomy kit, removing sterile field and placing on bedside table, adding contents of sterile basin to sterile field, and placing basin onto bedside table alongside the opened trach kit.			
Documents suctioning and trach care correctly in patient's chart.			

Figure 6-3. Tracheostomy care and suctioning task trainer simulation sample checklist items. (PPE = personal protective equipment.)

Behavioral Rating Scales

Behavioral rating scales allow evaluator to detect differing levels of performance along a continuum of performance. Types and examples of behavioral rating scales familiar to the reader include:

- Graphic rating scales—Likert and visual analog scales
- Numerical rating scales—Pain scales
- Descriptive rating scales—Satisfaction surveys
- Comparative rating scales—User ratings

The reliability and accuracy of rating scale assessments are dependent upon rater familiarity with the scale, clinical expertise, and rater training in the use of the scale (Ilgen et al., 2005).

Table 6-1 includes several scales that have been used in simulation-based education. These scales have been well validated and been shown to be reliable for the population they were developed for; however, further evaluation and the reporting of psychometric measures, as well as other steps, need to be taken to ensure validation with different populations (Adamson et al., 2013). These scales also require training prior to adoption and use.

Reflections

In classical learning, reflection is a method of analyzing a person's experiences with a task in order to improve the way they function in that task. A reflection or reflective simulation is a focused, flexible, and critical learning process that recaptures, explores, and interprets a practice-based activity (i.e., scenario) to develop, enhance, and modify the necessary KSAs that can be transferable to real-life situations. Reflection means analyzing your own experiences to improve the way you learn or work.

Self-monitoring is performed by participants during or after a simulation experience (Lioce et al., 2020). This process, which requires active involvement by the learner and guidance by the facilitator, assists the learner in identifying gaps in their knowledge and demonstrates areas where they need further improvement (Decker et al., 2008; Kuiper & Pesut, 2004; Rodgers, 2002). Refer to Chapter 2.

Rubrics

Rubrics are guidelines that instructors use for evaluating learners' assignments. Instructors use rubrics as a tool to define their expectations and contain the different criteria to be evaluated and the desired quality to aspire to. These include three components: (a) evaluation criteria or the different criteria required to complete the assignment, (b) quality definitions or a rating scale or marker to determine quality or demonstration of a skill, and (c) a scoring strategy or the points or scoring for each criterion (Reddy & Andrade, 2010). The expectations are set by the instructor and are determined by the criteria from which the student has a clear expectation of what is required to demonstrate proficiency in the material. Rubrics should list the objectives or concepts that the learner's assignment should contain and a scale of possible points that are to be assigned to each. The scoring scale should also include a set of descriptors for several levels of performance or quality in order to eliminate bias and provide more reliable scoring. Wiggins (1998) suggests that indicators can be included with each descriptor to provide examples for each level. These levels of quality can utilize different ratings (e.g., excellent, good, needs improvement) or numerical scores (e.g., 4, 3, 2, 1), which can then culminate in a total score or grade (e.g., A, B, C).

Rubrics can be used for any course assignment as either a summative or formative assessment. In formative assessments, they can easily lead to remediation opportunities by evaluating the steps required to meet each criterion and having the student self-assess and develop their own remediation plan to move them to fulfillment of the rubric.

Figure 6-4 offers an example of a rubric that can be used in evaluating a learner's ability to conduct a threshold auditory brainstem response (ABR). This example rubric evidences the three components recommended by Reddy and Andrade (2010) and could serve as a summative or formative assessment, which would lead to the need for remediation or not. The prebrief describes the scenario to the learner, and the rest of the form describes the evaluator's expectations and the value of each component. This rubric is used with a computerized manikin and an ABR testing system. The learner is required to complete an assessment of the infant's hearing acuity and is evaluated according to the scoring on the rubric. This allows the examiner to assess the learner's ability to conduct a threshold ABR and determine if they require remediation of this skill.

Incorporating the Transparent Assignment Framework

After designing the learning objectives, assessments, and activities associated with an SBLE, outcomes may be improved by sharing the purpose, task, and criteria for success with the student. Specifically, educators can apply the Transparent Assignment Framework to SBLEs (Winkelmes et al., 2016). Transparent teaching and learning focuses on how and why students are learning content, concepts, and skills in a particular way. It also helps students understand how they will use what they performed or learned later in their profession. Though this approach has not been investigated specifically in SBLEs, research across a variety of undergraduate courses yielded significantly greater learning benefits in key areas of student success, including employer-valued skills, academic confidence, and sense of belonging.

When applying the Transparent Assignment Framework to SBLEs, the educator may use an assignment template that includes three key elements. First, the educator provides the purpose of the SBLE. The skills that will be practiced and the knowledge that will be gained are included in this section. Also, a summary of how this SBLE connects to professional roles and responsibilities is included in the purpose section of the SBLE overview. The next section focuses on the task and provides information on what to do and how to do it. The educator specifies actions that will be taken, steps that will be conducted, and components of the SBLE. Finally, the criteria section explains what excellence looks like. The criteria section may include a rubric, a checklist, examples, or descriptions. By providing the criteria for success in advance, educators support the learner in preparation and self-evaluation.

Transparent SBLE expectations may be communicated with learners in advance through learning management system announcements, email announcements, written documents, or overview videos. The transparent framework may also be applied during the prebrief as the educator shares the purpose of the SBLE, the tasks to be completed, and the criteria for success. After the SBLE, the educator may utilize the criteria for success when assessing and offering feedback to learners.

Threshold ABR Rubric

Name: ______________________________ Date: ______________________________

Prebrief

A 1-month-old infant has come to your clinic after referring on their newborn hearing screening while in the hospital. They referred on the right ear but passed on the left ear using DPOAEs. Using the information obtained from the parent, the results from their hearing screenings, the results that you obtain, and any other information provided to you, determine this infant's type and degree of hearing loss. Review your AC results and determine if they are appropriate for this evaluation. Mark the peaks and calculate the infant's AC thresholds. Using the BC waveforms provided, determine the type and degree of loss for this infant. To be able to conduct this assessment, set up the ABR equipment and prepare the infant for you to conduct a one channel (ipsi) threshold ABR for the right ear of your infant.

Time

Start Time ________ Stop Time ________ Time (5 pts) ________ (5)

- Subtract one point for every 2 minutes past 30 minutes

Set up Parameters

Stimulus and Response Parameters (1 pt each)

_____ Electrodes: Non-Inverting (Active/Positive) Fz Inverting (Reference/Negative) – A2/M2 Ground – Fpz/Shoulder
_____ Stimulus: Tone Burst
_____ Frequency choices and rationale
_____ Rate: 37-41/sec
_____ Intensity: Choice using worksheet
_____ Filter settings: 30-100 – 1500 Hz
_____ Polarity (alternating split/condensation or rarefaction)
_____ Window size: 20-24 ms ________ (8)

Analyze the Response

_____ Examine in EEG (1 pt)
_____ Determine residual noise values (≤ 0.05) (2 pts)
_____ Calculate cross correlation value (≥ 0.70) (2 pts)
_____ Number of rejections (1 pt)
_____ Create and review a noise tracing from the two tracings (1 pt)
_____ Determine the presence/absence of repeatable waveform (2 pts)
_____ Correctly mark Wave V for all AC at both 0.5 and 2.0 kHz (4 pts)
_____ Determine where to go from first waveform - increase 20/decrease 10 dB (4 pts)
_____ Using the worksheet, plot the presence/absence of Wave V at each intensity tested (2 pts)
_____ Using the BC results provided, correctly mark Wave V for all BC at both o.5 and 2.0 kHz (4 pts)
_____ Using the worksheet, determine threshold at 2000 and 500 Hz for both AC and BC (4 pts)
_____ Convert thresholds from dB nHL to dBeHL (2 pts)
_____ Determine degree of loss (4 pts)
_____ Determine type of loss (4 pts) ________ (37)

Total ________ (50)

Examiner: ____________________ REMEDIATION/NO REMEDIATION

COMMENTS:

Figure 6-4. An example rubric used to evaluate audiology students when performing a threshold ABR. (DPOAE = distortion product otoacoustic emissions; EEG = electroencephalogram.)

Interpreting, Reporting, and Using Assessment Information

Effective assessment begins with learning goals, which are achieved through learning opportunities and then assessed. However, the process of assessment continues through the use of the results. SBLE assessments can be used to measure individual student performance, identify gaps in learning to inform curriculum and program evaluation, and improve the SBLE. Patterns of assessment results help educators identify gaps in learning. For example, if students do not meet expectations for patient education during an SP encounter, the educators may look at the curriculum to ensure that adequate instruction is provided in didactic and clinical contexts prior to the SBLE. Assessment of the learning experience by the educators and the learners is beneficial for quality improvement. The assessment results may be used to modify specific components of the SBLE to improve the overall experience for learners.

BOX 6-2

Rubric Questions

Student work can be graded using a set of scoring guidelines or rubric. Rubrics answer the following questions (Wiggins, 1998, p. 154):

- "By what criteria should performance be judged?
- Where should we look and what should we look for to judge performance success?
- What does the range in the quality of performance look like?
- How do we determine validly, reliably, and fairly what score should be given and what that score means?
- How should the different levels of quality be described and distinguished from one another?"

BOX 6-3

Rubric Design

Rubrics are never finished!

When designing a rubric, the instructor must determine the appropriate criteria and indicators to evaluate the competency of the learner. However, it is a difficult task to move from general to specific descriptors. These specific descriptors must be appropriate to the task, detailed, and helpful to the learner. The evaluator may have a general concept of what is to be appraised but then work backward to determine the specific descriptors, as it is the descriptors that reflect the characteristics in the task. These descriptors will emerge from the reviews of multiple examples, and every review completed will focus the descriptors improving both content and understanding. Therefore, we need to understand that the rubric will not be complete until it has been used to evaluate the learner, and this process will be used to sharpen the rubrics descriptors.

Summary

Aligned assessments provide a mechanism for educators to determine to what extent the purposes of the SBLE were met for the learner, for the program, or even for future patients. Using a backward design process, educators determine in advance how they will know if the intent of the SBLE is achieved. When carefully designed, assessments are useful to the learner, educator, and program, allowing for growth of the learner and continuous improvement of the SBLE.

References

Adamson, K., Kardong-Edgren, S., & Willhaus, J. (2013). An updated review of published simulation evaluation instruments. *Clinical Simulation in Nursing, 9*, e393-e400.

Anderson, L. W., Krathwohl, D. R., Airasian, P. W., Cruikshank, K. A., Mayer, R. E., Pintrich, P. R., Raths, J., & Wittrock, M. C. (2001). *A taxonomy for learning, teaching and assessing: A revision of Bloom's taxonomy of educational objectives*. Longman.

Anson, W. (2015). Assessment in healthcare simulation. In J. C. Palaganas, J. C. Maxworthy, C. A. Epps, & M. E. Mancini (Eds.), *Defining excellence in simulation programs* (pp. 509-533). Wolters Kluwer.

Bensfield, L. A., Olech, M. J., & Horsley, T. L. (2012). Simulation for high-stakes evaluation in nursing. *Nurse Educator, 37*(2), 71-74. https://doi.org/10.1097/NNE.0b013e3182461b8c

Black, P., & Wiliam, D. (2009). Developing the theory of formative assessment. *Educational Assessment, Evaluation and Accountability, 21*(1), 5. https://doi.org/10.1007/s11092-008-9068-5

Cason, M. L., & Lee, F. W. (2019). Evaluation of simulation activities. In L. Wilson & R. A. Wittmann-Price (Eds.), *Review manual for the Certified Healthcare Simulation Educator (CHSE) exam* (2nd ed., pp. 251-266). Springer.

Cruess, R. L., Cruess, S. R., & Steinert, Y. (2016). Amending Miller's pyramid to include professional identity formation. *Academic Medicine, 91*(2), 180-185. https://doi.org/10.1097/ACM.0000000000000913

Decker, S., Sportsman, S., Puetz, L., & Billings, L. (2008). The evolution of simulation and its contribution to competency. *Journal of Continuing Education in Nursing, 39*(2), 74-80.

Dudding, C. C., & Nottingham, E. E. (2018). A national survey of simulation use in university programs in communication sciences and disorders. *American Journal of Speech-Language Pathology, 27*(1), 71-81. https://doi.org/10.1044/2017_AJSLP-17-0015

Estis, J. M., Rudd, A. B., Pruitt, B., & Wright, T. (2015). Interprofessional simulation-based education enhances student knowledge of health professional roles and care of patients with tracheostomies and Passy-Muir valves. *Journal of Nursing Education and Practice, 5*(6), 123. https://doi.org/10.5430/jnep.v5n6p123

Gaba, D. M. (2004). The future vision of simulation in health care. *BMJ Quality & Safety, 13*(Suppl 1), 2.

Ilgen, D. R., Hollenbeck, J. R., Johnson, M., & Jundt, D. (2005). Teams in organizations: from input-process-output models to IMOI models. *Annual Review of Psychology, 56*, 517-543. https://doi.org/10.1146/annurev.psych.56.091103.070250

INACSL Standards Committee. (2016). INACSL Standards of Best Practice: Simulation participant evaluation. *Standards of Best Practice: Simulation, 12*(Suppl.), S26-S29. https://doi.org/10.1016/j.ecns.2016.09.009

INACSL Standards Committee, Bowler, F., Klein, M. & Wilford, A. (2021). Healthcare Simulation Standards of Best Practice Professional Integrity. *Clinical Simulation in Nursing, 58*, 45-48. https://doi.org/10.1016/j.ecns.2021.08.014

Jeffries, P. R. (2005). A framework for designing, implementing, and evaluating simulations used as teaching strategies in nursing. *Nursing Education Perspectives, 26*(2), 96-103.

Jeffries, P. R., & Rizzolo, M. A. (2006). *Designing and implementing models for the innovative use of using simulation to teach nursing care of ill adults and children: A national, multi-site, multi-method study.* National League for Nursing.

Jeffries, P. R., Rodgers, B., & Adamson, K. (2015). NLN Jeffries Simulation Theory: Brief narrative description. *Nursing Education Perspectives, 36*(5), 292-293. https://doi.org/10.5480/1536-5026-36.5.292

Kardong-Edgren, S., Adamson, K. A., & Fitzgerald, C. (2010). A review of currently published evaluation instruments for human patient simulation. *Clinical Simulation In Nursing, 6*(1), e25-e35. https://doi.org/10.1016/j.ecns.2009.08.004

Kibble, J. D. (2017). Best practices in summative assessment. *Advances in Physiology Education, 41*(1), 110-119. https://doi.org/10.1152/advan.00116.2016

Kuiper, R. A., & Pesut, D. J. (2004). Promoting cognitive and metacognitive reflective reasoning skills in nursing practice: Self-regulated learning theory. *Journal of Advanced Nursing, 45*(4), 381-391. https://doi.org/10.1046/j.1365-2648.2003.02921.x

Kulasegaram, K., & Rangachari, P. K. (2018). Beyond "formative": Assessments to enrich student learning. *Advances in Physiology Education, 42*(1), 5-14. https://doi.org/10.1152/advan.00122.2017

Leighton, K., Ravert, P., Mudra, V., & Macintosh, C. (2015). Updating the Simulation Effectiveness Tool: Item modifications and reevaluation of psychometric properties. *Nursing Education Perspectives, 36*(5), 317-323. https://doi.org/10.5480/15-1671

Lioce, L., Lopreciato, J., Downing, D., Chang, T. P., Robertson, J. M., Anderson, M., Diaz, D. A., Spain, A. E., & Terminology and Concepts Working Group (Eds.). (2020). *Healthcare simulation dictionary* (2nd ed.). Agency for Healthcare Research and Quality. https://doi.org/10.23970/simulationv2

McGaghie, W. C., Miller, G., Sajid, A., & Telder, T. (1978). *Competency-based curriculum development in medical education: An introduction.* World Health Organization.

McLaughlin, K., Gregor, L., Jones, A., & Coderre, S. (2006). Can standardized patients replace physicians as OSCE examiners? *BMC Medical Education, 6*(1), 12. https://doi.org/10.1186/1472-6920-6-12

Mikasa, A., Cicero, T., & Adamson, K. (2013). Outcome-Based Evaluation Tool to evaluate student performance in high-fidelity simulation. *Clinical Simulation in Nursing, 9*, e361-e367. https://doi.org/10.1016/j.ecns.2012.06.001

Miles, M. B., Huberman, A. M., & Saldana, J. (2020). *Qualitative data analysis: A methods sourcebook* (4th ed.). SAGE Publications.

Miller, G. E. (1990). The assessment of clinical skills/competence/performance. *Academic Medicine: Journal of the Association of American Medical Colleges, 65*(9 Suppl.), S63-S67. https://doi.org/10.1097/00001888-199009000-00045

National League for Nursing. (2005a). Core competencies of nurse educators. www.nln.org/profdev/corecompetencies.pdf

National League for Nursing. (2005b). Hallmarks, indicators, glossary, & references. www.nln.org/excellence/hallmarks_indicators.htm

National Research Council. (2012). *A framework for K-12 science education: Practices, crosscutting concepts, and core ideas.* The National Academies Press. https://doi.org/10.17226/13165

Novotny, J., & Griffin, M. T. Q. (2006). *A nuts-and-bolts approach to teaching nursing* (3rd ed.). Springer.

Reddy, Y. M., & Andrade, H. (2010). A review of rubric use in higher education. *Assessment & Evaluation in Higher Education, 35*(4), 435-448. https://doi.org/10.1080/02602930902862859

Rizzolo, M. A., Kardong-Edgren, S., Oermann, M. H., & Jeffries, P. R. (2015). The National League for Nursing project to explore the use of simulation for high-stakes assessment: Process, outcomes, and recommendations. *Nursing Education Perspectives, 36*(5), 299-303. https://doi.org/10.5480/15-1639

Rodgers, C. R. (2002). Defining reflection: Another look at John Dewey and reflective thinking. *Teachers College Record, 104*, 842-866.

Rosen, M. A., Salas, E., Silvestri, S., Wu, T. S., & Lazzara, E. H. (2008). A measurement tool for simulation-based training in emergency medicine: The Simulation Module for Assessment of Resident Targeted Event Responses (SMARTER) approach. *Simulation in Healthcare: Journal of the Society for Simulation in Healthcare, 3*(3), 170-179. https://doi.org/10.1097/SIH.0b013e318173038d

Rush, S., Firth, T., Burke, L., & Marks-Maran, D. (2012). Implementation and evaluation of peer assessment of clinical skills for first year student nurses. *Nurse Education in Practice, 12*(4), 219-226. https://doi.org/10.1016/j.nepr.2012.01.014

Sadler, D. R. (1998). Formative assessment: Revisiting the territory. *Assessment in Education: Principles, Policy & Practice, 5*(1), 77-84. https://doi.org/10.1080/0969595980050104

Scalese, R. J., & Issenberg, S. B. (2008). Simulation-based assessment. In E. S. Holmboe & R. E. Hawkins (Eds.), *Practical guide to the evaluation of clinical competence* (pp. 179-200). Mosby-Elsevier.

Suskie, L. (2018). *Assessing student learning: A common sense guide* (3rd ed.). John Wiley & Sons.

Thomas, P. A. (2016). Goals and objectives. In P. A. Thomas, D. E. Kern, M. T. Hughes, & B. Y. C. Chen (Eds.), *Curriculum development for medical education* (3rd ed., pp. 50-64). Johns Hopkins University Press.

VandeWaa, E., Rudd, A. B., Estis, J. M., & Gordon-Hickey, S. (2019). Safe medication administration in patients with communication disorders: A simulation-enhanced interprofessional education approach. *Journal of Allied Health, 48*(4), 257-262.

Wiggins, G. (1998). *Educative assessment: Designing assessments to inform and improve student performance.* John Wiley & Sons.

Wiggins, G., & McTighe, J. (2005). *Understanding by design* (2nd ed.). Association for Supervision and Curriculum Development.

Wiggins, G., & McTighe, J. (2011). *The understanding by design guide to creating high-quality units.* Association for Supervision and Curriculum Development.

Winkelmes, M.-A., Bernacki, M., Butler, J., Zochowski, M., Golanics, J., & Weavil, K. H. (2016). A teaching intervention that increases underserved college students' success. *Peer Review: Emerging Trends and Key Debates in Undergraduate Education, 18*(1-2), 31.

Witheridge, A., Ferns, G., & Scott-Smith, W. (2019). Revisiting Miller's pyramid in medical education: The gap between traditional assessment and diagnostic reasoning. *International Journal of Medical Education, 10*, 191-192. https://doi.org/10.5116/ijme.5d9b.0c37

Wittmann-Price, R. A., & Price, S. W. (2019). Educational theories, learning theories, and special concepts. In L. Wilson & R. A. Wittmann-Price (Eds.), *Review manual for the Certified Healthcare Simulation Educator (CHSE) exam* (2nd ed., pp. 165-196). Springer.

Zraick, R. I. (2012). Review of the use of standardized patients in speech-language pathology clinical education. *International Journal of Therapy and Rehabilitation, 19*(2), 112-118. https://doi.org/10.12968/ijtr.2012.19.2.112

PART III

Professional Issues and Advocacy

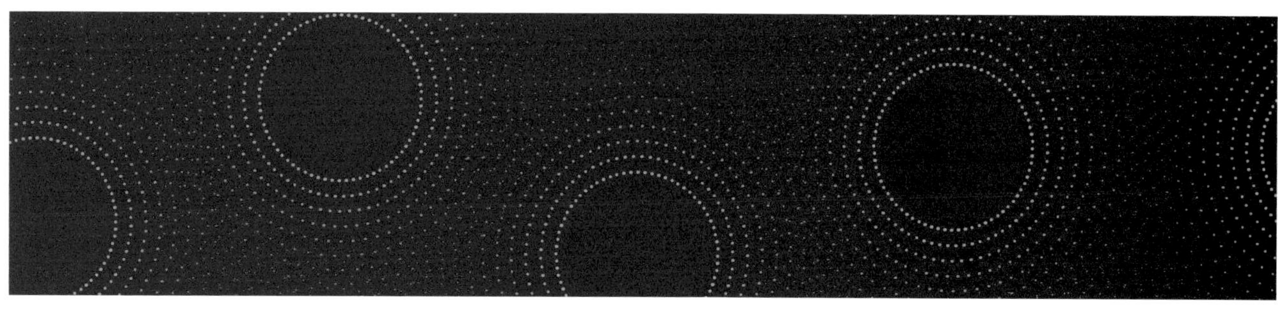

Faculty and Professional Development

Alison R. Scheer-Cohen, PhD, CCC-SLP and Suzanne Moineau, PhD, CCC-SLP

Who dares to teach must never cease to learn.
—John Cotton Dana (1912)

Educators play a central role in simulation-based education. Literature on simulation for clinical education emphasizes the importance of effective training as part of the simulation experience. Jeffries (2005) states that "effective teaching and learning using simulations are dependent on teacher and student interactions, expectations, and roles of each during these experiences" (p. 97). Jeffries (2005) further describes the importance of the educators' comfort level in the use of simulation, which can be increased through faculty development. Faculty development plays a crucial role in all phases of simulation—development, implementation, and execution.

It is helpful to have a base knowledge about simulation before implementing the pedagogy into academic or clinical curricula and training programs. This base knowledge should include education around the history and relevance of the use of simulation in training practitioners in the fields of health care and education; an overview of how to integrate simulation into the academic and clinical curricula; coverage of regulations around the use and limitations of simulation toward meeting competencies and counting clinical hours; a presentation and possible demonstration of the tools that can be used (e.g., manikins, task trainers, computer-based programs, virtual and augmented reality platforms, standardized patients [SPs]/simulated participants); an outline of the simulation process and design; and explanation of the assessment and evaluation procedures postsimulation. It is preferable to provide opportunities for educators to observe the implementation of a simulation and to review simulation materials during this initial training phase. Figure 7-1 represents the seven components of base knowledge.

Hub-and-Spoke Model of Professional Development

This chapter will review the essential components of professional development offerings from the perspective of the trainer and the trainee (e.g., clinical educator, facilitator, simulation designer, faculty). To frame the discussion on faculty development, a definition from medicine will be used. Sheets and Schwenk (1990) consider faculty development "to be any planned activity designed to improve an individual's knowledge and skills in areas considered essential to the performance of a faculty member" (p. 141). There are two main

Dudding, C. C., & Ginsberg, S. M. (Eds.).
Simulation-Based Learning in Communication Sciences and Disorders: Moving From Theory to Practice. (pp. 105-123).

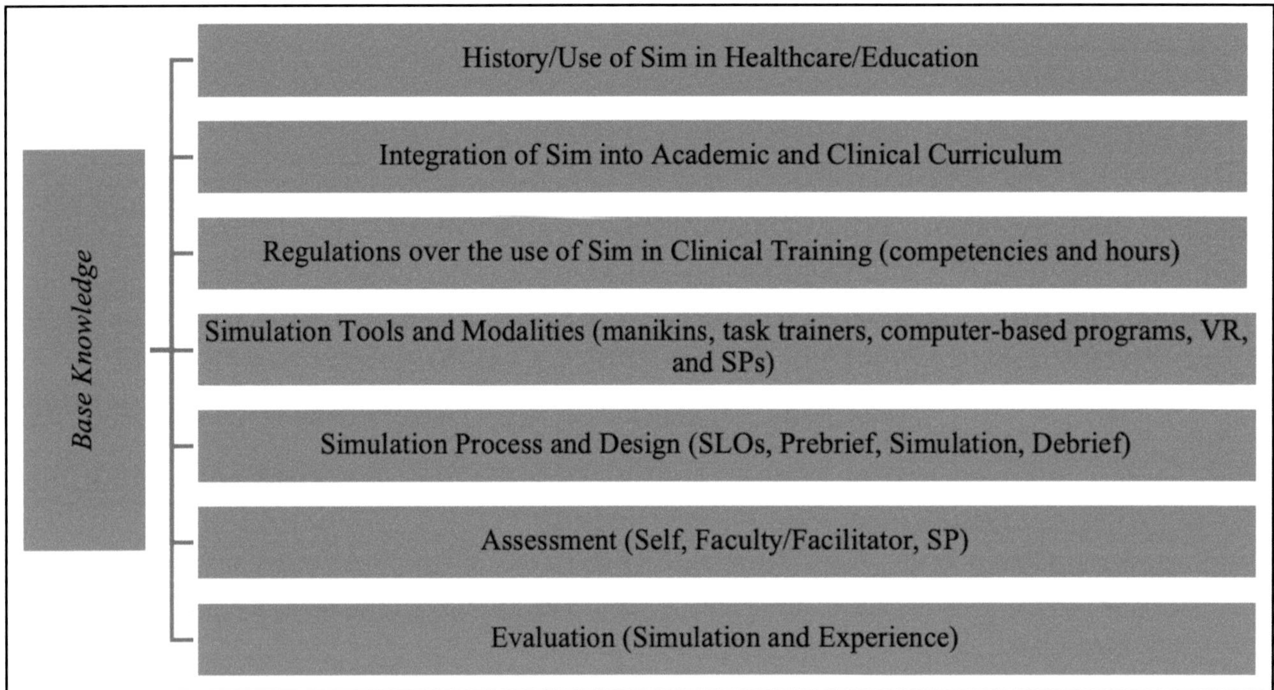

Figure 7-1. Components of base knowledge for simulation-based education. (SLO = specific learning objective; VR = virtual reality.)

components to this definition—the knowledge, skills, and attitudes and the format of development or training program.

The reader will find the hub-and-spoke model for faculty development (Bidwai & Mercer, 2015) to be a useful model for designing and evaluating opportunities for education in simulation. The hub in this model refers to the knowledge, skills, and attitudes required of educators engaged in the development, implementation, and execution of simulations. For example, educators must know the purpose of the debrief; understand planning and executing the debrief; and appreciate the importance of reflecting on the utility and outcomes of the debrief. The spokes of this model are the learning strategies or training components (e.g., self-guided learning, didactic instruction, train-the-trainer models, mentoring). Figure 7-2 depicts a sample hub-and-spoke model for faculty development and training.

The Hub: Knowledge, Skills, and Attributes

A professional faculty development program in simulation should aim to grow and transform the knowledge (K), skills (S), and attributes (A) of the participant, known collectively as KSAs. For this chapter, these key terms will be defined as follows (Freeth et al., 2003 as cited in Steinert et al. [2006], p. 501; Kirkpatrick, 1994; McAllister, 2006):

- **Knowledge**—Acquisition of concepts, procedures, and principles
- **Skills**—Acquisition of thinking/problem solving, psychomotor, and social skills
- **Attributes**—Attitudes and personal characteristics that influence performance

A professional faculty development program in simulation will grow and transform the KSAs of the participants.

Knowledge

As faculty, we often use learning models to scaffold our teaching in an effort to progress students from a level of knowledge to evaluation. One such example is Bloom's taxonomy that offers a hierarchy of learning objectives: remembering, understanding, applying, analyzing, evaluating, and creating (Bloom et al., 1956). This taxonomy, familiar to many educators, is one hierarchical method that could be used to quantify the progression of knowledge-based learning in simulation. There have been a number of revisions and expansions of Bloom's work, some of which are helpful in considering levels of knowledge as it applies to simulation training. Krathwohl (2002) expands upon the dimensions of Bloom's revised taxonomy (Anderson et al., 2001) and describes a continuum of knowledge plus interaction of dimensions. This continuum of knowledge begins with factual knowledge (e.g., terminology, details, elements), followed by conceptual knowledge (e.g., principles, theories, models), then procedural knowledge (e.g., subject-specific skills, criteria for appropriate procedures), and finally metacognitive knowledge (e.g., self-knowledge). Likewise, educators developing knowledge of a novel teaching and learning practice, such as simulation, may begin with more factual knowledge when being introduced to simulation (e.g., looking up the term debrief), continue with conceptual knowledge (e.g., best practices in debriefing), then procedural knowledge (e.g., Debriefing with Good Judgment),

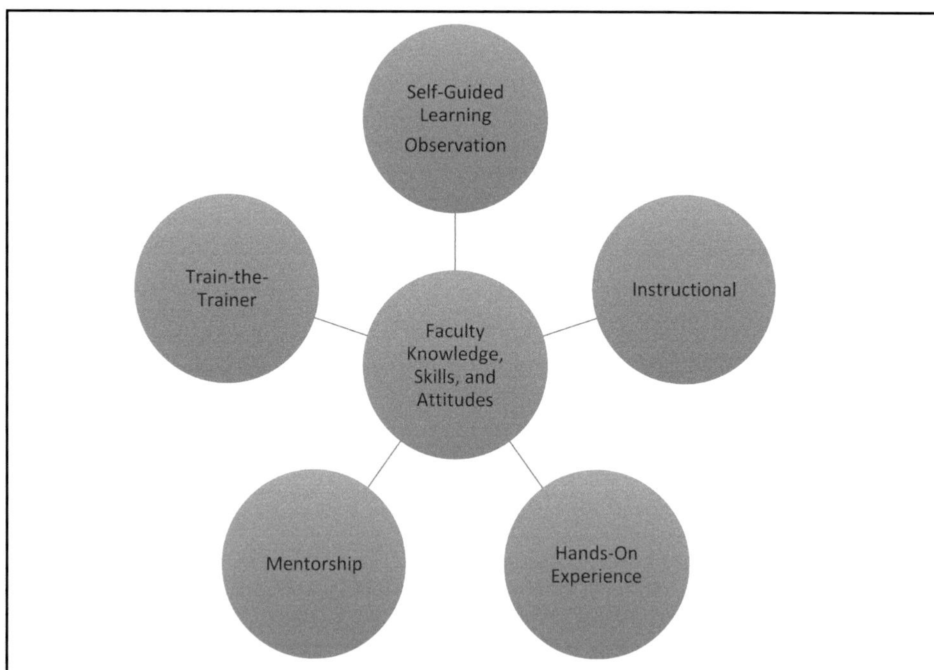

Figure 7-2. A hub-and-spoke model for faculty development in simulation-based education. (Adapted from Bidwai, A., & Mercer, S. [2015]. Reviewing the impact of a one-day fully immersive simulation faculty development course. *Standard Posters*, A54.1–A54.)

and progress to metacognitive knowledge after further research (e.g., determining which style of debriefing to use). As the faculty member learns more about simulation and grows interested in its use, knowledge will intersect with the cognitive dimensions (i.e., remembering, understanding, applying, analyzing, evaluating, and creating). Later in this chapter, the reader will explore a variety of independent and collaborative ways (i.e., the spokes) that an educator can acquire knowledge for simulation-based education and specific academic and clinical scenarios.

Skills

To apply knowledge and develop new skills, a learner must practice. Skill development in simulation may include how to provide feedback to learners during a simulation experience, how to conduct debriefing sessions using a particular model, and designing outcomes and objectives. Practice leading to skill development can take many forms, such as practicing a prebrief session or implementing a particular approach to providing feedback to learners. An effective professional development program will include practice opportunities that increase transfer of learning through variability of practice and increasing the complexity of the skills required (van Merriënboer & Kirschner, 2018). Varying levels of support and guidance, as well as self-reflection, are also helpful for learners to advance from one stage of development to the next (Kellgren, 2019).

Attributes

Attributes, as discussed in Chapter 2, refers to the characteristics of the learner that influences performance. These characteristics may include, but are not limited to, a person's cognitive style, learning preferences, and attitudes. An educator's perception of simulation-based education is an important factor in their willingness to implement a high-impact teaching and learning practice. As the use of simulation-based education becomes more prevalent in communication sciences and disorders (CSD) programs, it will be important to address faculty and educator perceptions. Using a published or informal survey or questionnaire of experience and attitudes toward simulation can be helpful in identifying an educator's willingness or hesitancy to adopt the pedagogical approach in their setting. Wade (2012) found that when educator attitudes were positive, they were more likely to consider the use of simulation in educational learning experiences. If attitudes are negative and express concerns about using the practice, these may be considered barriers to successful implementation of simulation within a curriculum. DeCarlo et al. (2008) found a variety of factors that may influence the attitudes of hospital-based nurses to participate in simulation. In a survey, three of the common barriers identified were (a) "being videotaped," (b) "[being] unfamiliar with the equipment," and (c) "stressful environment"—these barriers were influenced by previous experience with and prior exposure to simulation (DeCarlo et al., 2008, p. 94). Increasing familiarity and confidence with simulation may help reduce perceived barriers and increase accessibility. This is where quality professional development training is useful. A well-designed training program can help to overcome some of the perceived barriers to successful implementation of a simulation-based learning experience (SBLE). Through the integration of knowledge and skills within a simulation training experience, an educator will develop attitudes, which may be positive, neutral, or negative, toward this form of education and training that will carry over to the learners.

TABLE 7-1

Elements of Simulation Professional Development Related to Knowledge, Skills, and Attitudes

ELEMENTS OF SIMULATION FACULTY DEVELOPMENT	TARGET AREA OF IMPROVEMENT
Observation	Knowledge
Didactic	Knowledge
Interactive learning experiences	Knowledge Skills
Practice	Skills
Expert feedback	Skills
Mentoring	Skills Attitudes
Networking	Attitudes

Adapted from Peterson, D. T., Watts, P. I., Epps, C. A., & White, M. L. (2017). Simulation faculty development: A tiered approach, *Simulation in Healthcare*, *12*(4), 254-259. https://doi.org/10.1097/SIH.0000000000000225.

The Spokes: Format and Training Methods

The next consideration for professional development in simulation is the format and modality of the training activity (i.e., the spokes). Given the wide range of KSAs necessary for effective, high-quality SBLEs, it is not surprising that the methods to train educators also vary by outcomes, profession, and setting, as seen in Table 7-1. These methods include observation of simulations, didactic learning through workshops or continuing education courses, participation in trainings focused on specific components of a simulation (e.g., debriefing, evaluation methods), or receiving training from an experienced colleague. These methods can be carried out by educators in a specific setting (e.g., university, medical simulation lab) or as part of a larger offering (e.g., workshop at a national conference). Some faculty development in simulation has been presented in books or journals, at local and national conferences, and, increasingly, online.

Educators can choose a method of faculty development that fits their goals and learner needs. Let's consider an example of how the method of educator training may evolve according to the level of the learner (see Table 7-1). Consider a faculty member who is new to simulation-based education as a teaching and learning practice. They will likely begin the professional training by participating in a learning experience focused on acquiring knowledge on simulation education. This might include live or video-based observation of a simulation within or outside of CSD or didactic or instructional learning in the foundations and theories of simulation. As the faculty member advances in their level of knowledge about simulation education, they may learn about and seek out new simulation practices (e.g., case development, debriefing, student evaluation) through more interactive learning experiences with more opportunities for practice and skill development. To advance in the area of skills related to simulation, the faculty member should participate in simulated learning experiences that provide opportunity for practice, as well as feedback, from someone experienced in simulation from development to execution. Repeated practice in facilitating a simulation will advance general and specific skills. Feedback and mentoring during this process can also aid in skill growth. It is recommended that those interested in conducting simulations are mentored by an experienced simulation educator either through formal programs such as the Society for Simulation in Healthcare (SSH) mentorship programs or through less formal means by working with a Certified Healthcare Simulation Educator (CHSE) in their facility or university. Additionally, colleagues with simulation experience across campus in related disciplines and across universities can be very helpful to consult with in beginning the process of learning about simulation technology.

Train-the-trainer models are another form of mentorship in which the trainer teaches other faculty about simulation-based learning practices in education with the expectation that they will champion the training of other educators (Jeffries, 2008). The S.T.E.P. Educator Preparation Plan is a simulation-specific train-the-trainer model of development (Jeffries, 2008). In this model, the educator will become a skilled facilitator prepared in a way to "guide the simulation-based learning experience to optimize opportunities for participants to meet expected outcomes" (Boese et al., 2013, p. S22). The plan includes (Jeffries, 2008):

"S = standardized materials;

T = train the trainer;

E = encourage the development of a simulation design and integration team;

P = plan to coordinate the simulation development and implementation activities (pp. 71-72)."

As the use of simulation-based education continues to expand among health professions, so does the number and types of available training programs. Organizations, universities, and companies dedicated to health care simulation offer a range of trainings from specific topics, such as case study design, to courses in simulation operations and the use of SPs, to a multiweek curriculum leading to a certificate. Many of these offerings are available online free of charge or at a modest cost. The motivated reader is encouraged to take advantage of these resources.

BOX 7-1

Certification and Accreditation in Simulation

The SSH offers certification in the following:

- CHSE/CHSE-A—Certified Healthcare Simulation Educator and Advanced
- CHSOS/CHSOS-A—Certified Healthcare Simulation Operations Specialist and Advanced

SSH also offers accreditation for simulation programs.

Novice to Expert

Literature from medicine and nursing is rich with models of skill development, some of which can be applied to faculty and professional development. Early on, Dreyfus and Dreyfus (1980) proposed a five-stage progressive model of skill acquisition (i.e., novice, competent, proficient, expert, master) that incorporates varying degrees of mental function (i.e., recollection, recognition, decision, awareness). Benner's (1984) model of moving from novice to expert added clinical experience to the equation. More recent work in this area finds that these models serve as guidelines for professional development in simulation-based education (Thomas & Kellgren, 2017). Researchers report that as educators gain experience with simulation, they develop KSAs that progress them from one level to the next for specific phases of simulation, types of simulation, and/or components of simulation (Thomas & Kellgren, 2017; Waxman & Telles, 2009; Waxman et al., 2011). Table 7-2 summarizes situations presented by these authors to guide educators in refining simulation skills.

Assessment and Evaluation in Professional Development

Quality professional development offerings, like quality SBLEs, include a plan to evaluate the learners' achievement of the intended KSAs as they relate to simulation. As with SBLEs, the assessment plan should have a theoretical model as its base. One such model is offered by Steinert et al. (2006). Steinert and colleagues' (2006) model includes four main levels, with sublevels: Level 1 Reaction, Level 2 Learning, Level 3 Behavior, and Level 4 Results, as shown in Figure 7-3.

An example of the application of this model for the evaluation of a workshop is as follows: Level 1, measure satisfaction of workshops using a Likert scale; Level 2a, include measurement of attitudes of attendees of the workshops; Level 2b, evaluate changes in knowledge and skill pre- and postworkshop; Level 3, focus on use of techniques learned in the workshop; Level 4A identify changes in curriculum; and Level 4b, assess attendees' change in performance on exams (Steinert et al., 2006). This type of systematic evaluation can also help faculty and educators identify their own future development or training needs. For example, a faculty member who wants to modify a curriculum would benefit from a workshop on how to implement simulation across a graduate program/Level 4A. Regardless of the model or types of evaluation methods employed, both consumers and producers of professional development offerings should comply with what best practices, including formative and summative assessments that are clearly linked to learning objectives.

Training Models Specific to Simulation

Along with the advances in simulation, and the expansion in use of simulation-based health care education, comes an increase in the types of training models. This section provides an overview of several prominent models of professional development with the purpose of demonstrating the various ways that the hubs and spokes of professional training may be configured. Peterson and colleagues (2017) offer a tiered approach to faculty development in simulation ranging from apprentice to expert. Each tier contains one or more of the elements as outlined in Figure 7-2 and specifies knowledge and skills (i.e., the hub) and strategies (i.e., spokes) required to progress from one tier to the next.

Debriefing is also a common focus of professional development programs. The literature contains several models for consideration. For example, Cheng et al. (2015) outline a model specific to debriefing that includes five main components: education and practice; summative assessment; formative assessment; feedback; and self-assessment. These best practices are then applied to a framework of stages of skill development that includes discovery, growth, and maturity (Cheng et al., 2020). These stages provide flexibility and account for the complex nature of skill development from beginner to expert. Fey et al. (2020) used learning models to structure a plan to refine debriefing skills. Specific debriefing strategies (e.g., scripts and tools, additional training) were outlined for three implementation phases (adoption, implementation, maintenance) and three developmental stages (discovery, growth, maturity). General and specific development and training offerings provide faculty with options that meet their wants and needs as they relate to simulation pedagogy.

TABLE 7-2

Descriptions of Stages of Professional Development

STAGE OF PROFESSIONAL DEVELOPMENT	THOMAS & KELLGREN (2017)	WAXMAN & TELLES (2009); WAXMAN ET AL. (2011)
Novice	• Knowledge of teaching and learning theories and practices (not specific to simulation) • Perform one simulation component at a time (e.g., only debriefing) • Still need to learn more about technology used in simulation (e.g., manikins)	*Level 1* • Basic technical training ◦ Example: Knowledge of terminology
Advanced beginner	• Learns about multiple components of simulation and begins to realize the complex interactions among the components (e.g., altering learning outcomes in the planning phase, can modify methods in the implementation phase, and results in a different execution of the simulation) • Follows rigid practices (e.g., use of a checklist for the stages of simulation) • Seek simulation-specific resources (e.g., peer-reviewed literature)	*Level 2* • Training in simulation methodology ◦ Example: Review of concepts specific to simulation and participation in components of a simulation

Competent	• Experience in various types of simulations
	• More flexible in practices (e.g., modifications made during a simulation; application of theory to practice)
	• Participate in additional learning experiences (e.g., see boxes throughout this chapter; co-author presentations or grants)
		Level 3
		• Specialized training
		  ◦ Example: Debriefing
		• Mentorship
		  ◦ Example: Faculty receive the mentorship of Level 4 experts

Proficient	• Diverse experiences as facilitators in simulation • Ability to focus more on the student performance and achievement of outcomes • Increased confidence • Provide leadership and mentorship in the area of simulation (i.e., emotional level)	*Level 4* • Faculty become trainers in the train-the-trainer model ◦ Example: Meet specific simulation competencies; commit to using and teaching the learning practice
Expert	• Advance simulation theory and practice • Support students and new faculty (e.g., novice or competent levels) • Institutional change (e.g., vision for use of simulation in the department, seek funding from college)	*Level 4* • Mentors for Level 3

Adapted from Thomas, C. M., & Kellgren, M. (2017). Benner's novice to expert model: An application for simulation facilitators. *Nursing Science Quarterly, 30*(3), 227-234. https://doi.org/10.1177/0894318417708410; Waxman, K. T., Nichols, A. A., O'Leary-Kelley, C., & Miller, M. (2011). The evolution of a statewide network: The Bay Area Simulation Collaborative. *Simulation in Healthcare, 6*(6), 345-351. https://doi.org/10.1097/SIH.0b013e31822eaccc; and Waxman, K. T., & Telles, C. L. (2009). The use of Benner's framework in high-fidelity simulation faculty development. *Clinical Simulation in Nursing, 5*(6), e231-e235, https://doi.org/10.1016/j.ecns.2009.06.001.

Level 1	**REACTION**	Participants' views on the learning experience, its organization, presentation, content, teaching methods, and quality of instruction
Level 2A	**LEARNING**—Change in attitudes	Changes in the attitudes or perceptions among participant groups towards teaching and learning
Level 2B	**LEARNING**—Modification of knowledge or skills	For *knowledge*, this relates to the acquisition of concepts, procedures and principles; for *skills*, this relates to the acquisition of thinking/problem-solving, psychomotor and social skills
Level 3	**BEHAVIOR**—Change in behaviors	Documents the transfer of learning to the workplace or willingness of learners to apply new knowledge and skills
Level 4A	**RESULTS**—Change in the system/ organizational practice	Refers to wider changes in the organization, attributable to the educational program
Level 4B	**RESULTS**—Change among the participants' students, residents or colleagues	Refers to improvement in student or resident learning/performance as a direct result of the educational intervention

Figure 7-3. Kirkpatrick's model for evaluating educational outcomes. (Reproduced with permission from Steinert, Y., Mann, K., Centeno, A., Dolmans, D., Spencer, J., Gelula, M., & Prideaux, D. [2006]. A systematic review of faculty development initiatives designed to improve teaching effectiveness in medical education: BEME Guide No. 8. *Medical Teacher, 28*[6], 497-526. https://doi.org/10.1080/01421590600902976)

For the learner, self-assessment of one's current skill level can assist in determining the requirements and experiences needed to continue to grow their skills. For the trainer, awareness of various skill levels is key in program development. Learners are also able to seek out workshops that are focused on a specific method of debriefing (Cockerham, 2015).

The role of facilitator is often a topic of professional development. The term *facilitator*, as it is used in simulation education, refers to an individual who is involved in the implementation and/or delivery of simulation activities. Given the importance of this role, INACSL Standards of Best Practice Simulation™: Facilitation (INACSL Standards Committee, 2016) has established nine criteria. Those interested in becoming a skilled facilitator should engage in professional development opportunities that address the KSAs as part of INACSL Standards for facilitators (INACSL Standards Committee, 2021):

1. Specific knowledge and skills in simulation pedagogy.
2. Utilizes a facilitative approach appropriate to the level of learning, experience, and competency of the learners.
3. Employs best practices in prebriefing activities.
4. Facilitate the experience to assist learners in achieving expected outcomes.
5. Conduct debrief in a manner that supports learners in achieving expected outcomes.

In addition to learning and performing skills, it is important that faculty development programs also address attitudes of the faculty educators toward simulation (Paige et al., 2015; Roh et al., 2016). After presenting two 90-minute workshops at the Association for Surgical Education Annual Meeting in 2012, Paige and colleagues were able to identify changes in self-efficacy (confidence) and attitudes pre- and posttraining. The opportunity for participants to provide qualitative feedback may further help identify neutral or negative attitudes toward simulation that could be addressed in future trainings.

Designing and implementing high-quality SBLEs is a complex matter. There may be barriers for educators to overcome when engaging in simulation (e.g., time, resources, funding). Professional development offerings that include opportunities for networking with other simulation educators may help in overcoming barriers to simulation-based education. Joining professional organizations and networking at professional development workshops allows simulation educators to share information, ideas, practice skills, perceptions, and feedback for simulation practices. Membership in an organization may also motivate new educators to implement simulation in their current setting.

Several authors have published curricula expanding on the hub-and-spoke model of professional development for simulation. The Maryland Clinical Simulation Resource Consortium offers a curriculum for professional development in simulation that includes the following (Beroz et al., 2020):

1. Education and simulation theory
2. Simulation design
3. INACSL Standards of Best Practice: Simulation™
4. Curriculum integration
5. Debriefing: beginning and advanced
6. Interprofessional education
7. Evaluation in simulation (p. 57)

This curriculum was developed to be adapted for simulation educators at the novice, competent, or expert level. Those at the level of novice would begin with education and simulation theory, standards of practice, and knowledge and skills of simulation methods. At the expert level, topics would include leadership, scholarship, and certification. Reported outcomes from the use of this curriculum included changes in confidence, learning, foundations of simulation (e.g., theory to practice, phases of simulation), and use of simulation (Beroz et al., 2020). There are other examples of curriculum-based approaches to simulation training available in the literature (e.g., Chauvin & Karpinski, 2014). Those interested in developing professional development programming are encouraged to seek out such resources.

Barriers to Professional Development in Simulation

Barriers to professional development need to be reduced or eliminated for educators to gain the knowledge and skills needed for simulation and participate in the educational practice. The top three barriers to professional development in simulation are time, space, and the availability of materials and/or equipment (Beroz, 2017). In spite of the importance of educator simulation training for specific learner outcomes, Beroz (2017) found that only 19% of nursing schools had a formal simulation orientation plan, excluding programs in which mentoring was the only faculty training option available. In a survey of programs in CSD, Dudding and Nottingham (2018) found that less than half of respondents engaged in formal training is simulation, most having participated in self-study or readings (71%).

Professional development takes additional time on the part of the educator. Educators may need to find coverage for classes or participate in workshops or continuing education outside of scheduled worktimes. Space and equipment are often needed to allow for hands-on practice within SBLEs. If medical equipment is needed for a health care simulation, the equipment needs to be available for use during training. Additionally, the equipment used for training needs to be stored when not in use. Other barriers include educator buy-in, staffing, and scheduling.

Several ways of reducing such barriers to professional training in simulation have been identified (Bidwai & Mercer, 2015; Lemieux et al., 2013):

- Providing financial support for membership and registration fees
- Demonstrating support from leadership
- Allowing dedicated time away from other job responsibilities
- Co-sponsoring of events that allow for sharing of space, equipment, and staff
- Offering a variety of instructional formats (hands-on, virtual, self-paced, on demand)

Developing Your Professional Development Program

Professional development is a dynamic process that may include a variety of formats (e.g., didactic, practice, evaluative), different size learner groups (e.g., self-study, large group), and interprofessional collaboration (Pololi et al., 2001). Different types of learning may help educators achieve specific outcomes at distinct times of learning. As an educator, it can be difficult to identify what type of learning model to look for in a training program, what knowledge and skills need to be refined, and whether the training meets your own learning objectives.

Steps for creating a professional development plan include:

1. Identify your professional activities, roles, and competencies for performance within those roles.
2. Determine your current skills and identify any gaps in knowledge and skills.
3. Create an action plan to address any gaps.
4. Monitor your progress.

Organizations dedicated to simulation-based education are excellent sources of professional development. One such example is the INACSL Simulation Education Program. The SSH offers extensive professional development programs, as well as a professional development roadmap to assist members in determining training needs. The National League of

BOX 7-2

Professional Development Resources

- Center for Medical Simulation: https://harvardmedsim.org/training/
- International Nursing Association for Clinical Simulation and Learning: https://learning.inacsl.org/resources
- National League of Nursing: https://www.nln.org/education
- Society for Simulation in Healthcare: https://www.ssih.org/Professional-Development

Nursing offers a faculty development toolkit with resources listed by level of expertise. Vendors and manufacturers of simulation equipment are known to provide free training for customers. Avkin, Inc. is one such company. During the COVID-19 pandemic, Avkin offered free training in the use of virtual SPs.

It is recognized that not everyone has the financial resources and time to enroll in conferences and workshops. Here are a few ways to continue your professional development on your own time and at little to no cost. Reading this book on simulation is a good example. There are extensive resources cited in the chapters, such as call-out boxes and reference lists. These will serve as a great starting point for obtaining foundational and intermediate knowledge. You may find that websites and journals listed within this text will be helpful to you in developing your knowledge base regarding the implementation of simulations.

Several organizations offer toolkits with access to resources based on an individual's level of expertise and needs. This allows for accessible, individualized, and independent or collaborative learning. It is important that programs focus on all areas of learning (i.e., knowledge, skills, and attributes) and can be provided in multiple modalities for increased access.

Observation and participation in SBLEs designed and executed by experts is another important way of learning. This form of mentorship training is highly encouraged by organizations such as INACSL and SSH. Educators are encouraged to record the SBLEs and self-reflect on parts that went well, parts to be improved, and questions that still need to be answered. Several professional organizations offer mentorship and networking that can take place virtually through the use of online platforms, such as discussion boards and video conference calls.

Here are some evidence-based take-home messages regarding professional development programs in allied health professions (Jeffries, 2015; McClean et al., 2008; Pololi et al., 2001):

- The outcomes of professional development should be realistic and measurable (i.e., task oriented) with clearly outlined competencies.
- Professional development should be tailored to suit the needs of individuals, disciplines, and the institution.
- Activities used in professional development programs should encourage experiential learning and reflection (e.g., expert and peer evaluation, portfolios).
- Professional development should strive for collaboration across disciplines and professions.
- Professional development takes many forms, from formal instruction leading to certification, to mentoring programs, to self-study. All have value within a professional development plan.

Summary

If you are reading this book about simulation-based education, your motivation and attitude toward simulation supports the use of simulation as an educational activity in the academic or clinical setting. This chapter aimed to help you identify your level of expertise with simulation. Based on your level of expertise in simulation-based education, your approach to developing knowledge, skills, and attributes through professional development may vary. Even after identification of the level of competence, educators may have a preferred method of faculty development. You might prefer self-guided learning over instructional workshops. Additionally, you may be limited to specific training opportunities given your profession, setting, or funding. Attending a live workshop may be cost- and time-prohibitive, but mentorship is more readily available in an educator's environment. Given the knowledge about facilitator training gained from this chapter, educators can apply models of faculty development in simulation and modify methods of knowledge, skill, and attitude acquisition to fit their individual wants and needs.

Practice Resources

The following section offers examples of simulations developed at California State University San Marcos. A total of seven simulation-based examples are provided across a variety of content areas and settings. The simulations vary in the type of technology used and as well as the level of complexity of the SBLE. These levels refer to the complexity of the simulations and serve as a guide for educators to use this in developing simulation. Table 7-3 provides a guide for the simulation examples included in this chapter; each simulation is described in area, setting, curriculum, modality, and complexity (i.e., Level 1, Level 2, Level 3).

TABLE 7-3

Guide for the Simulation Examples Included in This Chapter

SIMULATION	AREA	SETTING	CURRICULUM	MODALITY	LEVEL 1	LEVEL 2	LEVEL 3
OME/counseling	A&P and counseling	Outpatient HC	Academic	SP	√		
AAC	AAC	Education	Clinical	SP	√		
Aphasia/ProSem	Receptive and expressive language	Acute care	Academic	Manikin		√	
MBSImP	Swallowing	Fluoroscopy HC	Clinical	CB		√	
SimuTrach	Voice and swallow	Rehab HC	Clinical	TT with SP			√
Palliative care IPE	Cognition—IPE	ICU	Academic	SP			√

A&P = anatomy & physiology; AAC = augmentative and alternative communication; CB = computer-based; HC = health care; ICU = intensive care unit; IPE = interprofessional education; MBSImP = Modified Barium Swallow Impairment Profile; OME = oral motor examination; ProSem = professional seminar; SP = simulated participant or standardized patient; TT = task trainer.

BOX 7-3

Level 1: Oral Motor Examination/Counseling

Simulation Details

Area: Assessment of anatomy and physiology and counseling practices; *Setting*: Outpatient (health care-based sim); *Curriculum*: Academic courses; *Modality*: Simulated participants

Simulation Overview

The simulation was designed with the aim of training first-semester students to carry out an OME, while also training fourth-semester students to provide counseling around prognostic indicators. The setting of practice is an outpatient health care setting, and this simulation is implemented into two didactic, academic courses. The first-year and second-year students serve as simulated participants for one another. (Note: Simulated participants are not standardized participants.)

This simulation is carried out in either a classroom setting or in our on-campus clinic. The sequence is for the first-year student to carry out the OME on the second-year student and provide a brief summary of the findings and any recommendations, followed by the second-year student then providing education and counseling over the prognosis for the communication and swallowing functions as it relates to this neurological condition. Both educators are present during the simulation and provide feedback in situ (i.e., during the simulation). This simulation uses a time-out/time-in tool so that the students can stop and ask a question before resuming the simulation.

(continued)

BOX 7-3 (continued)

The Hub: Faculty Knowledge and Skills

This simulation is conducted toward fulfillment of the SLOs in two courses: Neuroscience for the Speech-Language Pathologist and Seminar: Counseling in Speech-Language Pathology. The simulation utilizes two instructors with academic knowledge and clinical skills related to neurologically based motor speech and swallowing disorders. The faculty should have a strong working knowledge of the neurological bases for abnormal findings on an OME, including knowledge of the direct and indirect pathways for motor execution and regulation. The faculty should also have clinical expertise in carrying out and interpreting the findings from OMEs. The faculty need to have a spirit of collaboration and work well together. This simulation requires that both instructors be familiar with the SLOs for both sets of students engaged in the simulation.

The Spoke: Faculty Development/Training Ideas

An educator new to simulation may choose to observe this SBLE as it is being facilitated by a more experienced educator. The novice educator may then participate in the SBLE in a limited manner, such as conducting the prebriefing activities. Over time, the educator would assume the majority of responsibility for facilitating the SBLE under the direction of the more experienced educator.

BOX 7-4

Level 1: Augmentative and Alternative Communication

Simulation Details

Area: AAC; *Setting*: Education; *Curriculum*: Clinical practice; *Modality*: Simulated participants

Simulation Overview

This simulation is carried out in either a classroom setting or in our on-campus clinic. Students are paired with a grandparent simulated participant and are required to provide education about the device and its use. The faculty member is present during the simulation and acts as a clinical supervisor to be able to provide on-site guidance to the students if needed. The faculty member assumes a realistic role as clinical supervisor to jump in and model as needed, or to be available for consultation prior to making any final recommendations to the grandparent.

The Hub: Faculty Knowledge and Skills

The simulation was designed with the aim of training first-year students to program an AAC device to be used by a child in a public school setting with carryover for use in the home with a grandparent. The setting is a public school classroom, and the simulation is implemented in one didactic, academic course. Simulated participants serve as the "grandparent."

The Spoke: Faculty Development/Training Ideas

A faculty member who has some knowledge of the foundations and theoretical underpinnings of simulation but wants more information on a specific skill, such as debriefing, could observe the debrief of this academic-based clinical simulation and follow up with additional self-guided learning specific to the debriefing process (e.g., research article, instructional webinar). The faculty member executing the simulation could provide one-on-one instruction of the debriefing process to the novice faculty member. For example, the two faculty could review an article on debriefing together and detail how to execute this process in a future simulation. Because the debrief was observed, specific examples of debrief questions, student responses, and instructor evaluation and feedback could be the focus of the discussion.

BOX 7-5

Level 2: Aphasia and Professional Seminar (ProSem)

Simulation Details

Area: Receptive and expressive language disorders in adults (i.e., aphasia) and health care practice; *Setting*: Acute care (health care-based Sim); *Curriculum*: Clinical practice; *Modality*: High-fidelity manikins

Simulation Overview

The simulation was designed with the aim of training first-year students to carry out a language screening on a newly admitted patient with an acute left hemisphere cerebrovascular accident who presents with aphasia. The setting of practice is an acute care hospital setting, and this simulation is implemented into clinical practice via simulation. High-fidelity manikins serve as the patient, and two clinical educators serve as the patient voices.

This simulation is carried out in the Simulation Theatre Suite in our on-campus clinic. We have two high-fidelity manikins that are running simultaneously. The students are paired and required to administer the Bedside Western Aphasia Battery to determine if the patient requires additional follow-up with a full language assessment battery. Each room has one speech-language pathologist supervisor and one (behind-the-scenes) clinical instructor serving as the manikin voice/patient. The two rooms share a registered nurse (RN).

The three up-front faculty assume realistic clinical roles for this simulation and are available for consultation over the patient's care and status.

The Hub: Faculty Knowledge and Skills

This simulation is conducted toward fulfillment of the SLOs in two courses: Language Disorders in Adults (LDA) and Professional Seminar I (ProSem). These courses are both offered in the first semester of the program and the students in both courses are the same. The simulation utilizes five faculty members: the two primary academic instructors for the courses, two clinical educators, and a nursing (RN) faculty member. All of the faculty should have a strong working knowledge of acquired language disorders in adults (i.e., aphasia) and clinical skills related to working in an acute care setting with patients who have had a stroke who present with cognitive–linguistic disorders. The faculty should be versed in the use of PPE, Health Insurance Portability and Accountability Act, environmental checks, safety measures, medical orders and charting, and scope of practice. The faculty should be familiar with aphasic error patterns, administration and interpretation of the Bedside Western Aphasia Battery, and strategies for communicating with someone with aphasia. This simulation is most effective when the faculty train together and have implemented the simulation previously. Therefore, observation of this simulation before participating is beneficial. The faculty need to have a spirit of collaboration and work well together. This simulation requires that all instructors are familiar with the SLOs for both courses.

The Spoke: Faculty Development/Training Ideas

A faculty member new to simulation could use this SBLE as a hands-on experience in two ways: (a) as a clinical faculty member who serves as the manikin voice or (b) acting as the clinical supervisor working in the hospital. Perhaps it would be useful to start as a manikin voice in a more observational role to the primary instructor in the simulation process (i.e., development, implementation, and execution) and transition to carrying out the phases of simulation (e.g., assisting with execution of debriefing and student evaluation). The primary faculty member for this simulation (i.e., course instructor of LDA or ProSem) could mentor the faculty member who is not as familiar with intermediate simulations, such as those using manikins. Mentorship might include feedback on specific skills, such as debriefing and student evaluation.

BOX 7-6

Level 2: Dysphagia

Simulation Details

Area: Swallowing; *Setting*: Radiology (health care–based simulation); *Curriculum*: Clinical practice; *Modality*: Computer-based program

Simulation Overview

The simulation was designed with the aim of training third-semester students in the use of imaging to assess and treat swallowing disorders. The setting of practice is in a fluoroscopy suite in radiology in a hospital setting, and this simulation is implemented into clinical practice via simulation. A computer-based program (MBSImP) is used for the clinical training.

This simulation is carried out in our on-campus clinic in small groups through debriefing over the cases. Each component part of the SLOs is reviewed in consecutive order with probing questions by the faculty member. Each student is responsible to turn in their written documentation of all parts of the SLOs. The students can count the hours toward the required 400 clinical clock hours as they are interpreting the results of the evaluation, making a diagnosis, planning treatment, and demonstrating how to implement it.

The Hub: Faculty Knowledge and Skills

This simulation is conducted towards fulfillment of the SLOs in the Dysphagia course. This simulation also satisfies clinical practice hours in the diagnosis and management of swallowing disorders. The simulation utilizes an instructor with academic knowledge and clinical skills related to dysphagia management. The faculty should have a strong working knowledge and practice around: the nature and etiologies of swallowing disorders, conducting and interpreting videofluoroscopic swallow studies, strategies and maneuvers used to improve swallowing function and/or bolus flow during a videofluoroscopic swallow studies, and evidence-based intervention approaches to treat dysphagia. The faculty member drafts SLOs and needs to be well versed in the use of MBSImP.

The Spoke: Faculty Development/Training Ideas

There are a variety of spokes that could be used to achieve the knowledge and skills to independently conduct this simulation in the future. A faculty member with an intermediate level of expertise in simulation could research computer-based technologies for simulation-based education. They could also begin to complete the MBSImP zones to become familiar with the training, protocols, scoring, and reporting components. MBSImP offers online courses and live webinars for didactic learning. Faculty can debrief on one or more cases as a hands-on experience. During this hands-on experience, they can be observed by the more experienced faculty member that has previously executed debriefing of MBSImP cases. This can be a source of mentorship that includes guidance through modeling, evaluation, and feedback of the less experienced facilitator.

BOX 7-7
Level 3: SimuTrach

Simulation Details

Area: Voice and swallow in the presence of a TT; *Setting*: Rehabilitation center (health care–based simulation); *Curriculum*: Clinical practice; *Modality*: Task trainer with a simulated participant

Simulation Overview

The simulation was designed with the aim of training fourth-semester students in management of voice and swallowing in patients with tracheostomy tubes. The setting of practice is in a rehabilitation unit in a local hospital setting, and this simulation is implemented into clinical practice via simulation. The Avkin Wearable Tracheostomy Task Trainer (Avtrach) is used in this simulation and is worn by a trained SiP.

This simulation is carried out using two SiPs in our on-campus clinic. The sequence is for the students to assess if the patient is suitable to proceed with the screening and treatment session. The students are then expected to be able to identify the need and request assistance for cuff deflation and suctioning. They begin with finger occlusion and then proceed to placement of the Passy Muir speaking valve, if appropriate, followed by achievement of voicing. Finally, the students are expected to complete a swallow screening with the assistance of the RN for suctioning. The speech-language pathologist faculty members are present throughout the simulation to assist the students, while the RN faculty member enters and exits as needed for support. The faculty assume realistic roles as clinicians, jumping in to provide support and being available for consultation in making interpretations and decisions. This simulation uses a time-out/time-in tool so that the students can essentially pull away from the simulation and ask a question before resuming with the client.

The Hub: Faculty Knowledge and Skills

This simulation is conducted toward fulfillment of the SLOs in the Grand Rounds course. This simulation also satisfies clinical practice hours in the diagnosis and management of voice and swallowing disorders in patients with tracheostomy tubes. The simulation utilizes three instructors with academic knowledge and clinical skills related to the management of patients with tracheostomy tubes including two faculty/clinical educators and a nursing faculty member. All of the faculty should have a strong working knowledge and practice skills related to airway safety in the presence of cuffed tracheostomy tubes, best practice in dysphagia management in patients with tracheostomy tubes, the use and placement of a Passy Muir speaking valve for achievement of voice (and swallowing) in patients with tracheostomy tubes, and familiarity with Avkin Wearable Tracheostomy Simulator. In addition, the faculty should be well versed in the use of PPE, conducting environmental and status checks, obtaining medical orders, and scope of practice between speech-language pathologists and RNs in the care of patients with tracheostomy tubes. This simulation is most effective when the faculty train together and have implemented the simulation previously. Therefore, observation of this simulation before participating is beneficial. The faculty need to have a spirit of collaboration and work well together. This simulation requires that all instructors are familiar with the SLOs.

The Spoke: Faculty Development/Training Ideas

Faculty participating in advanced simulation likely have completed multiple types of development and training. Therefore, preparing for this simulation might include acquisition of simulation-specific skills. For example, faculty may want to complete self-guided learning on case development (e.g., use of a "Scenario Overview" template and "Scenario Validation Checklist" in Appendices A and B, respectively, of Waxman et al., 2011). Instruction can come from Avkin; they offer consulting for faculty participating in simulation and trainings for SiPs.

Faculty less experienced with advanced simulation, such as the use of task trainers, could benefit from a train-the-trainer model. Faculty with more experience with this modality, who have received instruction from Avkin and participated in the simulation numerous times, can train other faculty in the knowledge and skills needed to execute this or a similar advanced simulation. This learning method might include sharing resources, individual instruction and discussion, practice with feedback, evaluation, and self-reflection.

BOX 7-8

Level 3: Institute of Palliative Care—Interprofessional Education

Simulation Details

Area: Cognition; *Setting*: ICU (health care–based simulation); *Curriculum*: Extracurricular academic; *Modality*: Simulated participant

Simulation Overview

The simulation was designed with the aim of training students in their final semester to work on interdisciplinary teams in the management of a patient with a traumatic brain injury and resulting cognitive deficits. The setting of practice is in an ICU in a local hospital setting and this simulation is implemented through an extracurricular activity. Two simulated participants are used for this simulation, including a patient and a family member.

This simulation is carried out in two parts: the first part requires the students to work through the paper case, which has probing questions to determine the plan of care for the patient. This is a time-consuming process and happens over three separate 4-hour sessions. The students provide their input from their discipline-specific lens and then collaborate to determine an effective and evidence-based course of action for the patient. The second part of the simulation requires the students to hold a family care conference where the students work as a team to deliver education and recommendations to the patient and their family member. A seasoned faculty member serves as the tutor for the three evenings where the students are engaged in solving the paper-based case. The tutor only assists if the students are getting off-track or need support to continue. The tutor uses the manual to direct the conversation as needed, or to provide a leading question for the students to consider. The tutor also assigns any homework related to "to dos" or "look ups" that the students may need to work through before they return to the next session. When the students are engaged in the care conference, only the tutor is present in the room and all of the other faculty are watching on monitors in a debriefing room.

The Hub: Faculty Knowledge and Skills

This simulation is conducted as an add-on to the curriculum on a volunteer basis for students who are interested in going into a health care setting post-graduation. The simulation utilizes faculty and students from kinesiology, medicine, nursing, social work, and speech-language pathology. All of the faculty should have a strong working knowledge and practice skills related to critical care management, traumatic brain injury, and behavioral profiles associated with Levels 4 and 5 on the Rancho Los Amigos Scale of Cognitive Functioning (RLAS). In addition, the faculty should be well versed in the use and practice of IPE in case management. As noted above, the faculty should be trained in the use of PPE, conducting environmental and status checks, obtaining medical orders, and roles and responsibilities of interdisciplinary teams. This simulation is most effective when the faculty train together and have implemented the simulation previously. This is a very complex simulation across many disciplines, and as such, observation of this simulation multiple times before leading is critical. The faculty need to have a spirit of collaboration and work well together. This simulation requires that all instructors are familiar with the SLOs.

The Spoke: Faculty Development/Training Ideas

As previously mentioned, observation of this simulation prior to being involved in execution of the simulation is imperative. The train-the-trainer model could be used to teach specific skills. For example, faculty could be trained to be the tutor or to lead the debrief. Perhaps a faculty member trained in simulation, but new to this particular simulation, could lead components of the simulation following training. For instance, the faculty is trained to be a tutor and acts as a tutor during the simulation, receiving feedback from faculty who have previously been the tutor. Mentorship from other faculty will also help faculty refine skills. Faculty from the School of Nursing may have different knowledge about simulation than faculty experienced in simulations in the Department of Speech-Language Pathology. This provides faculty with the opportunity to learn from each other about simulation-based education; facilitator KSAs; and how to approach this advanced simulation from different academic and clinical perspectives.

BOX 7-9

Society for Simulation in Healthcare

The SSH developed the Certified Healthcare Simulation Educator (CHSE) certification for educators involved in health care simulations. More information on the CHSE process, handbook, and examination can be found at https://www.ssih.org/Credentialing/Certification/CHSE.

The benefits of certification for faculty include:

- "Improves health care simulation education through the identification of best practices and recognition of practice
- Improves health care simulation education through providing standardization and a pool of knowledge of best practices
- Strengthens patient safety efforts through support of simulation modalities
- Provides external validation of individual educator KSAs
- Strengthens organizational, community, and learner confidence in the quality of education
- Garners local support, resources, and commitment
- Fosters a feedback loop between education and practice
- Encourages performance improvement and knowledge expansion of the individual educator
- Programs with certified simulation professionals receive a competitive edge in the community, program offerings, and grant funding
- Recognizes expertise in simulation above and beyond domain expertise" (SSH, 2020, para. 11)

BOX 7-10

American Speech-Language-Hearing Association

The ASHA website has a Frequently Asked Questions page with about the use of clinical simulation in audiology and speech-language pathology. The FAQs include information about obtaining clinical clock hours using simulation, the supervision of simulation, specific practices (e.g., debriefing), and types of simulation (e.g., computer-based; SPs).

https://www.asha.org/certification/certification-standards-for-slp-clinical-simulation/

ASHA also has publications that discuss the use of simulation in CSD. "Health Care Simulation in Clinical Education" (Dudding & Ingram, 2018) can be found at https://academy.pubs.asha.org/2018/08/health-care-simulation-in-clinical-education/.

Additional educational opportunities in the area of clinical simulation can be accessed at the annual ASHA Convention and through Special Interest Group resources (e.g., *Perspective* articles, workshops, online communities). For more information, see https://www.asha.org/sig.

BOX 7-11

Council of Academic Programs in Communication Sciences and Disorders

CAPCSD has a series of podcasts (https://www.capcsd.org/podcasts/) concerning simulation-based education:

- Simulations in Communication Sciences and Disorders
- The Importance of Debriefs in Simulations
- Audiology Simulation Resources
- Using Standardized Patients to Develop Professional Competence

BOX 7-12

Association for Standardized Patient Educators

The ASPE (n.d.) lists five domains for standards of best practice:

1. Safe work environment
2. Case development
3. SP training
4. Program management
5. Professional development

The ASPE website provides a variety of resources for educators using simulation-based methodology.

For example:

Core curriculum modules in a variety of formats. For more information on the core curriculum offerings: https://www.aspeducators.org/core-curriculum.

Core competencies across three levels (i.e., foundation, intermediate, senior) for individuals involved in health care simulations. Core competencies include Audio-Visual Technology, Health Care, Management & Operations, Simulation, Education, Information Technology, Research & Evaluation, and Theatrics & Staging. See https://simghosts.org/page/capability_framework for additional details.

ASPE also offers a Resource/Mentor/Mentee to members: https://www.aspeducators.org/aspe-mentors.

References

Anderson, L. W., Krathwohl, D. R., Airasian, P. W., Cruikshank, K. A., Mayer, R. E., Pintrich, P. R., Raths, J. D., & Wittrock, M. C. (Eds.). (2001). *A taxonomy for learning, teaching, and assessing: A revision of Bloom's taxonomy of educational objectives*. Allyn & Bacon.

Association of Standardized Patient Educators (n.d.). *The ASPE standards of best practice*. https://www.aspeducators.org/standards-of-best-practice-

Benner, P. (1984). *From novice to expert: Excellence and power in clinical nursing practice*. Addison-Wesley.

Beroz, S. (2017). A statewide survey of simulation practices using NCSBN simulation guidelines. *Clinical Simulation in Nursing, 13*(6), 270-277. https://doi.org/10.1016/j.ecns.2017.03.005

Beroz, S., Schneidereith, T., Farina, C. L., Daniels, A., Dawson, L., Watties-Daniels, D., & Sullivan, N. (2020). A statewide curriculum model for teaching simulation education leaders. *Nurse Educator, 45*(1), 56-60. https://doi.org/10.1097/NNE.0000000000000661

Bidwai, A., & Mercer, S. (2015). 0134 Reviewing the impact of a one-day fully immersive simulation faculty development course. *BMJ Simulation and Technology Enhanced Learning, 1*(Suppl. 2), A54.

Bloom, B. S., Engelhart, M. D., Furst, E. J., Hill, W. H., & Krathwohl, D. R. (1956). *Taxonomy of educational objectives: The classification of educational goals. Handbook I: Cognitive domain*. David McKay Company.

Boese, T., Cato, M., Gonzalez, L., Jones, A., Kennedy, K., Reese, C., Decker, S., Franklin, A. E., Gloe, D., Lioce, L., Meakim, C., Sando, C. R., & Borum, J. C. (2013). Standards of best practice: Simulation standard V: Facilitator. *Clinical Simulation in Nursing, 9*(6), S22-S25.

Chauvin, S., & Karpinski, A. (2014) Board #207—Program innovation LA-SIM: A statewide interprofessional simulation faculty development program. *Simulation in Healthcare: Journal of the Society for Simulation in Healthcare, 9*(6), 445. https://doi.org/10.1097/01.SIH.0000459346.49662.c1

Cheng, A., Eppich, W., Kolbe, M., Meguerdichian, M., Bajaj, K., & Grant, V. (2020). A conceptual framework for the development of debriefing skills: A journey of discovery, growth, and maturity. *Simulation in Healthcare: The Journal of the Society for Simulation in Healthcare, 15*(1), 55-60. https://doi.org/10.1097/SIH.0000000000000398

Cheng, A., Grant, V., Dieckmann, P., Arora, S., Robinson, T., & Eppich, W. (2015). Faculty development for simulation programs: Five issues for the future of debriefing training. *Simulation in Healthcare, 10*(4), 217-222. https://doi.org/10.1097/SIH.0000000000000090

Cockerham, M. E. (2015). Effect of faculty training on improving the consistency of student assessment and debriefing in clinical simulation. *Clinical Simulation in Nursing, 11*(1), 64-71. https://doi.org/10.1016/j.ecns.2014.10.011

DeCarlo, D., Collingridge, D. S., Grant, C., & Ventre, K. M. (2008). Factors influencing nurses' attitudes toward simulation-based education. *Simulation in Healthcare: The Journal of the Society for Simulation in Healthcare, 3*(2), 90-96. https://doi.org/10.1097/SIH.0b013e318165819e

Dreyfus, S. E., & Dreyfus, H. L. (1980). *A five-stage model of the mental activities involved in directed skill acquisition*. Defense Technical Information Center. https://doi.org/10.21236/ADA084551

Dudding, C. C., & Nottingham, E. E. (2018). A national survey of simulation use in university programs in communication sciences and disorders. *American Journal of Speech-Language Pathology, 27*(1), 71-81. https://doi.org/10.1044/2017_AJSLP-17-0015

Fey, M. K., Auerbach, M., & Szyld, D. (2020). Implementing faculty development programs: Moving from theory to practice. *Simulation in Healthcare: The Journal of the Society for Simulation in Healthcare, 15*(1), 5-6. https://doi.org/10.1097/SIH.0000000000000429

Freeth, D., Hammick, M., Koppel, I., Reeves, S., & Barr, H. (2003) A critical review of evaluations of interprofessional education. *Higher Education Academy Learning and Teaching Support Network for Health Sciences and Practice*. Higher Education Academy, Health Sciences and Practice Network. https://doi.org/OccasionalPaperNo2

INACSL Standards Committee. (2016). INACSL Standards of Best Practice: Simulation facilitation. *Clinical Simulation in Nursing, 12*, S16-S20. https://doi.org/10.1016/j.ecns.2016.09.007

INACSL Standards Committee. (2021). Healthcare Simulation Standards of Best Practice. *Clinical Simulation in Nursing, 58*, 66. https://doi.org/10.1016/j.ecns.2021.08.018

Jeffries, P. R. (2005). A framework for designing, implementing, and evaluating: Simulations used as teaching strategies in nursing. *Nursing education perspectives, 26*(2), 96-103.

Jeffries, P. R. (2008). Getting in STEP with simulations: Simulations take educator preparation. *Nursing Education Perspectives, 29*(2), 70-73.

Jeffries, P. R., Dreifuerst, K. T., Kardong-Edgren, S., & Hayden, J. (2015). Faculty development when initiating simulation programs: Lessons learned from the National Simulation Study. *Journal of Nursing Regulation, 5*(4), 17-23. https://doi.org/10.1016/S2155-8256(15)30037-5

Kellgren, M. (2019). *Simulation facilitator competency: Validity and reliability of a self-assessment tool* [Doctoral dissertation, University of Wisconsin Milwaukee]. UWM Digital Commons. https://dc.uwm.edu/etd/2086

Kirkpatrick, D. L. (1994). *Evaluating training program*. Berrett-Koehler Publishers.

Krathwohl, D. R. (2002). A revision of Bloom's taxonomy: An overview. *Theory Into Practice, 41*(4), 212-218. https://doi.org/10.1207/s15430421tip4104_2

Lemieux, N., Nicholas, C., & Cohen, C. (2013). Board 194—Program innovations abstract making connections: overcoming nstitutional barriers to interprofessional educational innovation through a faculty development program in simulation based education: *Simulation in Healthcare, 8*(6), 457-458. https://doi.org/10.1097/01.SIH.0000441459.81036.a6

McAllister, S. (2006). *Competency based assessment of speech pathology students' performance in the workplace* [Doctoral Thesis, The University of Sydney]. Sydney Digital Theses. http://hdl.handle.net/2123/1130

McLean, M., Cilliers, F., & Van Wyk, J. M. (2008). Faculty development: Yesterday, today and tomorrow. *Medical Teacher, 30*(6), 555-584. https://doi.org/10.1080/01421590802109834

Paige, J. T., Arora, S., Fernandez, G., & Seymour, N. (2015). Debriefing 101: Training faculty to promote learning in simulation-based training. *American Journal of Surgery, 209*(1), 126-131. https://doi.org/10.1016/j.amjsurg.2014.05.034

Peterson, D. T., Watts, P. I., Epps, C. A., & White, M. L. (2017). Simulation faculty development: A tiered approach. *Simulation in Healthcare: The Journal of the Society for Simulation in Healthcare, 12*(4), 254-259. https://doi.org/10.1097/SIH.0000000000000225

Pololi, L., Clay, M. C., Lipkin Jr., M. Hewson, M., Kaplan, C., & Frankel, R. M. (2001). Reflections on integrating theories of adult education into a medical school faculty development course. *Medical Teacher, 23*(3), 276-283. https://doi.org/10.1080/01421590120043053

Roh, Y. S., Kim, M. K., & Tangkawanich, T. (2016). Survey of outcomes in a faculty development program on simulation pedagogy: Outcomes in a faculty development program. *Nursing & Health Sciences, 18*(2), 210-215. https://doi.org/10.1111/nhs.12254

Sheets, K. J., & Schwenk, T. L. (1990). Faculty development for family medicine educators: An agenda for future activities. *Teaching and Learning in Medicine, 2*(3), 141-148. https://doi.org/10.1080/10401339009539447

Steinert, Y., Mann, K., Centeno, A., Dolmans, D., Spencer, J., Gelula, M., & Prideaux, D. (2006). A systematic review of faculty development initiatives designed to improve teaching effectiveness in medical education: BEME Guide No. 8. *Medical Teacher, 28*(6), 497-526. https://doi.org/10.1080/01421590600902976

Thomas, C. M., & Kellgren, M. (2017). Benner's novice to expert model: An application for simulation facilitators. *Nursing Science Quarterly, 30*(3), 227-234. https://doi.org/10.1177/0894318417708410

van Merriënboer, J. J., & Kirschner, P. A. (2018). *Ten steps to complex learning: A systematic approach to four-component instructional design*. Routledge.

Wade, S. (2012). *Faculty attitudes toward the utilization of high-fidelity human patient simulation in nursing education* [Master's thesis, South Dakota State University]. Electronic Theses and Dissertations.

Waxman, K. T., Nichols, A. A., O'Leary-Kelley, C., & Miller, M. (2011). The evolution of a statewide network: The Bay Area Simulation Collaborative. *Simulation in Healthcare: The Journal of the Society for Simulation in Healthcare, 6*(6), 345-351. https://doi.org/10.1097/SIH.0b013e31822eaccc

Waxman, K. T., & Telles, C. L. (2009). The use of Benner's framework in high-fidelity simulation faculty development. *Clinical Simulation in Nursing, 5*(6), e231-e235. https://doi.org/10.1016/j.ecns.2009.06.001

Research and Advocacy

Meredith L. Baker-Rush, PhD, MS, CCC-SLP/L, CHSE, FNAP

Earlier chapters have established that the design and use of simulation for clinical education are grounded in best practices, guidelines, and standards. These practices, to a large extent, are a result of systematic and rigorous research in simulation. Utilizing simulation for educational and practice-based skills is a growing activity in many professional areas, and, as such, it is important to stress that research in simulation demands the same rigors in methodology, efficacy, validity and reliability, data, and system integration as other research endeavors.

A survey of current research in simulation will reveal a wide range of purposes and research methods. Research may be quantitative or qualitative in nature or may use both approaches in mixed methods designs. Researchers might be seeking to answer questions such as the following:

- What are the benefits and limitations of simulation for clinical education?
- How do simulations change the knowledge, skills, or attributes of the learners?
- What type of simulation works best for specific types of learning objectives?
- What are the practices that, when applied to simulation-based education, lead to the best outcomes?

Scholarship of Teaching and Learning

The nature of these types of questions leads us to a discussion of research known as *scholarship of teaching and learning* (SoTL). The aim of SoTL research is to bring a scholarly lens to the behaviors, events, culture, values, and learning within the respective discipline as it applies to learning. Boyer's *Model of Scholarship* (1990) expanded the definition of scholarship from discovery, integration, and application to also include the scholarship of teaching (Bernstein & Bass, 2005; Boyd, 2013; Boyer, 1990; Nibert, 2001).

While there is not an agreed-upon definition of SoTL (Felten, 2013; Trigwell, 2013), Ginsberg and colleagues (2017) offer the following:

> SoTL is inherently action, practitioner research that is contextually-based. Such research is focused on pedagogical refinement or continuous improvement in a context that is continuously changing. As such, researchers acknowledge that SoTL inquiry varies by place, time, stakeholder, and sub-discipline. (p. 3)

Dudding, C. C., & Ginsberg, S. M. (Eds.).
Simulation-Based Learning in Communication Sciences and Disorders: Moving From Theory to Practice. (pp. 125-138).

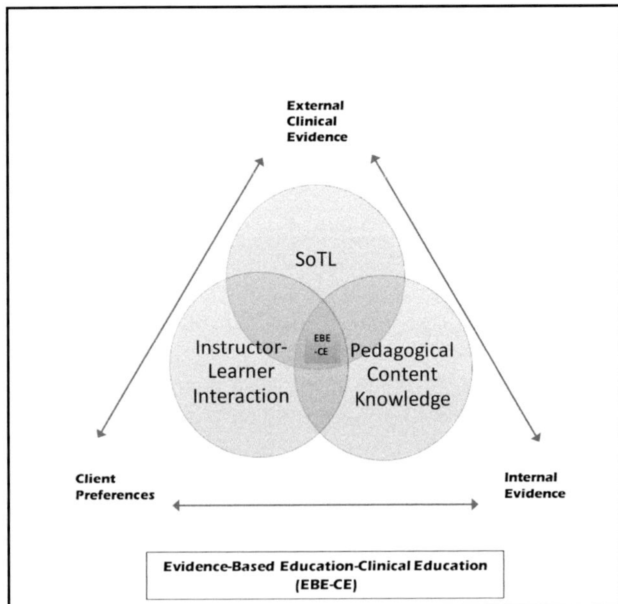

Figure 8-1. Evidence-based education-clinical education. (Reproduced with permission from Ginsberg, S. M., & DeRuiter, M. [2019]. Research methods. In E. McCrea & J. Brasseur [Eds.], *The clinical education and supervisory process in speech-language pathology and audiology* [pp. 411-426]. SLACK Incorporated.)

In developing SoTL research inquiries, Hutchings (2000) identifies a series of questions that can be useful to us in developing questions that may guide us. As we consider the questions that we may ask ourselves about the impact and merits of simulations in communication sciences and disorders (CSD) education, we might consider (a) "what works" questions that seek to identify the effectiveness of those educational methods we are currently employing (or perhaps are typically employed); (b) "what is" questions that represent an attempt to not measure effectiveness as much as describe the process or the experience; (c) "visions of the possible" inquiries that seek to explore how we might manage teaching and learning; and (d) "formulating new conceptual frameworks," in which we investigate ways that our thinking might be shaped and guided by new theories and perspectives on teaching and learning (Hutchings, 2000, pp. 4-5). In considering these questions we may begin to think about how we might develop inquiries or investigations that would move our understanding of the best practices for the use of simulations forward in an evidence-based manner.

Evidence-Based Education

When we use SoTL research to guide our pedagogical practices, it means that we are using evidence-based education (EBE) for teaching. EBE, as the name would imply, refers to the use of educational strategies that are based on objective evidence, just as clinical strategies use evidence-based practice (EBP) based on objective evidence (Ginsberg et al., 2012). Educators use EBE to inform the design or guide the modification of instructional strategies. EBE, originally oriented toward classroom teaching and learning, relies on (a) SoTL literature, (b) pedagogical content knowledge (Shulman, 1998), which reflects the instructor's insights teaching the specific content, and (c) insights related interactions between the teacher and learners (Ginsberg et al., 2012). A model of evidence-based education-clinical education was developed to account for clinical education contexts and takes into account the fact that clinical educators must balance not only how they teach in the clinical context (EBE) but that they must also simultaneously overlay the clinical aspects of the client's needs (EBP) in order to achieve an effective therapeutic outcome for the client and an effective educational outcome for the student at the same time (Ginsberg & DeRuiter, 2020). Figure 8-1 depicts the factors that must be considered in order for clinical education to be effective. This model may be useful in guiding the development of specific aspects of SoTL research inquiries related to classroom and clinical education. The more evidence we gather regarding the educational process and the use of simulations, the greater our likelihood of improving our teaching and our students' learning.

Participatory Action Research

Participatory action research (PAR) seeks to find meaning, understanding, and improvement within the community affected by the research. It can be a useful way to think about designing a SoTL study in your own classroom or clinic. The hallmark of PAR is that the researchers are often members of the participant pool and utilize reflection to aid in the analysis and understanding of the culture, local context, and social relationships that occur within that setting (Baum et al., 2006; MacDonald, 2012). Furthermore, it embraces the reflective thought of the researchers and participants alike, seeking to create a change. PAR enjoys a lengthy history in education and is particularly well suited to educational contexts (Eisner, 1998). PAR is often thought of as qualitative; however, it may include qualitative and quantitative components based on the level of desired involvement on the part of all participants (Baum et al., 2006).

PAR's purpose in the context of simulation research in CSD is to improve the effectiveness of our teaching and clinical outcomes (Bogden & Biklen, 2003). The action is further researched by the participant/researchers using a re-evaluation and reflective cycle. Some use the steps such as "plan-do-check-act-repeat" or "plan-act-observe-analyze-repeat" when describing action research. PAR is also unique in the attention to the concept of power and power relationships as part of the research itself (Baum et al., 2006). In PAR, the participants are equal partners in all aspects of the study, deciding what needs to be studied and how data will be collected, analyzed, and acted upon. In PAR, it is accepted that "the observer has an impact on the phenomena being observed and brings to their inquiry a set of values that will exert influence on the study" (Baum et al., 2006, p. 854), and, therefore, the shared power is a large aspect of the research. Through action research, educators may find a greater understanding and insight to learner experiences and processes, enrich their confidence in teaching, and build a method for ongoing reflection on their teaching knowledge (Megowan-Romanowicz, 2010). A benefit of PAR is that it allows the voices of all participants, including students, to be heard clearly. Gathering insights, engaging in reflection, and considering changes may allow for improved outcomes for learner learning and educator growth.

PAR can play an important role in the validation of practices, cases, processes, and teaching methods employed in simulation-based education. The researcher and the learners are involved in the planning, action, observation, and analyzing of the data collected and make collective recommendations for change. In addition, standardized patients (SPs), simulation educators, technician specialists, and assistants may serve as additional members of the research team and aid in the ongoing process of improvement and action. For example, a course instructor trains an advanced graduate CSD student to serve as an SP for an adult language assessment scenario with first-semester graduate students. The instructor, along with the SP and first-semester students, collaborate to design a study that assesses the impact of the simulation experience on their clinical reasoning skills. In this way, PAR not only gathers data about the use of simulation for learning from the instructor's perspective, it also includes data from the participants' perspectives. This allows for a greater inclusion of various cultures, local contexts, and social relationships in the process of reflection and action. This type of inquiry addresses the "what is?" question posed earlier (Hutchings, 2000).

Overview of Research Methodologies

This section serves as an overview for those interested in utilizing and/or conducting research in the area of simulation. There are a variety of approaches that may be used to conduct research. The approach that a researcher takes in conducting research will be dictated largely by the research question that you ask. If they are seeking to identify correlations between variables, then quantitative research is going to be the most appropriate design. However, if they are seeking to develop insights into how a process impacts learning, then qualitative research is the most effective approach. Mixed methods study designs are complex but allow both types of approaches. There is not one preferred or recommended method to conduct research in simulation. Table 8-1 highlights key features of quantitative, qualitative, and mixed methodologies.

Quantitative Methods

Quantitative is the most common research methodology, sometimes considered "true" or "hard" science. Quantitative research relies on data and statistical analysis to describe, test relationships, and determine cause and effect by breaking down concepts into discrete and specific variables that can be tested against hypotheses (Creswell & Creswell, 2018; Rahman, 2017).

There are a number of design methods used in quantitative research. These include experimental, nonexperimental, longitudinal, correlational, and descriptive (Creswell & Creswell, 2018; Goertzen, 2017; Leedy & Ormrod, 2019; Rahman, 2017). A study may be structured as an experimental or quasi-experimental design (Meline, 2010). Experimental design requires that individuals are randomly assigned to groups, such as randomly assigning students within a course into two or more groups. Quasi-experimental designs are used when it is not possible to randomize the participants. This design is often used when comparing learning outcomes for groups of students enrolled in different courses.

Quantitative research has benefits and limitations. Benefits include, but are not limited to, identifying correlational relationships among variables, increased control against threats to validity, developing a theoretical framework, facilitating generalizability, and using statistical methods (Creswell & Creswell, 2018; Goertzen, 2017; Leedy & Ormrod, 2019; Rahman, 2017). Limitations include a potential of researcher bias as well as lacking the ability to obtain the "why" as it relates to the findings (Goertzen, 2017; Rahman, 2017).

Qualitative Methods

Qualitative research is a systematic approach that seeks to improve understanding of a phenomena or behavior. It is theoretically based in the constructivist and/or transformative worldview (Creswell & Creswell, 2018). Qualitative research differs from quantitative methods in that it acknowledges the worldviews and beliefs of the researchers and uses these to shape the study (Creswell, 2007). Qualitative research can take many forms and gathers data, mostly in word form, from a variety of sources, including interviews, surveys, and recorded observations, making it well suited for simulation research. A well-known scholar in qualitative research, John Creswell (2007), has described five distinct approaches to qualitative research:

1. Narrative
2. Grounded theory
3. Ethnographic
4. Case study
5. Phenomenological

Table 8-2 provides more details on each of these approaches, including the types of data collection associated with each approach.

TABLE 8-1

Key Features of Quantitative, Qualitative, and Mixed Methodologies

	QUANTITATIVE	QUALITATIVE	MIXED METHODS
RESEARCH QUESTION TYPES	• What variables correlate with improved outcomes?	• Why does a phenomenon occur? • How does the process work? • What was the experience of the participant?	• What variables correlate with improved outcomes and why is there a correlation?
RESEARCH DESIGNS	• Experimental • Nonexperimental • Longitudinal • Correlational	• Narrative • Grounded theory • Ethnographies • Case study • Phenomenology	• Convergent • Explanatory sequential • Exploratory sequential • Complex design with subdesigns entrenched within
USE OF THEORY	• Causality • Founded by theory	• Grounded theory • Phenomenological • Ethnographic	• Social science • Participatory social justice • Multiple
TYPES OF DATA	• Performance • Attitude • Observational • Census • Closed-ended	• Interviews • Observations • Documents • Audiovisual • Open-ended	• Multiple
TYPES OF ANALYSES	• Statistical analyses	• Thematic analysis	• Multiple

Adapted from Creswell, 2015; Creswell & Creswell, 2018; Goertzen, 2017; Leedy & Ormrod, 2019; Libarkin & Kurdziel, 2002; Pan, 2008; Rahman, 2017; Saldana, 2013; and Tashakkori and Creswell, 2017.

TABLE 8-2

Qualitative Research Designs

RESEARCH DESIGN	DEFINITION
Narrative	Collection of stories about lives, researcher retells the story
Grounded theory	Researchers develop general, abstract theory founded in the viewpoints of participants in the study
Ethnographies	Longitudinal research shared patterns (behavior or language) of a group in a natural setting
Case study	In-depth analysis of a single case, cases are bounded by time and activity
Phenomenology	Reports of lived experiences, contains strong philosophical foundations

Adapted from Creswell, J. W., & Creswell, J. D. (2018). *Research design: Qualitative, quantitative and mixed methods approaches* (5th ed.). SAGE Publications and Patton, M. (2015). *Qualitative research and evaluation methods* (4th ed.). SAGE Publications.

BOX 8-1

Steps in Evidence-Based Education

1. Identify a question that you have regarding the simulation in education.
2. Find the best evidence for your topic.
3. Read and critically evaluate the literature that you find.
4. Assess the strength of the evidence.
5. Consider the relevance of the literature in association with your question.

Like quantitative methods, qualitative research comes with strengths and limitations. The methodology's strengths include the ability to obtain insights into the meaning associated with the phenomena from the individuals or groups who experience it, the ability to generate theory and policy based on data, the ability to explain why phenomena occur, and the ability to conduct analyses that are grounded within the data context (Creswell & Creswell, 2018; Leedy & Ormrod, 2019; Libarkin & Kurdziel, 2002). Areas of weaknesses are the vulnerability to researcher bias and limited generalizability (Creswell & Creswell, 2018; Leedy & Ormrod, 2019; Libarkin & Kurdziel, 2002). Qualitative research often requires considerable time for data analysis.

Mixed Methods

Mixed method designs are well suited for simulation research in that investigators are often interested in the what, how, and why of simulation-based learning. Mixed method design investigations look into what phenomena occur and how they occur. There is a clear purpose as to why both qualitative and quantitative methods are employed in this approach (Creswell & Creswell, 2018; Tashakkori & Creswell, 2017).

Mixed methods research is a systematic combination of both quantitative and qualitative methods. Mixed methods may be conceptualized as a combination of all aspects of quantitative and qualitative research with the added benefit that mixed methods neutralize the advantages and disadvantages of each individual method by enhancement and complement for the differences (Creswell & Creswell, 2018; Regnault et al., 2018). Mixed methods contain the following characteristics: two types of research questions, two types of sampling procedures, two types of data collection, two types of data, two types of data analysis, and two types of conclusions (Tashakkori & Creswell, 2017). Mixed methods may rely on a variety of designs, including conducting either the quantitative or qualitative aspect of data collection first, often with an eye toward informing the subsequent data collection measures.

The limitations of mixed methods include, but are not limited to, increased duration of the study, complexity, significant volume of data, multiple types of data, and the potential skill level of the researcher (Creswell & Creswell, 2018; Leedy & Ormrod, 2019).

Utilizing Research Literature in Simulation Education

For some, the thought of reading or engaging in research can be overwhelming and, perhaps, scary. It brings to mind thoughts of an unfamiliar language and a graduate course in statistics. Practitioners mistakenly believe they must have a doctorate to read, let alone do, research. This section will focus on best practices in the evaluation of research literature as it relates to simulation-based education. It is embedded in the same principles of gathering evidence for EBP and EBE. Davies (1999) calls on all educators to be able to take the steps outlined in Box 8-1 in order to utilize EBE. These steps are applicable to those interested in implementing best practices in simulation.

Identify a Question

An important first step in EBP and EBE is to identify the clinical problem or educational strategy for which you are seeking evidence. The PICO method is a widely used method for framing a question of interest. Asking a focused question will save you time by making your literature search more efficient. There is evidence that using a framework such as the PICO method results in better overall reporting quality (Rios et al., 2010). PICO stands for population, intervention, comparator/comparison, and outcome (Richardson et al., 1995). By way of example, suppose you are interested in the best way to conduct a debrief session as part of an interprofessional simulation experience. The PICO might look something like this:

- **P:** Learners from audiology and nursing programs
- **I:** GAS (gather, analyze, summarize) debriefing tool
- **C:** PEARLS (Promoting Excellence and Reflective Learning in Simulation); Debriefing with Good Judgment
- **O:** Student understanding of Interprofessional Education Collaborative (IPEC) Core Competencies

Possible PICO Question: Which of these two debriefing methods yields better information regarding student knowledge of IPEC competencies?

Following this exercise, the educator will want to look for evidence in the literature so that ultimately, they can make an informed decision about what they want to use in their simulation.

Find the Evidence

Now that you have framed and defined the area of interest or problem you are trying to solve, it is time to look into the existing research. The purpose of the research literature search is to help in identifying the gaps in knowledge and inform best practices. There are several search engines that are available for that purpose. As you begin, develop a list of search terms and set your parameters for the search. In the previous example, the search terms could be *simulation* and *debriefing* and *interprofessional* (do not use acronyms). The PICO is helpful for identifying search terms. The use of "and" is part of the *Boolean phrase* that is part of most database search engines. Using "and" means that the search engine will identify any literature that contains both the terms/phrases. Note, if the term "or" is used, the search will only pull literature that has either *simulation* or *debriefing* or *interprofessional*, but not a combination of all terms. The search engine/database will then generate a list of individual research articles for you to access. It is valuable to remember that research completed in allied health and related fields, including education, may inform our thinking about the PICO question.

The American Speech-Language-Hearing Association (ASHA; n.d.) recommends a number of resources for finding external evidence. Many of these are clinically oriented, but you may also find resources related to education as well. Additionally, consider looking in Google Scholar and the Directory of Open Access Journals. As your work is likely to encompass issues related to SoTL and simulation, consider expanding your search beyond the clinical realm and seeking out open access SoTL journals. In the field of CSD, *Teaching and Learning in Communication Sciences & Disorders* is an open access journal that focuses on pedagogy and publishes research on the use of simulation in our field. Table 8-3 lists a variety of resources, including those suggested by ASHA, that may be useful to you in identifying external evidence. Remember that some resources, such as those from open access journals, are free, while others will require either a fee or a subscription. If you work at a university, educational institution, or health care facility, your workplace may have the access you need to get the latter type of article. If you do not work someplace that has subscription access to the resources that you are looking for, consider asking your local university, such as the one that sends you students for internships, if they would be willing to download a few articles for you. There are many ways to conduct a search and start learning about what resources are available to you. There are many additional methods, tools, resources, and ways to navigate a literature search. It is recommended to connect with a local librarian to help with more advanced searches and techniques as you continue to develop your research skills.

Read and Evaluate the Research Evidence

As you read the literature, it is imperative to interpret and evaluate the content of the research. The quality of the research is crucial to determining the relevance and application of the results to your question. Once the existing research is identified, it is time to challenge the literature. To challenge, in the realm of research, is to bring a critical lens, deep analysis, and inquisitive thought as to how we look at constructs, methods, interpretations, and applications of fact. There are a number of checklists available to help readers evaluate the strengths and limitations of published research. As you read the article, ask yourself questions such as those listed in Figure 8-2, which will help you analyze the article's content not only for overall quality but also for applicability to your own context.

Assess the Strength of the Evidence

There are several ways in which to assess the relative strengths or merits of the research evidence that you are reading. It is important to keep in mind that your assessment criteria may differ depending upon what you are assessing: quantitative or qualitative research. Validity, reliability, and generalizability are terms that are commonly associated with the analysis of the strength of research, but they mean very different things in the two different methodologies. In simulation and simulation research, these constructs are vitally important to ensure consistency and accuracy. Let's break these down and apply them to simulation and simulation research.

TABLE 8-3

External Evidence Resources

RESOURCE	LOCATION
ASHAWire	https://pubs.asha.org/
speechBITE	https://speechbite.com/
ERIC	https://eric.ed.gov/
ASHA's Evidence Maps	https://www.asha.org/evidence-maps/
The Cochrane Library	https://www.cochranelibrary.com/
Campbell Collaboration	https://www.campbellcollaboration.org/
What Works Clearinghouse	https://ies.ed.gov/ncee/wwc
PubMed	https://pubmed.ncbi.nlm.nih.gov/
PsycNet	https://psycnet.apa.org/search/basic
JSTOR	https://www.jstor.org/
Google Scholar	https://scholar.google.com/
Directory of Open Access Journals	https://doaj.org/
Teaching and Learning in Communication Sciences & Disorders	https://ir.library.illinoisstate.edu/tlcsd/
Journal of Effective Teaching in Higher Education	https://jethe.org/index.php/jethe
Journal of the Scholarship of Teaching and Learning	https://scholarworks.iu.edu/journals/index.php/josotl/index
International Journal for the Scholarship of Teaching & Learning	https://digitalcommons.georgiasouthern.edu/ij-sotl/

Data source: American Speech-Language-Hearing Association. (n.d.). Where should you search for external evidence? https://www.asha.org/research/ebp/gather-evidence

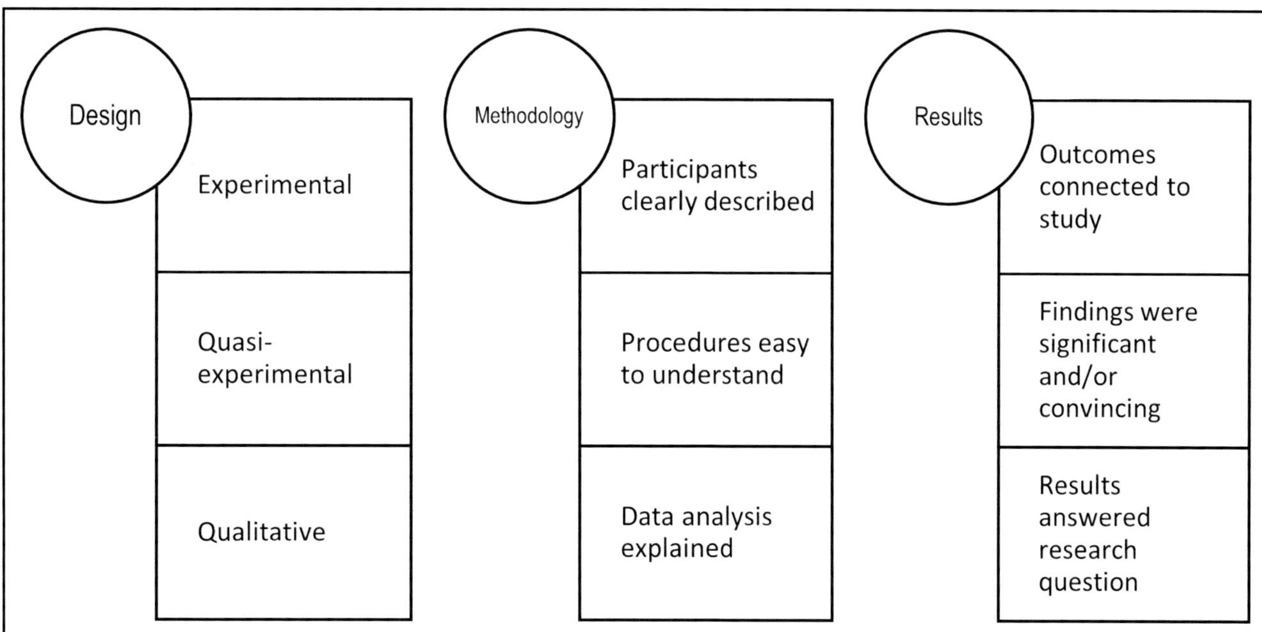

Figure 8-2. Evaluating pedagogical research evidence. (Reproduced with permission from Sarah M. Ginsberg. Adapted from Dollaghan, C. A. [2007]. *The handbook for evidence-based practice in communication disorders*. Paul H. Brookes Publishing Co and Subramanyam, R. [2013]. Art of reading a journal article: Methodically and effectively. *Journal of Oral and Maxillofacial Pathology, 17*[1], 65-70. https://doi.org/10.4103/0973-029X.110733)

TABLE 8-4

Types of Validity

CONSTRUCT	DEFINITION
Face validity	The extent to which a measurement appears at face value to assess a particular construct
Content validity	The extent to which a measurement instrument assesses the depth and breadth of a construct
Internal validity	The extent to which the results represent the truth from the sample
External validity	The extent to which the results are generalizable
Criterion validity	The extent to which the assessment strategy or plan is consistent with other assessment tools
Construct validity	The extent to which the assessment strategy or plan assesses a characteristic that is not observable but can be assumed to be present based on behavior; also known as the *assessment of a hypothetical construct*

Adapted from Creswell, J. W., & Creswell, J. D. (2018). *Research design: Qualitative, quantitative and mixed methods approaches* (5th ed.). SAGE Publications and Leedy, P. D., & Ormrod, J. E. (2019). *Practical research: Planning and design* (12th ed.). Pearson.

Quantitative Research

Validity is defined as the extent a construct is accurately measured (Leedy & Ormrod, 2019). There are several types of validity, such as face, content, internal, external, criterion, and construct validity. See Table 8-4 for definitions of the various types of validity that may be useful for you to consider as you read your research. Critical to the concept of validity in quantitative research are the threats to internal and external validity (Creswell, 2003). Internal validity is threatened when characteristics of the study, such as the methods, participants, or variables, are not well defined or consistent such that the interpretation of the data is incorrect. Threats to external validity include when the researchers make overly broad applications of the results, perhaps inferring they that they apply to all members of a population that was studied.

Reliability is defined as the ability for results to be replicated if the same methods and circumstances are utilized (Leedy & Ormrod, 2019). In simulation, reliability may be considered as replicability, meaning if a simulation was to occur over a series of dates/times, the simulation would be the same. A few types of reliability can be taken into consideration as you read the literature. *Interrater reliability* refers to the level of agreement when two different raters score the same item. In simulation, this may take the form of two different faculty members using a checklist and simultaneously scoring a learner's performance of demonstrated skills during a simulation. *Test–retest*, as the name implies, states that the test and retest scores should be consistent over multiple points in time. In simulation, test–retest reliability may be a simulation repeated with various groups of CSD learners, such as a group participating in the morning and another group participating in the afternoon. In this situation, the test–retest reliability would demonstrate similar results as the only change is the time of day the learners participate in the simulation. *Internal consistency reliability* refers to how well related items within an assessment result in similar findings. As an example, after a simulation activity is completed, the learner is asked to complete an online survey about the activity. One survey question asks the participant to provide a diagnosis based on the simulation encounter. Later in the same survey, the participant is asked to indicate their diagnostic statement based on the encounter. In this example, the internal consistency is seeking to identify if the responses for the two questions align.

> Generalizability is the degree to which the results of a research study reflect what the results would be "in the real world," with another sample of participants or with the variables operationalized in other ways. In other words, research results are generalizable when the findings are true generally speaking in most contexts with most people most of the time. (Frey, 2018, p. 725)

While the definition of and types of generalizability are not always agreed upon, there is a growing appreciation that the ability to apply findings to a person or persons not involved in the study is central to EBP and EBE (Polit & Beck, 2010). Polit and Beck (2010) suggest that statistical generalization, which draws upon the representativeness of the sample population, may be a useful dimension to consider for quantitative research.

Qualitative Research

Validity may be seen as one of the strengths of qualitative research, but it does not mean quite the same thing as it does in quantitative research. In this tradition, validity represents the "appropriateness" of the mechanisms of data collection and results relative to the research question (Leung, 2015, p. 326). Various terms including "truth" (Green & Thorogood, 2018, p. 388), "trustworthiness," "authenticity," and "credibility" (Creswell & Miller, 2000, p. 124) have been used to represent the concept of validity in qualitative work. Identifying specific procedures that were completed by the researchers may be indicators of their attempt to improve validity, such as using triangulation (using different sources to view the same phenomenon); "rich, thick description" that provides a clear and strong appreciation of the participants' perspectives; and using external reviewers, either peer debriefers or auditors, to review the accuracy of the data and interpretation across researchers (Creswell, 2003, p. 196).

Qualitative research is less focused on the notion of reliability, as it is assumed that the interview process and similar methods of data collection are a necessarily human interaction that may not be replicable by all researchers with all participants. In general, discussion regarding this research approach does not much include the term reliability. Some of the techniques associated with the rigor of a study's implementation may also be useful to improving the reliability of the study. For example, using external reviewers, as noted previously, can be used to verify that the data analysis and conclusions could have been arrived at by a researcher who was not present for the data collection process (Green & Thorogood, 2018; Leung, 2015). Another technique, known as *member checking*, gives the participants of the study an opportunity to corroborate with the researcher that the conclusions identified by them are consistent with the participants' perspectives (Creswell, 2003; Green & Thorogood, 2018).

The concept of generalizability in qualitative research is often debated and not always "expected" (Leung, 2015, p. 326). The reason for this may be that unlike quantitative research, which often seeks to collect data from as large a population as possible so as to give strength and merit to the statistical analysis, qualitative research often relies on data from smaller, more focused participant groups. Because qualitative studies do not use statistics, they may be seen as lacking the statistical rigor of analyzing hundreds of participants and determining significance. As a result, you will often read that generalizability is a limitation of the study, but this should not be taken at face value as a flaw with the research. Analytic generalization, which generates theory or findings based on specific details, and transferability, which applies findings to others based on similarities of shared characteristics, may be useful constructs (Leung, 2015; Polit & Beck, 2010). Finally, Denzin and Lincoln (2003) describe generalization of a study's findings as being "constantly tested by readers as they determine if it speaks to them about their experience or about the lives of others they know" (p. 229).

Consider the Relevance of the Literature in Association With Your Question

While strategies to enhance generalization exist, it is up to the informed reader to determine if the results and findings of a publication are transferrable to the question or population at hand. Referring back to the PICO you developed may help you to decide. Other considerations include:

- Does this study investigate a population similar to my learners?
- Does the study review a simulation learning strategy that I could use to meet the learner objectives?
- Are the study's outcomes related to my question?
- If the study does not perfectly match my question, can it provide relevant insights to guide EBP?

Conducting Research in Simulation

This section serves as a guide for those considering conducting SoTL research in simulation-based education. It begins with sharing developed standards and criteria for conducting research in simulation and addresses some key considerations, such as methodology, measurement, data, analysis, and dissemination. The last step of dissemination is a critical one, as making the results of this work publicly available to be scrutinized and consumed in the same way as clinical research is one of the hallmarks of SoTL research (Shulman, 1993). If you are not at all experienced in conducting research, this section will help you get started. If you are a seasoned researcher, this section will help you consider SoTL specifically as it relates to studying the use of simulations in teaching and learning.

Using the methods for searching and evaluating literature (e.g., PICO) can be useful in determining your research focus. For example, after reading the literature, challenging what is proposed, and rethinking the subject matter, you identify a hole or missing link in the subject matter. That is sometimes referred to as *finding the gap*, in which you identify those pieces of information or perspectives that have not yet been explored or that are not reported in the literature. For example, you begin to read about the use of SPs in rehabilitation medicine training. You discover that SPs are widely used in training physical therapists, nurses, medical learners, and pharmacists at a very high volume across the United States. You also notice that the use of SPs in speech-language pathology and audiology is significantly less than these other professions. Embracing an analytical way of thinking, you begin to look deeper in the literature comparing speech-language pathology and audiology and other professions' use of SPs. They may identify possible limitations (i.e., cost) that may inhibit speech-language pathology and audiology programs from starting an SP simulation center, whereas other programs (i.e., medical schools) have funding or resources. Another example is psychological safety. Psychological safety is a construct often discussed in published research on the topic of simulation. However, you find that research about the learner's feelings toward group participation and possible fears associated with group simulation experiences has not been investigated. This can be identified as a gap in the literature and can, in some cases, lead to the development of a research question (i.e., To what degree does fear impact learner participation in interprofessional simulation?).

Once you have identified the gap that you are interested in learning more about, you will need to develop a research question. The research question drives the methods; therefore, drafting a clear research question is critical to the next steps in research. There are several ways to generate a research question, but using criteria will aid in quality and ensuring key elements are considered. Recall that the type of question you ask will likely dictate the manner in which you design your research. For the sake of this chapter, further explanation of the exact research question will be deferred to specific research references such as Creswell, 2015; Creswell and Creswell, 2018; Goertzen, 2017; Leedy and Ormrod, 2019; and Tashakkori and Creswell, 2017. As you think in general terms, consider what the purpose of your research is, what you want to learn about, and what the context is for what you want to learn.

Research Standards

Research in simulation must adhere to the same standards and rigor as any other research endeavors. To that purpose, the Society for Simulation in Healthcare (SSH) Committee for Accreditation of Healthcare Simulation Programs (2016) provides accredited programs within the United States with standards and measurement criteria for conducting research. Internationally, several organizations offer best practices and guidelines in simulation-based research for simulation centers and researchers alike.

The Council of Academic Programs in Communication Sciences and Disorders created *Best Practices in Healthcare Simulations for Communication Sciences and Disorders* (Dudding et al., 2018) as a guide for those interested in utilization simulation for clinical education. It includes discussion on the nature and value of assessment in simulation-based education.

Methodology

Methodology of simulation research should adhere to the same levels of scientific rigor and federal, regional, institutional guidelines and practices, ethics, and human participant protections as stated throughout this chapter. The major types of research methodology (quantitative, qualitative, and mixed methods) are covered in an earlier section of this chapter. The International Nursing Association for Clinical Simulation and Learning (INACSL) provides extensive resources that can be helpful to you in designing and conducting simulation research (INACSL, n.d.) The SSH (n.d.) offers various resources for researchers:

- Tutorials on research basics
- Tools for planning and conducting research, including checklists
- Knowledge maps of existing literature
- Networking opportunities for researchers

Data Types and Measurement

Data in simulation research can take many forms, including, but not limited to, test scores, checklists, observations, self-reports, surveys, interviews, focus groups, prebriefs, debriefs, and narratives (Gravetter & Wallnau, 2007). The type of data collected is based on the methods of the research (e.g., qualitative or quantitative). For example, if the research is aiming to explore the learner's experience in a simulation, the researcher might employ questionnaires using a numbered Likert scale (quantitative) or conduct a focus group (qualitative). If the researcher is aiming to assess the learner's knowledge upon completion of a simulation, they may develop a multiple-choice test of knowledge (quantitative). It is important to mention that one method of research (e.g., qualitative, quantitative) or one type of data (e.g., surveys, focus groups, interviews) may not be enough to address the research question. The use of multiple data sets and methods can lead to new and unique directions for future research.

Reporting Guidelines for Simulation-Based Research

Dissemination and publication of research is an essential part of the research process. Various reporting guidelines have been established to aid in a standardized and consistent method of reporting clinical research, including but not limited to, the Consolidated Standards of Reporting Trials (CONSORT; Moher et al., 2010) and Strengthening the Reporting of Observational studies in Epidemiology (STROBE; von Elm et al., 2007). Cheng et al. (2016) developed a set of core extensions specific to reporting of simulation research. These extensions were necessary because of the unique aspects of simulation-based research. Compared to other clinical research, simulation-based research has a unique set of features that requires additional disclosure and transparency when publishing and disseminating. These features include (a) a wide variety of modalities may be used, (b) a variety of instructional design features in educational simulation research, (c) standardization of simulated environments and encounters that aid in reducing threats to internal validity, (d) use of multiple data collection methods (e.g., observation, score reports, video recordings), and (e) outcomes data relate only to the simulated experience; however, efforts are needed to discuss translation to the real-world setting (Cheng et al., 2016). Please note, these factors do not address any additional and specific publisher's requirements for journal submissions. Box 8-2 provides a noninclusive list of simulation journals. It is suggested that researchers seek out specific inclusion criteria for each respective journal prior to manuscript submission.

BOX 8-2
Simulation Journals

Key Simulation-Based Research Journals

Advances in Simulation
The British Medical Journal Simulation & Technology—Enhanced Learning
Clinical Simulation in Nursing
The Journal of Surgical Simulation
Simulation and Gaming
Simulation in Healthcare

Health Care Educational Journals

Academic Medicine
Advances in Health Sciences Education
Advances in Medical Education and Practice
Canadian Medical Education Journal
The Clinical Teacher
International Journal of Medical Education
Journal of Continuing Education in the Health Professions
Medical Education
Medical Education Development
Medical Education Online
Medical Teacher
Open Medical Education Journal
Teaching and Learning in Communication Sciences & Disorders
Teaching and Learning in Medicine

Interprofessional Journals

Journal of Allied Health
Journal of Interprofessional Care
Journal of Research in Interprofessional Practice and Education

Journals Related to Safety and Quality

BMJ Quality & Safety
International Journal for Quality in Health Care
Joint Commission Journal on Quality and Patient Safety
Journal of Nursing Regulation
Journal of Patient Safety

Single-Subject Research Design

While it is not feasible to discuss here all of the types of research designs that you might use, we want to be sure to mention single-subject research design (SSRD) as it may represent a simple design approach for those new to SoTL research. SSRD is commonly used in CSD and is also known as *within-subject design*; it is a quantitative, scientifically rigorous approach where each participant provides their own experimental control. SSRD is commonly mistaken for the use of case studies. ASHA hosts a Clinical Research Education Library (CREd) resource that provides excellent tutorials regarding SSRD (ASHA, 2014). Studies using this design have the following defining features (Horner et al., 2005; Kratochwill et al., 2010):

- An individual or case serves as the unit of intervention and analysis.
- The case serves as its own control.
- Dependent and independent variables are operationally defined.
- Experimental control is achieved through introduction and withdrawal/reversal, staggered introduction, or iterative manipulation of the independent variable.
- Outcome measurements occur repeatedly before, during, and after intervention within and across conditions.

We can consider an example of how this design might be used in a simulation experience. Let's imagine that I have a student in my diagnostic methods course who is having trouble identifying the appropriate standardized tests to administer based on the patient's presenting history. On a course examination that requires this kind of problem solving, they score a 62% correct. As the course instructor, I recommend that they spend some time with a computer simulation, such as Simucase, practicing the skill of identifying appropriate standardized assessments to administer to clients based on their symptoms. After they complete the assigned simulation practice, I readminister the course examination to see if their score improves. This is akin to a test–retest design and would give us some data that would indicate that learning improved based on the use of simulation technology.

Ethics in Simulation Research

Ethics refers to adhering to the professional, institutional, and federal standards for conducting human participant research and is a critical component of all research endeavors. It is especially relevant in simulation research in that most studies in simulation involve the use of human participants. The American Psychological Association (2021) offers five principals related to ethics in research:

1. Beneficence and nonmaleficence
2. Fidelity and responsibility
3. Integrity
4. Justice
5. Respect for an individual's rights and dignity

Ensuring research integrity is a high priority to researchers and institutions. There are two processes that are primarily used to provide training and oversight of human research. The first is that researchers participating in human research are required to complete training in human participant research. Such training educates the researcher on topics related to adherence to ethics, research integrity, collection, management and sharing of data, publication practices, and human participant rights and protections. The National Institutes of Health (NIH) and the Collaborative Institutional Training Initiative (CITI) are examples of approved human participant research training programs that are recognized by many institutions.

Governing research bodies and institutions of higher education have established institutional review boards (IRBs). In accordance with federal guidelines, the primary focus of IRBs is the protection of the rights and welfare of human research participants. Many IRBs have taken on the additional role of reviewing research methods and proposals to ensure high-quality research. Researchers are required to submit research proposals to IRBs prior to initiating research. Standard components of the IRB proposal include administrative information, type of review (e.g., full, expedited), study overview, participants, recruitment, compensation, risks and benefits, privacy and confidentiality, informed consent process, research collaborations, conflict of interest disclosures, and assurances. It is imperative that researchers check in with their respective IRB to ensure any researcher-based training and prerequisites (e.g., CITI, NIH, institution-specific training) are met prior to submitting an IRB application. Note that all research involving people, including students in our clinics and courses, requires IRB application. For additional information related to IRBs, please refer to the U.S. Food and Drug Administration's (2019) informational sheet on IRB frequently asked questions.

Advocacy

When we talk of advocacy, we think of advocating as the act or process of supporting, to argue in favor of something or someone. When we speak of advocacy for research in health care simulation, it means to sponsor, prepare, create, do, and support research endeavors in simulation-based learning. Advocacy includes supporting best practices in conducting simulation-based education as well as conducting simulation research. Organizations such as INACSL and SSH have established research agendas intended to advance the practice of simulation-based education. Some of the priorities include research aimed at:

- Advancing of the use of simulation-based education in health care
- Developing and evaluating tools for learner assessment
- Establishing best practices in interprofessional simulation
- Determining learner and patient outcomes
- Advancing best practices in the prebrief and debrief
- Determining transition to practice

These and other organizations have created sources of advocacy for research in simulation by establishing research journals, establishing research grants and funding opportunities, and offering guides for conducting and evaluating research. The interested reader is referred to SSH Research Tools for a complete listing of resources (https://www.ssih.org/SSH-Resources/Research-Information). Mentoring of researchers and educators is an important part of the field for simulation-based educators. In addition to providing informational resources, organizations provide opportunities for researchers in simulation to network and collaborate.

Funding of research is another important way to advocate for quality research in simulation-based education. Funding opportunities can be found with the help of professionals in the Office of Sponsored Programs located within many institutions of higher education. Readers can also search organizational websites such as SSH; Agency for Healthcare Research and Quality; National Patient Safety Foundation; INACSL; International Network for Simulation-based Pediatric Innovation, Research, and Education;

American Association for the Advancement of Science; and the U.S. government. Additional information on how to write a research grant may be found within the above websites as well as with the American Psychological Association and the American Medical Association.

As educators in CSD continue to embrace the advantages of simulation-based education within their curriculum, the need for high-quality research as it applies to our disciplines increases. As relative newcomers to the use of simulation, it is important for us to gain a knowledge base from the work of other disciplines, such as medicine and nursing. In light of the rapid growth of health care simulation and the onset of the pandemic of 2020, Park et al. (2020) created a simulation manifesto in which they advocate that health care simulation is a practice and the practice embraces three tenets: safety, leadership, and advocacy. It is within this manifesto that the discussion surrounding how health care simulation has been an act of accommodation, rather than collaboration, is provided. Research on knowledge, skills, attributes, interprofessionalism, and so on are all areas that warrant consideration for research in an effort to aid in the advocacy for more collaborative approaches in the practice of health care simulation.

Leadership and advocacy warrant discussion. Leadership involves aspects of ethics, judgment, safety, and many more attributes. It also speaks to the creative, forward-thinking elements that are found in simulation. The creative avenues in which teaching and learning occur in simulation warrants our investigation and the dissemination of findings. Finding gaps in practices, teaching, learning, modality, and assessments allows leaders in the field of simulation to step forward and model quality evidenced-based research. Mentoring novices in the use of simulations is an important aspect of leadership. Ultimately, it is to the benefit of our academic and clinical programs, learners, and those we serve that engage in quality research within our own fields of study; and that we conduct this research with a foundation of knowledge and best practices. It is the hope that this chapter serves as a starting point for your research path in simulation-based education.

Summary

Research in simulation is a necessary aspect of understanding behaviors, development of programs (educational and practice), evaluating methods of simulation implementation and execution, quality assurance, and assessment of results. All who engage in simulation (e.g., consumer, advocate, participant, publisher) are included in an open invitation to participate in research. Research endeavors afford the ability to use theoretical foundations in the ongoing evolution of simulation science and practice. Through the use of a variety of methods, theories, and resources, simulation researchers may continue to generate a body of literature to aid in the advocacy and growth of simulation practices in education and practice.

References

American Psychological Association. (2021). Ethical principals of psychologists and code of conduct. https://www.apa.org/ethics/code

American Speech-Language-Hearing Association. (n.d.). Where should you search for external evidence? https://www.asha.org/research/ebp/gather-evidence/

American Speech-Language-Hearing Association. (2014). CREd library, research design and method single-subject experimental design: An overview. https://academy.pubs.asha.org/2014/12/single-subject-experimental-design-an-overview/

Baum, F., MacDougall, C., & Smith, D. (2006). Participatory action research. *Journal of Epidemiology and Community Health, 60*(10), 854-857. https://doi.org/10.1136/jech.2004.028662

Bernstein, D., & Bass, R. (2005). The scholarship of teaching and learning. *Academe, 91*(4), 37-43. http://ww.jstor.org/stable/40253429

Bogden, R. C., & Biklen, S. K. (2003). *Qualitative research in education: An introduction to theory and methods.* Allyn & Bacon.

Boyd, W. (2013) Does Boyer's integrated scholarships model work on the ground? An adaption of Boyer's model for scholarly professional development. *International Journal for the Scholarship of Teaching and Learning, 7*(2), 25. https://digitalcommons.georgiasouthern.edu/il-sotl/vol7/iss2/25

Boyer, E. L. (1990). *Scholarship reconsidered: Priorities of the professoriate.* Jossey-Bass.

Cheng, A., Kessler, D., Mackinnon, R., Chang, T. P., Nadkarni, V. M., Hunt, E. A., Duval-Arnould, J., Lin, Y., Cook, D. A., Pusic, M., Hui, J., Moher, D., Egger, M., Auerbach, M., & the International Network for Simulation-based Pediatric innovation, Research, and Education Reporting Guidelines Investigators. (2016). Reporting guidelines for health care simulation research: Extensions to the CONSORT and STROBE statements. *Advances in Simulation, 1.* https://doi.org/10.1186/s41077-016-0025-y

Creswell, J. (2003). *Research design: Qualitative, quantitative and mixed methods approaches* (2nd ed.). SAGE Publications.

Creswell, J. W. (2007). *Qualitative inquiry and research design: Choosing among five approaches* (2nd ed.). SAGE Publications.

Creswell, J. (2015). *A concise introduction to mixed methods research.* SAGE Publications.

Creswell, J. W., & Creswell, J. D. (2018). *Research design: Qualitative, quantitative and mixed methods approaches* (5th ed.). SAGE Publications.

Creswell, J. W., & Miller, D. L. (2000). Determining validity in qualitative inquiry. *Theory Into Practice, 39*(3), 124-130.

Davies, P. (1999). What is evidence-based education? *British Journal of Educational Studies, 47*(2), 108-121.

Denzin, N. K., & Lincoln, Y. S. (2003). *Collecting and interpreting qualitative materials* (2nd ed.). SAGE Publications.

Dudding, C. C., Brown, D. K., Estis, J., Szymanski, C., & Zraick, R. I. (2018). *Best practices in healthcare simulations in communication sciences and disorders.* Council of Academic Programs in Communication Sciences and Disorders. http://www.capcsd.org/wp-content/uploads/2018/05/Simulation-Guide-Published-May-18-2018.pdf

Eisner, E. (1998). Does experience in the arts boost academic achievement? *Art Education, 51*(1), 7-15.

Felten, P. (2013). Principles of good practice in SoTL. *Teaching and Learning, 1*(1), 121-125.

Frey, B. (2018). Generalizability. In B. Frey (Ed.), *The SAGE encyclopedia of educational research, measurement, and evaluation* (Vol. 1, p. 725). SAGE Publications. https://www.doi.org.ezproxy.emich.edu/10.4135/9781506326139.n284

Ginsberg, S. M., & DeRuiter, M. (2020). Conscious clinical education: The evidence-based education-clinical education model. *Seminars in Speech and Language, 41*(4), 279-288. https://doi.org/10.1055/s-0040-1713779

Ginsberg, S. M., Friberg, J. C., & Visconti, C. F. (2012). *Scholarship of teaching and learning in speech-language pathology and audiology: Evidence-based education.* Plural Publishing.

Ginsberg, S. M., Friberg, J., Visconti, C. F., DeRuiter, M., & Hoepner, J. K. (2017). On the culture of scholarship of teaching and learning. *Teaching and Learning in Communication Sciences & Disorders, 1*(1), 1-5. https://doi.org/10.30707/TLCSD1.1

Goertzen, M. J. (2017). Chapter 3: Introduction to quantitative research and data. *Library Technology Reports, 53*(4), 12-18.

Gravetter, F., & Wallnau, L. (2007). *Statistics for the behavioral sciences* (7th ed.). Thompson Wadsworth.

Green, J., & Thorogood, N. (2018). *Qualitative methods for health research.* SAGE Publications.

Horner, R. H., Carr, E. G., Halle, J., McGee, G., Odom, S., & Wolery, M. (2005). The use of single subject research to identify evidence-based practice in special education. *Exceptional Children, 71*, 165-179.

Hutchings, P. (2000). Introduction. In P. Hutchings (Ed.), *Opening lines: Approaches to the scholarship of teaching and learning* (pp. 1-10). Carnegie Foundation for the Advancement of Teaching.

INACSL Research Committee. (n.d.). Resources. International Nursing Association for Clinical Simulation and Learning. https://www.inacsl.org/resources/for-researchers/

Kratochwill, T. R., Hitchcock, J., Horner, R. H., Levin, J. R., Odom, S. L., Rindskopf, D. M., & Shadish, W. R. (2010). *Single-case designs technical documentation.* What Works Clearinghouse.

Leedy, P. D., & Ormrod, J. E. (2019). *Practical research: Planning and design* (12th ed.). Pearson.

Leung, L. (2015). Validity, reliability, and generalizability in qualitative research. *Journal of Family Medicine and Primary Care, 4*(3), 324-327. https://dx.doi.org/10.4103%2F2249-4863.161306

Libarkin, J., & Kurdziel, J. (2002). Research methodologies in science education: The qualitative-quantitative debate. *Journal of Geoscience Education, 50*(1), 78-86.

MacDonald, C. (2012). Understanding participatory action research: A qualitative research methodology option. *Canadian Journal of Action Research, 13*(2), 34-50.

Megowan-Romanowicz, C. (2010). Inside out: Action research from the teacher-researcher perspective. *Journal of Science Teacher Education, 21*, 993-1011.

Meline, T. (2010). *A research primer for communication sciences and disorders.* Allyn & Bacon.

Moher, D., Hopewell, S., Schulz, K. F., Montori, V., Gøtzsche, P. C., Devereaux, P. J., Elbourne, D., Egger, M., & Altman, D. G. (2010). CONSORT 2010 explanation and elaboration: Updated guidelines for reporting parallel group randomized trials. *BMJ, 340*. https://doi.org/10.1016/j.ijsu.2011.10.001

Nibert, M. (2001). Boyer's model of scholarship. *Pacific Crest Faculty Development Series.* https://my.queens.edu/cafe/Best%20Practices%20Documents/Boyer's%20Model%20of%20Scholarship%20Overview.pdf

Park, C., Clark, L., Gephardt, G., Robertson, J. M., Miller, J., Downing, D. K., Koh, B. L. S., Bryant, K. D., Grant, D., Pai, D. R., Gavilanes, J. S., Bastida, E. I. H., Li, L., Littlewood, K., Escudero, E., Kelly, M. A., Nestel, D., & Rethans, J. -J. (2020). Manifesto for healthcare simulation practice. *BMJ Simulation and Technology Enhanced Learning, 6*(6), 365-368. https://doi.org/10.1136/bmjstel-2020-000712

Polit, D. F., & Beck, C. T. (2010). Generalization in quantitative and qualitative research: Myths and strategies. *International Journal of Nursing Studies, 47*(11), 1451-1458. https://doi.org/10.1016/j.ijnurstu.2010.06.004

Rahman, S. (2017). The advantages and disadvantages of using qualitative and quantitative approaches and methods in language "testing and assessment" research: A literature review. *Journal of Education and Learning, 6*(1), 102-112.

Regnault, A., Willgross, T., Barbic, S., & the International Society for Quality of Life Research Mixed Methods Special Interest Group. (2018). Towards use of mixed methods inquiry as best practice in health outcomes research. *Journal of Patient Reported Outcomes, 2*(19). https://doi.org/10.1186/s41687-018-0043-8

Richardson, W. S., Wilson, M. C., Nishikawa, J., & Hayward, R. S. (1995). The well-built clinical question: A key to evidence-based decisions. *ACP Journal Club, 123*(3), A-12.

Rios, L. P., Ye, C. & Thabane, L. (2010). Association between framing of the research question using the PICOT format and reporting quality of randomized controlled trials. *BMC Medical Research Methodology, 10*(11). https://doi.org/10.1186/1471-2288-10-11

Shulman, L. S. (1993). Teaching as community property: Putting an end to pedagogical solitude. *Change, 25*(6), 6-7.

Shulman, L. S. (1998). Theory, practice, and the education of professionals. *The Elementary School Journal, 98*(5), 511-526. https://doi.org/10.1086/461912

Society for Simulation in Healthcare. (n.d.). SSH research tools. https://www.ssih.org/SSH-Resources/Research-Information

Society for Simulation in Healthcare. (2016). Research standards and measurement criteria. https://www.ssih.org/Credentialing/Accreditation/Full-Accreditation

Tashakkori, A., & Creswell, J. (2017). The new era of mixed methods. *Journal of Mixed Methods Research, 1*(3), 3-7. https://doi.org/10.1177/2345678906293042

Trigwell, K. (2013). Evidence of the impact of scholarship of teaching and learning purposes. *Teaching and Learning Inquiry, 1*(91), 95-105.

U.S. Food and Drug Administration. (2019). Institutional Review Boards Frequently Asked Questions. https://www.fda.gov/regulatory-information/search-fda-guidance-documents/institutional-review-boards-frequently-asked-questions

von Elm, E., Altman, D. G., Egger, M., Pocock, S. J., Gøtzsche, P. C., Vandenbroucke, J. P., & STROBE Initiative. (2007). Strengthening the reporting of observational studies in epidemiology (STROBE) statement: Guidelines for reporting observational studies. *BMJ, 335*(7624), 806-808. https://doi.org/10.1136/bmj.39335.541782.AD

Forward Facing

Carol C. Dudding, PhD, CCC-SLP, F-ASHA, CHSE and Kevin Phaup, MFA

A good hockey player plays where the puck is. A great hockey player plays where the puck is going to be.
—Wayne Gretzky (as cited in Zoll, n.d.)

Challenges in Higher Education

It can be useful to consider what the thinkers and policy makers are saying about the future of higher education in the United States. The Educause Horizon Report 2020 has broadened its focus beyond trends in educational technologies to include social, technical, economic, and political forces impacting higher education (Brown et al., 2020). Social trends cited by the Horizon Report 2020 include the increase in mental health issues among students, changing student demographics, and a national call for equity and fair practices.

As educators, we are aware of the increase in mental health issues among students. Reports indicate that approximately one-third of undergraduate students exhibit signs of depression, anxiety disorders, or suicidality (Oswalt et al., 2020). While the full effects of COVID-19 pandemic on the mental health of students remains to be studied, initial reports indicate an increased level of anxiety and depression among college students in China as a result of the pandemic (Chang et al., 2020). A web-based survey of U.S. college students suggests that as many as half of students report a mental health issue as a result of the pandemic (Eisenberg et al., 2020). There is some evidence that the acute stress brought on by the pandemic may be responsible for students majoring in health care fields deciding not to pursue a career in health care post-graduation (Zhang et al., 2021). Universities are tasked with supporting and providing services for these students both in the short and long term.

Another social factor is the change in student demographics, known in higher education as the *enrollment cliff*. Due to the decreasing birth rate, it is anticipated that there will be a 15% decline in freshman enrollments by the year 2025 (Kline, 2019). It is not just the declining birth rate that is impacting enrollment. Demographics are changing in that more and more people enrolling in college are nontraditional students. Many of these students are interested in online

Dudding, C. C., & Ginsberg, S. M. (Eds.).
Simulation-Based Learning in Communication Sciences and Disorders: Moving From Theory to Practice. (pp. 139-146).

and part-time offerings that will allow them to continue to earn an income. More students are seeking nondegree offerings that help them do their existing jobs better. Employers are interested in what graduates can do as opposed to what courses they have completed. University administrators are recognizing the changing demands of the workforce and are expanding certificate programs and creating opportunities for lifelong learning (Brown, 2020).

Throughout the United States and across the world, we have heard calls for equity and fair practices. Universities in the United States are charged with examining their practices for explicit and implicit institutional biases that limit equal access to our programs. Many university programs have focused goals and objectives for expanding the diversity, equity, and inclusion of faculty and students. They are requiring changes in curriculum and how instruction is delivered in order to be culturally responsive and support all students (Brown, 2020). Inequities are often linked to limited access, and so it is prudent to consider ways in which technology can help provide access to quality experiences for all members of the university community.

Technical factors identified by the Educause Horizon Report 2020 as impacting higher education include the use of big data analytics, which has brought with it concerns about privacy and security of the vast amounts of data entrusted to the universities (Brown et al., 2020). Artificial intelligence (AI) and open-source educational platforms are poised to change the way students experience the learning environment in terms of both educational delivery methods and student support services. Reflection on your own undergraduate and graduate education will reveal the unmistakable impact that technology has had on our higher education system. Gone are the card catalogs and hours spent searching the library stacks. To a great extent, gone too are the computer labs. If predictions are correct, textbooks and campus bookstores are likely to become extinct. University classrooms have seen a proliferation of new technologies, including the use of smartphones for real-time polling, holograms for teaching anatomy, and video blogs to host group discussions. But with those changes comes a generation of digital natives—students who always have had cellphones, computers, and digital learning. Technology is the cornerstone of their social and educational experiences.

Economic factors to be addressed include the cost of higher education and the burden of student debt on society. As funding for public institutions of higher education decreases, and the cost of a university education increases, the amount of student debt also increases. It is estimated that the current amount of student debt in the U.S. is $1.5 trillion dollars, causing many to reevaluate the value of higher education (Looney et al., 2020). The Educause Horizon Report 2020 includes the impact of climate change on higher education as an economic factor (Brown et al., 2020). It is predicted that students and faculty will seek flexible learning environments that do not require them to commute to campus. Indeed, the events of the COVID-19 pandemic showed us the benefits of teaching and attending classes from home. This will likely shift the college experience from a physical campus-based experience to a web-based virtual community.

Economic, global, and political factors are impacting how administrators in higher education are positioning themselves for the future. Deans begin using terms like "return on investment" and "workforce skills." Universities are starting or expanding online education as an integral part of university offerings. This makes sense in that online education, if properly sourced and managed, has the potential to address the issues of cost and flexibility. A number of existing online programs have also adapted their curriculum to be attractive to adult learners needing to retool for their current jobs by offering credentials instead of degrees and offering credit for life experiences. Another way universities will continue to transform is through alliances and partnerships with other entities. Indeed, we have seen a move toward partnering with key businesses to sponsor and/or fund research labs and buildings.

Challenges to Clinical Education

This brings us to the question of how these factors will impact clinical education programs in audiology and speech-language pathology. In keeping with the topic of this book, we ask what is the role of simulation in addressing these factors impacting higher education? In order to address these questions, we need to consider them in a broader context. In the case of clinical education, the broader context includes changes in the health care and K-12 education systems, a rapidly evolving knowledge base, integration of technology into service delivery (e.g., mobile health apps, teletherapy), and evolving global, social, and economic demands.

Current clinical education models in medicine, nursing, and allied health programs, including speech-language pathology and audiology, rely heavily on preceptors/supervisors in off-campus sites for obtaining clinical skills and experiences. For years, program directors in communication sciences and disorders (CSD) have been reporting a scarcity of off-campus placements as one of the challenges to expanding our academic programs. This model of clinical education was further challenged during the COVID-19 pandemic when many hospitals and educational sites closed to our students. University programs were forced to quickly transition to the use of teletherapy and simulation technologies to provide students with the required experiences for graduation. This global event confirmed that our current system of reliance on off-campus sites is unsustainable. Additionally, our current model of clinical education comes at a high cost to universities in terms of faculty, staff time, and finances. A growing number of preceptors in medicine and nursing are requiring payment in order to accept students. We have seen recent evidence of this occurring in our professions. It would seem that one solution would be to expand clinical experiences in our on-campus clinics. To do so would entail a new set of challenges in terms of staffing, space, costs, and the ability to offer students a broad and expansive range of experiences.

A group of 61 deans of allied health programs took part in a research project to address the future of clinical education (Romig et al., 2017). In addition to identifying the aforementioned challenges, they offered guidance as we move forward toward a transformation of our clinical education programs. This group of administrators recommended a shift in focus from assessing what students know to what students do. That is, they recommend a shift toward a competency-based education. They recommended that we seek out and establish more collaborative partnerships and interprofessional education/practice opportunities. That is, rather than a one-to-one apprenticeship model, we develop collaborative models where students from different programs receive high-quality experiences in an environment that employs a team approach that most represents actual practice under the guidance of several preceptors of different backgrounds. A collaborative model would also allow for cross-training between disciplines. This model could only be effective in a competency-based curriculum where the focus is on developing clinical decision-making skills to promote evidence-based practice in our students (Cowan et al., 2005; McAllister et al., 2010, 2011). It would also require a loosening of licensing, accreditation, and certification standards on the part of professional organizations. Another recommendation of the group is to secure change in reimbursement systems that would allow our partnering sites to be reimbursed for services provided by student-practitioners (Romig et al., 2017).

Simulation-Based Education to Meet the Challenges

What we have learned in navigating the social, economic, demographic, and technical changes impacting clinical education is that with challenges come opportunities. The Association of Academic Health Centers (n.d.) has put forth an educational model for 21st century medicine, along with a statement of "urgency to undertake new, more efficient, and more effective paradigms for health professions education" (para. 1).

The model, while not unique in its focus, is easily adapted to serve as a framework for moving forward in clinical education in audiology and speech-language pathology. Such a model includes (Association of Academic Health Centers, n.d.):

- Making interprofessional education, collaborative practice, and team-based care the norm in CSD training programs
- Educating a workforce to meet the needs of the modern practice environments
- Reducing the length and cost of education in CSD
- Using massive open online courses and online platforms to increase access to information and provide global perspectives on the issues
- Incorporating the use of simulation and virtual technologies into clinical education

While it is beyond the scope of this chapter to offer prescriptive use of simulation technologies for clinical education in CSD, the reader is encouraged to take advantage of the resources and examples provided throughout this book. There are numerous resources available to you through professional organizations dedicated to the use of simulation for clinical education, online and in-person professional development offerings, certificate programs, and formal and informal mentoring. As you continue gaining the knowledge, skills, and attributes necessary for best practices in simulation-based education, keep in mind that simulations are "a technique—not a technology" (Gaba, 2004, p. i2) and, therefore, are within your grasp as another tool for providing high-quality clinical education experiences for students.

Skating to Where the Puck Will Be

This section is written from the viewpoint of an industrial designer. This offers the reader a unique approach to considering technical trends in the future, especially opportunities for advancement in the use of simulation in CSD. The section begins with an overview of existing and emerging technologies and uses within immersive simulations. It is not intended to thoroughly define the entire spectrum, but rather to establish a baseline for educators to make comparisons. It offers general definitions of terminology and technology while highlighting strengths of immersive simulations to enhance learning, training, and working experiences. This discussion leverages the comparison from a variety of disciplines to demonstrate the possibilities and the efficacy of utilizing extended reality simulation in clinical education. It aims to provide programs with a forward-facing orientation as our programs change to meet the challenges of future clinical education, rapidly changing work environments, and paradigm shifts in how we operate within a changing higher education system.

Benchmarking Immersive Technologies

Industrial design makes up the vast majority of commercial design, often described as the space between graphic design and architecture. Think about the objects of life, your phone, car, furniture, kitchen appliances, and tools. All of these were touched by an industrial designer. To address this large space, designers are constantly learning. Each new project or innovation requires an initial phase of discovery, a period of research that encompasses a variety of aspects, such as historical, ethnographic, market, and aesthetics. In order to innovate, designers first establish a thorough understanding of what already exists, the term we use to describe this is *benchmarking*.

Simulations that go beyond screen-based simulation, such as immersive simulations, virtual environments, and role play, are contained broadly in the term *extended reality* (XR). XR is an umbrella term that encompasses virtual reality (VR), augmented reality (AR), and mixed reality (MR). These are three related but unique immersive technologies that combine the actual (physical) world with a virtual (augmented) world.

VR uses a headset to completely immerse the user into a virtual world, removing them from the real world. During this experience users cannot see their actual surroundings. VR can be described as "real in effect although not in fact" and "can be considered capable of being considered fact for some purposes" (Wilson, 1997, p. 1057). Common VR hardware on the market today range from simple devices, like Google Cardboard and smartphones, to popular VR headsets, like the Oculus and HTC Vive.

AR overlays virtual elements onto the real world through the use of headsets or screens. In this format users can still see their actual surroundings combined with augmented visual elements. AR can be described as any system that has the following three characteristics: combines real and virtual, is interactive in real time, and is registered in three dimensions (Azuma, 1997). There are fewer AR headsets on the market than VR, with Microsoft HoloLens and Magic Leap leading that sector. However, the use of mobile (smartphone) AR is saturating the market and is far more ubiquitous than VR. AR technology saw record growth in 2019. Commercial support for AR is positioned to be strong, with big tech names like Microsoft, Amazon, Apple, Facebook, and Google making serious commitments. As of May 2019, the installed user base for AR-supporting mobile devices reached 1.5 billion (Makarov, 2021).

MR combines elements of physical and virtual worlds. MR refers to the class of all displays in which there is some combination of a real environment and VR (Drascic & Milgram, 1996). One of the most prevalent and meaningful ways we see this in health care is the combination of a real physical experience with a virtual or augmented one. MR takes simulations one step closer to actual experiences by combining visual and auditory effects with tactile experiences. For example, an MR experience might begin by placing a surgeon in a virtual operating room with a virtual patient through the use of a VR headset (visual and auditory). Simultaneously, the surgeon uses replicas of surgical tools and equipment (tactile) that are programed to sync with the virtual experience displayed and heard through the VR headset. These technologies are the basic existing building blocks for immersive simulations. As one might expect, they are constantly changing. Fueled by an industry built on gaming, these technologies are rapidly evolving as tools for teaching, training, and working more efficiently.

Amazing as these technologies are in providing unimaginable immersive experiences, they do have some drawbacks that hinder their progress. One of the most prominent, but rapidly improving, is the size of the headsets. The cumbersome equipment might be acceptable for users gaming in their basement, but professionals in the workplace feel quite awkward donning the current VR or AR headsets. There are also psychological and physical factors for users to overcome, particularly with the fully immersive VR experience. Novice VR users are often intimidated by the disconnect from their environment and onlookers. Additionally, many VR users experience physical issues, with nausea and vertigo ranking among the top reported. Smart glasses are not a new idea, as we saw with the Google Glass flop in 2012. However, while there are challenges for this device in the consumer market, they still hold value for training that requires hands-free and highly focused tasks. For example, smart glasses technology is being used in military and medical training.

AI and machine learning are also game changers in simulation development. As I (KP) can attest to in my own research, early iterations of these technologies presented challenges in terms of cost and the level of expertise required for programming. Recent changes in these areas are making AI and machine learning more accessible and affordable, changing what is capable of new developers in simulations. The "A" representing artificial in AI is broadly accepted as "made by people," as pointed out by Professor Kristinn R. Thorisson, Department of Computer Science, Reykjavik University, in his commentary on Wang's essay (Wang, 2019). The "I" representing intelligence was first understood as the mental or intellectual capacity displayed by humans. Broadly speaking, AI can be conceptualized as combining human intelligence with human-made software in a way that allows for problem solving. Machine learning is a branch of AI that aims at enabling machines to "learn" to perform their jobs skillfully by using intelligent software (Wang, 2019). Machine learning uses a series of algorithms to make decisions. As software and hardware become active and responsive thinkers, our XR experiences become more robust and interactive. The combination of AI and machine learning in the health care field will be significant. Deloitte Research concludes that AR and AI will transform the traditional health care business model offering AR/MR-enabled hands-free solutions and AI-based diagnostic tools (Deloitte Center for Health Solutions, n.d.-a). The development of new tools using the technology inevitably means new training. Advancements of technology require advancements in education, the production of simulations, the capabilities of those simulations, and the adaptation of this type of training in every university.

Changing the Way We Work, Learn, Play, and Shop

Shared Augmented Reality Workspaces

Imagine a world where your colleagues show up as holograms. That is exactly what's happening with spatial AR. The next wave in the work-life future, and, likely, more broadly accepted in response to the global pandemic, spatial AR is connecting avatars (digital representation of people) to meeting rooms all over the globe. A variety of companies like Mattel, LG, T-Mobile, and Ford, to name a few, are taking advantage of the technology as a connective tool for collaboration. The medical industry can certainly benefit from this type of experience connecting specialists to hospital rooms from all over the globe in a matter of seconds. In 2019, a class of undergraduate students at James Madison University developed a simulation known as OnCall (James Madison University X-Labs, n.d.). OnCall used spatial AR to connect college students in a VR hospital emergency department environment where they had to work across disciplines to diagnose a patient with vertigo. Students of different disciplines were electronically paged to join in the VR space to provide their input as they worked to diagnose and solve complex challenges. These are just a few examples of how connectivity through XR platforms is on the rise and what they offer us in our new distributed workforce conundrum.

Augmented Reality in the Automotive Industry

The automotive industry is the perfect platform for AR technology, with the windshield serving as a literal fixed screen continuously in the driver's field of view. This feature, sometimes referred to as a heads-up display, projects speed, blind spot warnings, and navigation with the windshield serving as a transparent display. When we think about the windshield as a display instead of a plane of glass, it begins to shape ideas about where else we can utilize these displays and illuminate the need for headsets or smartphones for viewing augmented elements. All the major car manufactures are testing concepts of AR adoption into their near future models. Even before we see this technology roll out in cars on the lot, we are seeing start-ups like Swiss-based WayRay, which has designed Deep Reality Display technologies for vehicles and aircraft. The holographic AR heads-up displays are designed for both drivers and passengers, conventional vehicles, self-driving cars, consumers, and businesses.

Augmented Reality in Retail and Business

IKEA was quick to jump on the AR bandwagon, helping their customers imagine furniture styles in their homes through mobile AR. With a smartphone or tablet, IKEA customers can "place" sofas, dining tables, beds, and more into their space, allowing them to check style and fit without ever leaving the house. We see similar trends in fashion and make-up where consumers can "try on" clothing or make-up. Companies like Sephora have AR dressing rooms or mirrors where consumers can cycle through different looks and get recommendations based on facial or body scans. Market research anticipates that the use of AR in retail will reach $85 billion in 2025 (Singh, 2019). This is not surprising given the ubiquitous nature and reliance on our mobile devices. Retail experiences employing AR have been shown to elicit greater immersion and enjoyment for the consumer when compared to viewing a retailer's website (Kowalczuk et al., 2021).

Training

VR and AR have taken off in retail and other businesses as an efficient and cost-effective method of training employees. Companies can ensure consistency in training by standardizing the training across locations, making sure every employee has the same quality of training. It is also freeing up work hours and saving companies money at the same time. Walmart has been using VR since 2017 as a training tool and describes it as an upgrade to their training. The company claims,

> Instilling confidence is exactly what makes VR so effective as a training tool. Because the effect of VR training is like an experience in real life, associates have the freedom to make mistakes and learn by doing, all while in a safe environment. (Incao, 2018, para. 11)

In addition to saving money, better training, and instilling confidence, VR is also reducing injuries and perhaps saving lives. Corporate giant Tyson is utilizing VR as a training tool to simulate things that are difficult or impossible to practice in real life (O'Donnell, 2018).

Other industries taking advantage of immersive technologies include:

- Real estate
- Professional athletics
- Military
- Surgical and medical training

Immersive Technologies in Health Care Delivery and Training

Roadblocks

After laying out many examples of immersive technologies, the question is what is hindering adoption of these in clinical health care education. The first, and most obvious, challenge is cost. Deloitte Center for Health Solutions' (n.d.) *Closing the Digital Gap* report lists cost as one of the top three challenges in implementing digital technologies. However, there are two factors to consider regarding cost: upfront investment and long-term savings. Initial expenses/investment associated with immersive technology, both hardware and software, can be prohibitive for programs getting on board. To complicate the issue, all of this is constantly changing, and to stay up to date requires frequent purchasing and constant maintenance. In contrast, programs need to consider the long-term savings and benefits, and not just monetary ones. Once these technologies are operational, they need the staff and resources and training to remain current.

Bringing Existing Technology Into Clinical Education

In the case of clinical health care education and its future utilizing immersive technologies, we do not need to reinvent the wheel. The fact is, as demonstrated throughout this section, clinical health care education can just plug right into existing technologies. For those considering adopting innovative and immersive technologies into clinical education, consider Deloitte's (n.d.) framework for incorporating digital solutions in health care, a framework that is not too far off from one that industrial designers might use to drive their design process.

The framework uses the acronym SMART:

- **S**traightforward and easy to use
- **M**easurable impact
- **A**gile solutions
- **R**eliant on industry collaboration
- **T**ailored to end-user needs

As experienced clinical educators, four of the five components of the framework are probably familiar in how we approach teaching and training students. The big outlier here is R "reliant on industry collaboration," although it might also read as reliant on cross-disciplinary collaboration within your university. Developing new ideas, even on existing technologies, not to mention something that is truly cutting edge, requires some significant investments at the levels that universities are often not equipped to provide. Therefore, collaborations with industry can be a win for both parties as they can develop ideas at lower cost. Academic collaborations may bring new viewpoints and insights to the design process that companies are not even thinking about. Deloitte (n.d.) goes on to say that one of the key steps to accelerate this digital transformation is to develop digital leadership skills and improve the digital literacy of staff and patients. Educators can be these digital leaders through industry collaboration, risk taking, and forward thinking. As a result, our students will step into the roles of future staff prepared to lead others in the next generation of health care. It is not just a matter of using these technologies for teaching, but also acknowledging that the current and future workplace in health care is one that is immersed in technology.

Vision for Simulations in Communication Sciences and Disorders

What do uses of immersive simulations look like for speech-language pathology and audiology training programs specifically? The uses are practically endless, but here are a few ideas to prime the pump. There have already been uses for task trainers for preterm infant feeding in nursing that offer solid evidence as a path forward. Broadfoot and Estis (2020) published a study in which an infant doll (i.e., task trainer) proved a successful method to effectively train entry-level clinical and nonclinical students to screen feeding skills in preterm infants. Immersive simulation has also been used to train students in procedures that are high risk, prohibiting the use of standardized patients for training. One example is the passing of a nasoscope as part of the assessment of swallowing. Some institutions of higher education may have access to a simulation lab and expensive manikin or task trainer that allow practice of this procedure; however, it is unlikely that there is broad access to these resources at most graduate programs in speech-language pathology. Immersive technology can be used to simulate the experience in a manner that is both accessible and affordable to programs (Phaup et al., 2019). If we consider evidence from companies like Tyson Foods, we can be confident that VR/AR allows us to train in real-world scenarios. It is not just about the physical task of scoping a patient, something we might be able to replicate in fairly crude physical models; it is also about the environment, the pressures, the patient's behavior or complications, and the need to make clinical judgments in the moment. Across numerous studies in multiple fields, XR is as effective of a training mechanism as the commonly accepted methods. The value of XR then lies in providing training in circumstances, which exclude traditional methods, such as situations when danger or cost may make traditional training impossible.

BOX 9-1

Virtual Health

Virtual health uses telecommunication and networked technologies to connect clinicians with patients (and with other clinicians and stakeholders) to remotely deliver health care services and support well-being. Virtual health appears to have the capacity to inform, personalize, accelerate, and augment people's ability to care for one another. Virtual health helps stakeholders access relevant data easily, improve quality of care, and deliver value (Deloitte Center for Health Research, n.d.-b).

Now More Than Ever

The global COVID-19 pandemic resulted in the shutdown of businesses, schools, and service industries. This event will be marked in history as a time when resistance to technology based on age, preference, fear, effort, or access was instantly overcome. Families communicated over digital video technologies such as Facetime (Apple) and Messenger (Meta). The global economy experienced a major shift to online shopping. Families used apps to purchase and schedule groceries for pick up. Workers adjusted to working remotely from makeshift home offices. Educators took to video conferencing platforms such as Zoom to deliver instruction. Medical professionals, allied health practitioners, and patients were drawn to the convenience of telemedicine.

While the lasting effects of the pandemic remain to be seen, it has likely forever impacted how we access and experience health care. Immersive technologies, such as the VR and AR applications discussed in this chapter, are likely to become a standard part of hospital and clinical practices. Deloitte's report *Closing the Digital Gap* makes the following observation (Deloitte Center for Health Solutions, n.d.-a):

> Over the past decade many customer-facing industries, such as hospitality, transport, communications, retail and banking, have been transformed almost beyond recognition by the adoption of digital technologies, particularly in relation to self-service access to services and improving the customer experience. Today, healthcare is at least ten years behind these industries in transforming the ways services are provided. (p. 8)

As dedicated health care professionals, it would be a disservice to those we serve not to train our students, the future of our professions in audiology and speech-language pathology, in the use of emerging technologies that they will likely experience in the workplace. As we move toward competency-based education, training programs and providers of professional development are prudent to incorporate high-quality simulation technologies into the clinical education of students.

Call to Action

This chapter was originally titled "Future Directions"; however, it was pointed out that CSD is in the position of catching up with medicine, nursing, and other allied health fields in the area of simulation. So, we face forward knowing that it is in the best interest of our university programs and students to educate ourselves and others about the appropriate role of simulation in clinical education. Every educator needs to have access to simulation as a learning tool with the goal of graduating professionals equipped to meet the changing needs of education and health care. This will only happen if we move beyond early adopters, those one or two faculty within our programs trained in the use of simulations for clinical education, to a comprehensive and integrated approach that thoughtfully integrates simulation throughout the curriculum. This will require an investment in time, personnel, training, and resources to move our training programs and professions toward a competency-based education model.

References

Allen, S. (2020). 2020 Global health care outlook report. Deloitte Global Public Health. https://www2.deloitte.com/content/dam/Deloitte/global/Documents/Life-Sciences-Health-Care/gx-lshc-2020-global-health-care-outlook.pdf

Association of Academic Health Centers. (n.d.). Advancing the education model for 21st century medicine. https://www.aahcdc.org/21st-Century-AHCs/Advancing-the-Education-Model-for-21st-Century-Medicine

Azuma, R. T. (1997). A survey of augmented reality. *Presence: Teleoperators and Virtual Environments*, *6*(4), 355. https://doi.org/10.1162/pres.1997.6.4.355

BRP. (2017). *Digital commerce survey*. https://www.windstreamenterprise.com/wp-content/uploads/2018/01/2017-digital-commerce-survey-results.pdf

Broadfoot, C., & Estis, J. (2020). Simulation-based training improves student assessment of oral feeding skills in preterm infants. *Teaching and Learning in Communication Sciences & Disorders*, *4*(3). https://ir.library.illinoisstate.edu/tlcsd/vol4/iss3/8

Brown, M., McCormack, M., Reeves, J., Brook, D. C., Grajek, S., Alexander, B., Bali, M., Bulger, S., Dark, S., Engelbert, N., Gannon, K., Gauthier, A., Gibson, D., Gibson, R., Lundin, B., Veletsianos, G., & Weber, N. (2020). *2020 Educause horizon report teaching and learning edition*. LearnTechLib. https://www.learntechlib.org/p/215670/

Chang, J., Yuan, Y., & Wang, D. (2020). [Mental health status and its influencing factors among college students during the epidemic of COVID-19]. *Nan Fang Yi Ke Da Xue Xue Bao*, *40*(2), 171-176. https://doi.org/10.12122/j.issn.1673-4254.2020.02.06

Cowan, D. T., Norman, I., & Coopamah, V. P. (2005). Competence in nursing practice: A controversial concept—A focused review of literature. *Nurse Education Today*, *25*(5), 355-362. https://doi.org/10.1016/j.nedt.2005.03.002

Deloitte Center for Health Solutions. (n.d.-a). Closing the digital gap: Shaping the future of UK healthcare. https://www2.deloitte.com/content/dam/Deloitte/uk/Documents/life-sciences-health-care/deloitte-uk-life-sciences-health-care-closing-the-digital-gap.pdf

Deloitte Center for Health Solutions. (n.d.-b). Insights. https://www2.deloitte.com/us/en/insights.html

Drascic, D., & Milgram, P. (1996). Perceptual issues in augmented reality. *Proceedings of SPIE—The International Society for Optical Engineering, 2653*. https://doi.org/10.1117/12.237425

Eisenberg, D., Lipson, S. K., Heinze, J., & Zhou, S. (2020). The Healthy Minds Study: Fall 2020 data report. Healthy Minds Network. https://healthymindsnetwork.org/wp-content/uploads/2021/02/HMS-Fall-2020-National-Data-Report.pdf

Gaba D. M. (2004). The future vision of simulation in health care. *BMJ Quality & Safety*, *13*(Suppl 1), i2-i10. https://doi.org/10.1136/qhc.13.suppl_1.i2

Incao, J. (2018). How VR is transforming the way we train associates. Walmart. https://corporate.walmart.com/newsroom/innovation/20180920/how-vr-is-transforming-the-way-we-train-associates

James Madison University X-Labs. (n.d.). Scope of practice. https://www.jmu.edu/news/2019/01/30-mm-virtual-reality.shtml

Kline, M. (2019, Fall). The looming higher ed enrollment cliff. *Higher Education HR Magazine*. https://www.cupahr.org/issue/feature/higher-ed-enrollment-cliff/

Kowalczuk, P., Siepmann, S., & Adler, J. (2021). Cognitive, affective, and behavioral consumer responses to augmented reality in e-commerce: A comparative study. *Journal of Business Research, 124*, 357-373. https://doi.org/10.1016/j.jbusres.2020.10.050

Looney, A., Wessel, D., & Yilla, K. (2020, January 28). Who owes all that student debt? And who'd benefit if it were forgiven? Brookings. https://www.brookings.edu/policy2020/votervital/who-owes-all-that-student-debt-and-whod-benefit-if-it-were-forgiven/

Makarov, A. (2021). 10 augmented reality trends in 2021: The future is here. Mobi Dev. https://mobidev.biz/blog/augmented-reality-future-trends-2018-2020

McAllister, S., Lincoln, M., Ferguson, A., & McAllister, L. (2010). Issues in developing valid assessments of speech pathology students' performance in the workplace. *International Journal of Language and Communication Disorders, 45*(1), 1-14.

McAllister, S., Lincoln, M., Ferguson, A., & McAllister, L. (2011). A systematic program of research regarding the assessment of speech-language pathology competencies. *International Journal of Speech-Language Pathology, 13*(6), 469-479.

O'Donnell, R. (2018). Tyson foods reduces worker injuries, illnesses and VR safety training. HRDive. https://www.hrdive.com/news/tyson-foods-reduces-worker-injuries-illnesses-with-vr-safety-training/532452/

Oswalt, S. B., Lederer, A. M., Chestnut-Steich, K., Day, C., Halbritter, A., & Ortiz, D. (2020). Trends in college students' mental health diagnoses and utilization of services. 2009-2015. *Journal of American College Health, 68*(1), 41-51. https://doi.org/10.1080/07448481.2018.1515748

Phaup, K., Dudding, C. C., Kamarunas, E., & Barnes, J. (2019, November). *A showcase of applications of virtual reality in communication sciences & disorders*. American Speech-Language-Hearing Association Convention (seminar), Orlando, FL.

Romig, B. D., Tucker, A. W., Hewitt, A. M., & Maillet, J. O. (2017). The future of clinical education: Opportunities and challenges from allied health deans' perspective. *Journal of Allied Health, 46*(1), 43-56.

Singh, S. (2019). Augmented reality market worth $85.0 billion by 2025. Markets and Markets. https://www.marketsandmarkets.com/PressReleases/augmented-reality.asp

Wang, P. (2019). On defining artificial intelligence. *Journal of Artificial General Intelligence, 10*(2), 1-37. https://doi.org/10.2478/jagi-2019-0002

Wilson, J. R. (1997). Virtual environments and ergonomics: Needs and opportunities. *Ergonomics, 40*(10), 1057-1077. https://doi.org/10.1080/001401397187603

Zhang, L., Qi, H., Wang, L., Wang, F., Huang, J., Li, F., & Zhang, Z. (2021). Effects of the COVID-19 pandemic on acute stress disorder and career planning among healthcare students. *International Journal of Mental Health Nursing, 30*(4), 907-916. https://doi.org/10.1111/inm.12839

Zoll, A. (n.d.). *Mini biography: Wayne Gretsky*. IMDb. https://www.imdb.com/name/nm0002115/bio

Glossary

ADDIE (analysis, design, development, implementation, and evaluation): A design model commonly used by instructional designers and educators.

advocacy in simulation: Supporting best practices in conducting simulation-based education as well as conducting simulation research through the sponsorship, preparation, creation, and support of research endeavors.

assessment: Gathering, analyzing, and interpreting evidence to determine how well learning outcomes are met (Suskie, 2018).

attributes: The desirable professional characteristics of the learners, including attitudes, learning styles, and beliefs and values.

augmented reality (AR): A type of extended reality in which digital objects are superimposed on the real-world objects through the use of headsets or screens.

avatar: A three-dimensional computer-generated persona.

backward design process: Also called backward planning or backward mapping. A process used to design learning experiences and instructional techniques. The process begins with the creation of learning objectives that are used to create lessons and assessments.

behavioral rating scales: An evaluation tool used to detect differing levels of performance along a continuum of performance.

behaviorist approach: A set of learning theories based on the premise that all behaviors are learned through interactions with environmental stimuli and that learning is based on observable behaviors and conditioning. This theory was made popular by Skinner, 1974.

checklists: Weighted or unweighted lists of specified behaviors scored dichotomously and judged to be present or absent (Anson, 2015).

clinical decision making (CDM): A series of decisions where data are gathered, interpreted, and evaluated in order to make an evidence-based decision regarding clinical intervention.

clinical simulation: A form of simulation designed to represent a real-life clinical event for the purpose of practice, learning, and/or evaluation.

cognitive load theory: The premise that new information is first dealt with by our working memory before being consolidated into long-term memory. Types include extrinsic, intrinsic, and germane cognitive load.

competency: A range of knowledge and behaviors that indicate a level of function commensurate with expected ability to perform professional action and judgment across a variety of professional settings and contexts.

competency-based education model: Education model requiring competency-based outcomes and assessments that support the development of professional competency focusing on the ability to practice (output) vs. accumulating hours of supervised experience (input).

computer-based simulations: Learner-centered simulations that model real-life processes, often through the use of a monitor, keyboard, or other simple assistive devices.

conceptual fidelity: All elements of the scenario or case relate to each other in a realistic way and comply with actual standards of practice.

constructivist theory: A set of learning theories based on the premise that learners actively construct their new knowledge based on their experiences and active engagement in the learning process.

critical thinking: An intellectual process of active conceptualization, application, and synthesis of information gained through observation, experience, and reflection.

debrief: A learning strategy following the simulation activity in which participants receive feedback and engage in reflective thinking in order to improve future performance. Debriefing is essential for maximizing learning within the simulation-based learning experience.

deliberate practice (DP): Learners repeatedly practice a skill or task to improve their current level of proficiency and performance of cognitive or motor skills. It requires rigorous assessment of those skills, and specific instructional feedback on performance.

digitized manikins: High-fidelity simulators or computerized manikins that mimic physiologic functions and allow learners to practice conducting tests or procedures.

evidence-based education (EBE): Educational strategies that are based on objective evidence.

experiential learning theory (ELT): A learner-centered theory that focusses on how the learner constructs their knowledge through concrete experience, reflective observation, abstract conceptualization, and active experimentation.

Dudding, C. C., & Ginsberg, S. M. (Eds.).
Simulation-Based Learning in Communication Sciences and Disorders: Moving From Theory to Practice. (pp. 147-150).

extended reality (XR): An all-encompassing termed to describe immersive technologies that incorporate both the physical and virtual world.

faculty development: Any planned activity designed to improve an individual's knowledge and skills in areas considered essential to the performance of a faculty member.

fidelity: How closely the simulation-based learning experience replicates the real-world experience and allows the learner to immerse themselves and suspend disbelief.

formative assessment: An assessment that provides feedback during the learning process and allows students to improve their own learning and achievement.

hybrid model of simulation: Simulations that include more than one modality (e.g., a standardized patient wearing a false tracheostomy tube).

immersion: The perception of being physically present in a nonphysical world.

immersive virtual reality: A computer-based three-dimensional representation that has the feeling of immersion.

institutional review board (IRB): An oversight committee formed by governing research bodies and institutions of higher education focused on the protection of the rights and welfare of human research participants.

interprofessional education (IPE): Students from two or more professions learning about, from, and with each other to enable effective collaboration and improve health outcomes (Interprofessional Education Collaborative, 2016).

interprofessional practice (IPP): Health care practitioners from different professional backgrounds working together as a team to deliver the highest quality of care. Also referred to as interprofessional collaborative practice (ICP). IPP/ICP requires skills in teamwork, communication, roles and responsibilities, and values and ethics.

knowledge: Propositional knowledge such as theory, facts, and principles; know-how; and insights gained through experience (Carter, 1985; Higgs & Jones, 2000; Higgs & Titchen, 2001; McAllister et al., 2011).

learner-centered approach: Learners construct meaning through integration of new knowledge and their own experiences. Also referred to as learner-oriented and student-centered.

manikins: Life-size human patient simulators are designed to be realistic and are available in a variety of preterm, infant, child, and adult models. High-technology simulators can simulate physiologic functions (e.g., cardiac function, pulse rate, respiratory patterns, pupil dilation, muscle tone, electroencephalography, cochlear hair cell movement) and may be programmed to respond accordingly to interventions. Vary in fidelity and cost (Dudding & Nottingham, 2018).

Miller's pyramid of competence: A method of assessment testing cognitive understanding and behavioral competency. with a hierarchical structure containing four levels.

mixed method: A research method that incorporates both quantitative and qualitative research methods.

mixed reality (MR): A simulative technology that brings together both real-world and digital elements by interacting with and manipulating both physical and virtual items and environments, using different sensing and imaging technologies.

Objective Structured Clinical Examination (OSCE): A method of summative clinical skills assessment requiring students to perform specific tasks within a prescribed period in a highly structured encounter. It assesses competency, based on objective testing through direct observation (Harden, 1988).

occupational competency: Competent performance of the tasks related to our professional practice. For example, we conduct assessments, analyze and interpret this data, and use this interpretation to create an intervention plan.

outcomes-based curriculum: An educational model that clearly articulates the specific outcomes and performance levels that the student must demonstrate.

participatory action research (PAR): Research that seeks to find meaning, understanding, and improvement within the community affected by the research through a researcher-rich participant pool that uses an iterative cycle of research, action, and reflection (Baum et al., 2006; MacDonald, 2012).

physical or environmental fidelity: How closely the physical context of the simulation reflects the real-life environment.

PICO: A method used to frame questions of interest using the organizational topics of population, intervention, comparator/comparison, and outcome.

prebrief: A period in which learners are oriented to the technology, introduced to the clinical case, and assigned roles for the simulation prior to engaging in the simulation experience (Dieckmann et al., 2007; Gaba, 2004; Jeffries, 2005).

professional competency: The competent exercise of complex professional judgment to inform action across all tasks and contexts of professional practice. Sometimes referred to as generic competencies, in that they are common to a number of professions. For example, we demonstrate reasoning, lifelong learning, communication, and professionalism.

professional tasks: Specific professional activities that draw on knowledge, skills, and attributes from which competency can be inferred.

psychological safety: A feeling within a simulation-based activity that participants are comfortable participating, speaking up, sharing thoughts, and asking for help as needed without concern for retribution or embarrassment (Lioce et al., 2020, p. 38).

qualitative method: A systematic approach that seeks to improve understanding of a phenomena or behavior and acknowledges the worldviews and beliefs of the researchers and uses these to shape the study using incalculable data collection techniques such as interviews, surveys, and recorded observations.

quantitative method: A research methodology that relies on numbers and statistical analysis to describe, test relationships, and determine cause and effect by breaking down concepts into discrete and specific variables that can be tested against hypotheses.

reflection: A method of analyzing a person's experiences with a task in order to improve the way they function in that task.

reflection-in-action: The immediate thinking during an experience; can be thought of as "thinking on your feet" (Schon, 1983).

reflection-on-action: The later analysis of the events in considering what went well and what did not (Schon, 1983).

rubric: Guidelines that instructors use for evaluating learner's assignments and to define expectations for different criteria to be evaluated, scoring strategies, and the desired quality to which to aspire.

schemas: Processes or patterns in which information has been organized and stored in long term memory and enable efficient retrieval and use in our working and help us manage cognitive load (Fraser et al., 2015).

scholarship of teaching and learning (SoTL): Research that brings a scholarly lens to the behaviors, events, culture, values, and learning within the respective discipline as it applies to learning. It is contextually based practitioner research that is focused on pedagogical refinement or continuous improvement in a context that is continuously changing (Ginsberg et al., 2017, p. 3).

self-evaluation: A method of evaluation affords the learner the opportunity to appraise their own performance through various self-analyzing techniques.

simulated participant: A term used to include all role players in any simulation context or activity with varying levels of experience. The simulated participant does not necessarily portray a patient. They may play roles such as clients, family members, and health care professionals. Simulated participants are sometimes referred to as confederates.

simulated patient (SiP): A broad term referring to a person who has been trained to portray a patient with a variety of different clinical conditions (Collins & Harden, 2011).

simulation-based learning experience (SBLE): The collection of carefully planned educational methods and procedures that make up a quality simulation-based learning experience. SBLEs consist of prebrief, simulation experience, and a debrief (Rudolph et al., 2014).

simulation-enhanced interprofessional education (sim-IPE): Simulation-based learning experiences integrating interprofessional education and collaboration.

simulators: Specialized devices that replicate components of a real-world task and are used as a part of the simulation activity (Lioce et al., 2020).

single-subject research design (SSRD): A research design commonly used in communication sciences and disorders, also known as within-subject design, that uses a quantitative, scientifically rigorous approach where each participant provides their own experimental control.

situated learning theory: Theory that states that knowledge needs to be presented in authentic contexts that are embedded within the activity, context, and culture in which it will be used (Lave, 1988).

skills: The application of knowledge and the demonstration of how the knowledge applies in each situation. Skills can be psychomotor, metacognitive, or emotional/social in nature.

standardized patient (SP): An individual trained to simulate a patient's illness, or a patient trained to present their disease in a realistic, standardized, and repeatable way.

References

Anson, W. (2015). Assessment in healthcare simulation. In J. C. Palaganas, J. C. Maxworthy, C. A. Epps, & M. E. Mancini (Eds.), *Defining excellence in simulation programs* (pp. 509-543). Wolters Kluwer.

Baum, F., MacDougall, C., & Smith, D. (2006). Participatory action research. *Journal of Epidemiology and Community Health, 60*(10), 854-857. https://doi.org/10.1136/jech.2004.028662

Carter, R. (1985). A taxonomy of objectives for professional education. *Studies in Higher Education, 10*(2), 135-149. https://doi.org/10.1080/0307507 8512331378559

Collins, J. P., & Harden, R. M. (1998). AMEE medical education guide No. 13: Real patients, simulated patients and simulators in clinical examinations. *Medical Teacher, 20*(6), 508-521 .

Dieckmann, P., Gaba, D., & Rall, M. (2007). Deepening the theoretical foundations of patient simulation as social practice. *Simulation in Healthcare, 2*(3), 183-193. https://journals.lww.com/simulationinhealthcare/fulltext/2007/00230/Deepening_the_Theoretical_Foundations _of _Patient .5 .aspx

Dudding, C. C., & Nottingham, E. E. (2018). A national survey of simulation use in university programs in communication sciences and disorders. *American Journal of Speech-Language Pathology, 27*(1), 71-81.

Fraser, K. L., Ayres, P., & Sweller, J. (2015). Cognitive load theory for the design of medical simulations. *Simulation in Healthcare, 10*(5), 295-307. https://doi.org/10.1097/SIH.0000000000000097

Gaba, D. (2004). The future vision of simulation in health care. *Quality & Safety in Health Care, 13*(1). https://pubmed.ncbi.nlm.nih.gov /15465951/

Ginsberg, S. M., Friberg, J., Visconti, C. F., DeRuiter, M., & Hoepner, J. K. (2017). On the culture of scholarship of teaching and learning. *Teaching and Learning in Communication Sciences & Disorders, 1*(1), 1-5. https://doi .org/10.30707/TLCSD1.1

Harden, R. M. (1988). What is an OSCE. *Medical Teacher, 10*, 19-22.

Higgs, J., & Jones, M. (2000). Clinical reasoning in the health professions. In J. Higgs & M. Jones (Eds.), *Clinical reasoning in the health professions* (2nd ed., pp. 3-14). Butterworth-Heinemann.

Higgs, J., & Titchen, A. (2001). *Practice knowledge and expertise in the health professions*. Butterworth-Heinemann.

Interprofessional Education Collaborative. (2016). *Core competencies for interprofessional collaborative practice: 2016 update*. Author.

Jeffries, P. (2005). A framework for designing, implementing, and evaluating simulations used as teaching strategies in nursing. *Nursing Education Perspectives, 26*(2), 96-103. https://pubmed .ncbi .nlm .nih .gov /15921126/

Lave, J. (1988). *Cognition in practice: Mind, mathematics and culture in everyday life*. Cambridge University Press. https://www.cambridge.org/core/books/cognition-in-practice/2AF0745B4B8636436A1DF8AAF374BB9E

Lioce, L. (Ed.), Lopreiato, J. (Founding Ed.), Downing, D., Chang, T. P., Robertson, J. M., Anderson, M., Diaz, D. A., Spain, A., (Assoc. Eds.), & the Terminology Concepts Working Group (2020). *Healthcare Simulation Dictionary* (2nd ed.). Agency for Healthcare Research and Quality. https://doi.org /10.23970/simulationv2

MacDonald, C. (2012). Understanding participatory action research: A qualitative research methodology option. *Canadian Journal of Action Research, 13*(2), 34-50.

McAllister, S., Lincoln, M., Ferguson, A., & McAllister, L. (2011). A systematic program of research regarding the assessment of speech-language pathology competencies. *International Journal of Speech-Language Pathology, 13*(6), 469-479.

Rudolph, J. W., Raemer, D. B., & Simon, R. (2014). Establishing a safe container for learning in simulation: The role of the presimulation briefing. *Simulation in Healthcare, 9*(6), 339-349. https://doi.org/10.1097/SIH.0000000000000047

Schon, D. A. (1983). *The reflective practitioner: How professionals think in action*. Basic Books.

Skinner, B. F. (1974). *About behaviorism*. Random House.

Suskie, L. (2018). *Assessing student learning: A common sense guide* (3rd ed.). John Wiley & Sons.

Weimer, M. (2013). *Learner-centered teaching: Five key changes to practice*. John Wiley & Sons. http://ebookcentral.proquest.com/lib/jmu/detail.action?docID=1119448

Financial Disclosures

Dr. Meredith L. Baker-Rush reported no financial or proprietary interest in the materials presented herein.

Dr. David K. Brown is a consultant for Intelligent Hearing Systems and owner of AudProf LLC.

Dr. Erin S. Clinard reported no financial or proprietary interest in the materials presented herein.

Dr. Carol C. Dudding reported no financial or proprietary interest in the materials presented herein.

Dr. Julie M. Estis reported no financial or proprietary interest in the materials presented herein.

Dr. Sarah M. Ginsberg reported no financial or proprietary interest in the materials presented herein.

Dr. Sue McAllister reported no financial or proprietary interest in the materials presented herein.

Dr. Suzanne Moineau reported no financial or proprietary interest in the materials presented herein.

Kevin Phaup reported no financial or proprietary interest in the materials presented herein.

Dr. Alison R. Scheer-Cohen reported no financial or proprietary interest in the materials presented herein.

Dr. Richard I. Zraick reported no financial or proprietary interest in the materials presented herein.

Index